D1345604

STUDIES ON THE DEVELOPMENT OF BEHAVIOR AND THE NERVOUS SYSTEM

Volume 2

ASPECTS OF NEUROGENESIS

CONSULTING EDITORS

STUDIES ON THE DEVELOPMENT OF BEHAVIOR AND THE NERVOUS SYSTEM

Volume 2

ASPECTS OF NEUROGENESIS

Edited by

GILBERT GOTTLIEB

Psychology Laboratory
Division of Research
North Carolina Department of Mental Health
Raleigh, North Carolina

ACADEMIC PRESS New York and London 1974

A Subsidiary of Harcourt Brace Jovanovich, Publishers

ACADEMIC PRESS, INC.
111 Fifth Avenue, New York, New York 10003

United Kingdom Edition published by
ACADEMIC PRESS, INC. (LONDON) LTD.
24/28 Oval Road, London NW1

LIBRARY OF CONGRESS CATALOG CARD NUMBER: 72-12194

PRINTED IN THE UNITED STATES OF AMERICA

CONTENTS

Problems of Neuronal Specificity in the Development of Some Behavioral Patterns in Amphibia

George Székely

A Plentitude of Neurons

Marcus Jacobson

Section 2 FETAL BRAIN FUNCTION: SENSORY AND MOTOR ASPECTS

Early Epigenesis of Recipient Functions in the Neocortex

B. A. Meyerson and H. E. Persson

LIST OF CONTRIBUTORS

Numbers in parentheses indicate the pages on which the authors' contributions begin.

R. M. BERGSTRÖM (205), Institute of Physiology, University of Helsinki, Helsinki, Finland

MARTIN BERRY (7), Department of Anatomy, The Medical School, Birmingham, England

STANLEY M. CRAIN* (69), Department of Physiology, Albert Einstein College of Medicine, Bronx, New York

A. F. HUGHES (223), Department of Anatomy, Case Western Reserve University, Cleveland, Ohio

MARCUS JACOBSON (151), Department of Biophysics, The Johns Hopkins University, Baltimore, Maryland

B. A. MEYERSON† (171), Department of Physiology, Karolinska Institutet, Stockholm, Sweden

H. E. PERSSON (171), Department of Physiology, Karolinska Institutet, Stockholm, Sweden

JINDŘICH SEDLÁČEK (245), Laboratory of Embryophysiology, Institute of Physiology, Charles University, Prague, Czechoslovakia

GEORGE SZÉKELY (115), Department of Anatomy, University Medical School, Pécs, Hungary

*Kennedy Scholar at the Rose F. Kennedy Center for Research in Mental Retardation and Human Development.

†Present address: Department of Neurosurgery, Karolinska Sjukhuset, Stockholm 60, Sweden.

PREFACE

In the first volume of this serial publication, the emphasis was primarily behavioral. In the present companion volume, the emphasis is neurological. Here are treated those problems of the development of the nervous system (neurogenesis) which seem most relevant to the genesis of behavior. As in Volume 1, there has been an explicit attempt to keep the presentation at a level which allows the interested reader to follow the discussion, even if the material is unfamiliar. This is not an easy job and not always successful, but one hopes it has been successful in the main.

The predominant theme of this volume has to do with how connections get established between, and within, different parts of the nervous system. The first four articles (Martin Berry; Stanley Crain; George Székely; Marcus Jacobson) deal rather microscopically with how synapses are formed, so there is considerable theoretical as well as factual discussion of the specificity of interneuronal connections, and the development of excitatory and inhibitory synapses, especially in relation to early behavior. The next two articles (B. A. Meyerson and H. E. Persson; and R. M. Bergström) continue the same theme but at the more macroscopic level of the electrophysiological functioning of intact, living fetuses. The final two articles (A. F. Hughes; J. Sedláček) introduce us to some of the more conspicuous and important things that happen in the nervous system during metamorphosis and birth, especially the critical role of hormones and biochemical factors during these stages.

The Editor is grateful for the counsel provided by the consultants. Mary Catharine Vick has continued to provide cheerful and efficient assistance with numerous editorial details, which is very much appreciated.

GILBERT GOTTLIEB

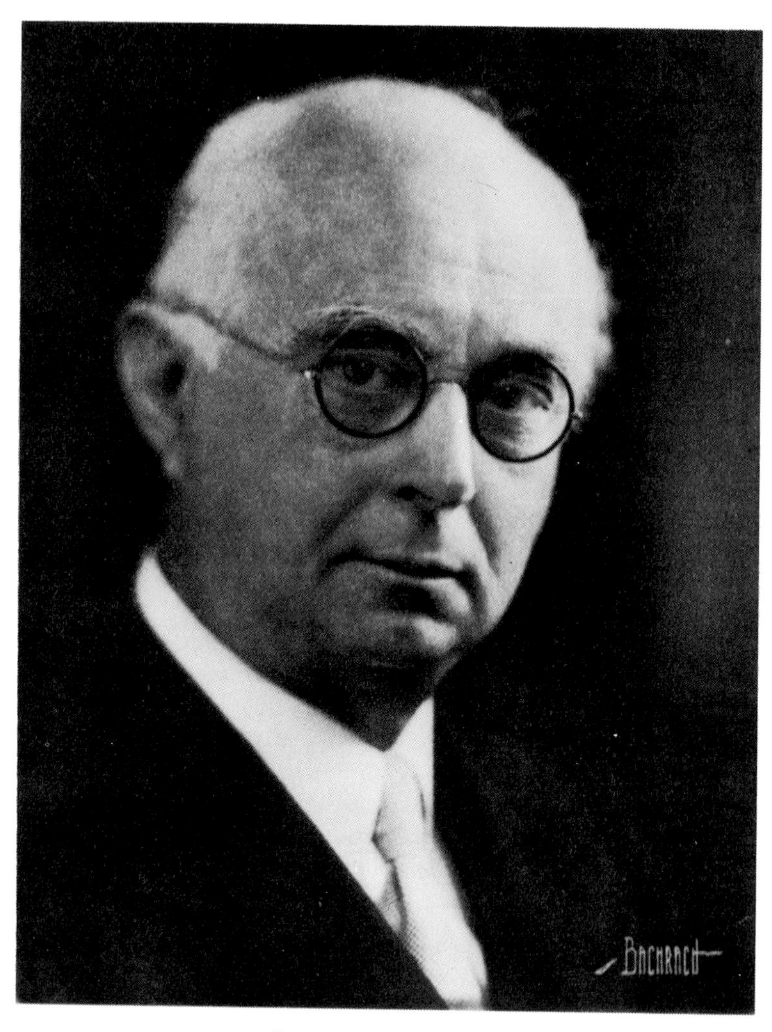

G. E. Coghill

DEDICATION TO G. E. COGHILL (1872–1941)

> It seemed to me basic to a scientific study of behaviour to know whether the behaviour pattern of an animal develops haphazard or in an orderly manner; and that, if it should be found that behaviour develops in an orderly manner, then there should be a corresponding order of development structurally and functionally in the nervous system. Should such correlation be found to occur, it seemed to me that the development of behaviour would offer a new basis for the interpretation of nervous structure and function, and that the development of the nervous system would throw new light on problems of behaviour.

So wrote Professor Coghill in the preface to his small monograph, *Anatomy and the Problem of Behaviour*, published in 1929 by the Cambridge University Press. Coghill pursued his goal of relating developmental neuroanatomy to the development of behavior by studying embryonic and larval salamanders of the genus *Ambystoma*; his publications on this subject extended from 1902 to 1943 (posthumous), almost always appearing in the *Journal of Comparative Neurology*.

The modern-day founder of behavioral embryology, W. Preyer, to whom the first volume in this series was dedicated, had the insight that behavior must be studied from its inception if we are to achieve a proper understanding of the genesis of psychological function. This insight took him to the study of the behavior of embryos. Coghill added a crucial dimension to Preyer's insight by attempting to correlate developmental changes in behavior to anatomical changes in the embryonic or larval nervous system.

Coghill, too, was greatly interested in psychology. As he writes in the preface:

> My earliest scientific interests were aroused by an introductory collegiate course in psychology.... This course of instruction left me in an inquiring state of mind concerning what seemed to me to be the fundamental principles of psychology—the nature and interrelation of sensation, perception and thought. Eventually this attitude ripened into a decision to enter upon graduate study in psychology. But before an opportunity came for me to carry out this decision I became aware that the natural approach to the kind of psycho-

logical information I wanted lay through the physiology of the nervous system. Obviously, also, the physiology of the nervous system must be approached through its anatomy. . . .

Coghill credited Clarence L. Herrick with directing his attention to salamanders as an appropriate form for the investigative purposes he had in mind. These creatures are easily observed in the embryonic and larval stages, they are equipped to swim in water as well as walk on land, and they are abundantly distributed in North America. Interestingly, the studies of *Ambystoma* larvae which occupied all of Coghill's professional life were originally intended to be merely preliminary and temporary stepping stones to research on mammals. Coghill's lifelong friend, C. Judson Herrick, Clarence's brother, also became infected with an enduring devotion to salamanders, even though he, too, planned to do more embracing comparative studies of the brain. (C. Judson and Coghill intermittently collaborated on developmental studies of *Ambystoma* over the years, but Herrick's primary interest lay in the evolution of the brain. Toward the end of his prolific career, Herrick wrote a long and abundantly illustrated monograph on *The Brain of the Tiger Salamander*, which was published in 1948, one year before his tender and highly literate portrait of *George Ellett Coghill, Naturalist and Philospher*.)

While Coghill's neurobehavioral perspective deepened Preyer's original insight on the utility of behavioral embryology for an understanding of psychogenesis, his neurobehavioral findings also added a new dimension to Preyer's great principle of motor primacy. Preyer's observations on the chick embryo led him to correctly deduce that early motility is nonreflexogenic, being generated in the spinal cord, independent of sensory instigation. Coghill's correlative studies of the behavior and nervous system in developing salamander larvae led him to the view that the initial sensory-stimulated movements (in *Ambystoma*) caused the entire functional neuromuscular apparatus to discharge rather diffusely and massively at first, with the capability for discrete, highly local, independent responses occurring secondarily in development. As Coghill often expressed it, sensory stimulation does not "capture" the motor system until late in development. On the neurological side of the problem, he saw ". . . first, the primacy of a motor mechanism of total integration; second, the development of mechanisms of partial integration through localized acceleration of growth; and third, progressive organization of the nervous system from the whole to the part." On the behavioral side, he reiterated: "Behaviour develops from the beginning through the progressive expansion of a perfectly integrated total pattern and the individuation within it of partial patterns which acquire various degrees of discreteness."

Coghill's principles of neural and behavioral development excited considerable research on a number of different embryonic forms, including man. Inevitably, disagreement arose over the application of Coghill's principles to vertebrates in general, with some investigators favoring the view that, in some species at least, total integration follows secondarily from the elaboration and concatenation of numerous individual reflexes in the course of development. As more and more species came under investigation, it became apparent that no single set of principles of motor development could satisfactorily encompass the diversity of behavioral development evident in a large number of distantly related species. Interestingly enough, Davenport Hooker and Tryphena Humphrey, highly experienced and outstanding investigators of human prenatal development, felt that Coghill's principles adequately described the course of behavior in the human fetus.

It must have been a source of considerable satisfaction to Coghill to observe that his principles were given wide currency in the psychological literature of the 1920s and 1930s, as the tremendous conceptual battle raged between reflexological behaviorism and holistic Gestalt psychology. Since Coghill's formulation cast doubt on the developmental primacy of reflexes and emphasized that the parts must always be subservient to the whole as regards the neural mechanism for total integration, he lent strong support to the Gestalt position.

Throughout his career, Coghill remained truly interdisciplinary in the scope of his reading and thinking. In the published version of his presidential address to the American Association of Anatomists in 1933, for example, over half of the references are to works written by psychologists. Coghill's own writings are models of clarity and scholarship, especially in letting the opposition speak for itself in matters of fact and theory, and in trying to meet conceptual or empirical difficulties in a straightforward and clear-headed way. Directly and indirectly, he clearly inspired more research in behavioral embryology than any one before or since his time, and our field would have advanced little without his grand theorizing. Though a small tribute to such an important figure, it is a pleasure to dedicate this volume to the memory of George Ellett Coghill.

Section 1

SYNAPTOGENESIS AND THE PROBLEM OF NEURONAL SPECIFICITY: STRUCTURAL AND FUNCTIONAL ASPECTS

INTRODUCTION

In addition to the recently discovered phenomena of neuroid conduction and the electric coupling of cells early in development, the connections between the various parts of the maturing nervous system, including the pathways between the sensory and motor surfaces, are mediated primarily by synapses. The two main types of synapse are axodendritic (axon–dendrite junctions) and axosomatic (axon–cell body junctions). For the nonspecialist, it is sometimes very difficult to perceive the enormous difference in levels of analysis as far as the study of the origin and development of synapses (synaptogenesis) is concerned. For example, the main evidence that a synapse may exist in a particular place in the developing nervous system is an ultrastructural picture taken by means of an electron microscope, examples of which are shown in the following article by Dr. Martin Berry. However, a picture (electronmicrograph) can not attest to the functional capability of a synapse. Evidence that a particular synapse is functional must come from electrophysiological recording, examples of which appear in Dr. Stanley M. Crain's article. Evidence that such a functional synapse actually participates in behavior is almost always indirect and circumstantial—it is rendered likely if the synapse is located in the region of the brain, spinal cord, or musculature that is known to participate in the behavior (the experiments described by Dr. George Székely, for example), but even then the specific contribution of the synapse to the behavior in question may be unclear. The obvious point is that the journey from the ultrastructural level to the behavioral level involves a very intricate route, one that is rarely traveled in a single investigation, except by cogent inference. The more levels at which data is *not* gathered, the more highly inferential become the conclusions, regardless of whether the direction of inference is "down" (reductionistic) or "up" (constructionistic). It is necessary to enter these cautionary remarks here because some of the articles which follow assume this degree of understanding on the part of the reader.

Synapses perform both excitatory and inhibitory functions, and it was once believed that excitation (and therefore excitatory-type synapses) develops first and that inhibition (and therefore inhibitory-type synapses) develops later in ontogeny. Since there is a predominance of axodendritic synapses early and an increasing number of axosomatic synapses late in development, and young animals seem more capable of "inhibition" as they grow older, there has been a tendency to link the former synapses to excitation and the latter to inhibition. The picture is no longer that clear—as more becomes known about the early structural and functional aspects of the nervous system, we may not be able to make this neat and otherwise attractive chronological and morphological distinction, especially in the giant leap from ultrastructure to behavior. These points are particularly germane to the discussions of excitation and inhibition in the chick embryo by Dr. Crain in this section.

The various theoretical approaches to the knotty problem of the specificity of interneuronal connections have been reviewed in an introductory and historical way in the first article of Volume 1 in this serial publication. While various theories have been put forth to account for the well-documented affinities which neurons have for each other within similar systems and subsystems, a strictly biochemical one is currently in ascendancy. The reaggregation of scrambled nerve cells in Crain's tissue cultures is yet another example which would seem to call for a biochemical or molecular matching between nerve cells—this seems to be the only way we could possibly account for such a striking phenomenon, at least with our present conceptual set and empirical opportunities. With the genetic code "cracked" and DNA and RNA lurking figuratively and literally in the background, the biochemical hypothesis beckons even more seductively. While no one doubts the phenomenon of neuronal specificity itself, least of all George Székely, according to his behavioral results, neurons must be getting themselves linked together by some means other than (or in addition to) the biochemical; possibly, as Dr. Székely seems to suggest, by electrical impulse pattern. Thus, the means by which nerve cells establish orderly relationships with each other during maturation continues to be a major puzzle in developmental neurobiology, and the study of embryonic behavior itself can contribute to an understanding of the problem.

With the previous articles as a background, Dr. Marcus Jacobson concludes this section by presenting a rather novel theory of neuronal specificity. He takes as a starting point the familiar idea that there are basically two "types" of neurons in the nervous system. As defined in recent years by Joseph Altman, these two types (macroneurons and microneurons) can be distinguished on the basis of differences in their structure, function, ontogeny, phylogeny, and "plasticity." Macroneurons have long axons which conduct impulses from the peripheral sensory surfaces into the central nervous system and, on the motor side, from the central nervous system out to muscle. Such neurons also connect the different areas of the brain. Microneurons, on the other hand, have rather short axons and are found inside the central nervous system where they interconnect extensively *within*—but not between—areas of the brain. Macroneurons are said to develop earlier in ontogeny than microneurons; by virtue of their later development and their profuse and highly local interconnection (i.e., their "associative" character), microneurons are believed to be more dependent on, and responsive to, exogenous factors such as hormones and sensory stimulation, and, most importantly, they have been mentioned by numerous writers (e.g., Ramón y Cajal, Flechsig, Hebb, J. Z. Young, Altman) to possibly underlie learning, memory, and intelligent behavior.

As pointed out in the introductory article to the first volume in this serial publication, an important unanswered question is whether sensory stimulation (or, more generally speaking, function) plays merely a maintenance role in neural maturation or whether it also plays a constructive role. According to Dr. Jacobson, sensory stimulation plays only the former role and does so with respect to the microneurons only. Specifically, Dr. Jacobson's theory holds that (*a*) sensory stimulation or function plays no role whatsoever either in the construction or in the maintenance of the synapses formed by macroneurons, but (*b*) that such stimulation does affect the synapses made by microneurons but solely in terms of maintaining previously formed connections. The main contention of his essay, "A Plenitude of Neurons," is that there is an overabundance of microneuronal synaptic contacts early in development, and the individual experience (in this case, sensory stimulation) of the organism determines which (and how many) of these numerous contacts are preserved. Thus, the theory makes the interesting prediction that adult animals will have fewer microneuronal synapses and fewer microneurons than young animals of the same species. Naturally, sensory stimulation—or spontaneous function for that matter—could play a constructive role in the process as well, for example, by bringing about the essential "finishing touches" (anatomical, biochemical, and/or functional) in the synapses which are maintained. This would not be as dramatic as sensory stimulation *making* the synapses form here or there in the brain, an issue which is at the heart of the Gaze-Jacobson controversy on the development of retinotectal connections in amphibians, but it would nonetheless represent a constructive change in the synapse wrought by function. Another question concerns the *macroneurons*, particularly the possible difference in the ontogenetic functional requirements of the macroneurons which connect different areas of the brain and the ones which conduct impulses into or out of the central nervous system. Dr. Jacobson's theory is apt to provoke further research on these and related questions of synaptogenesis.

DEVELOPMENT OF THE CEREBRAL NEOCORTEX OF THE RAT

MARTIN BERRY

Department of Anatomy
The Medical School
Birmingham, England

I. Introduction

The stage of development attained by the cerebral cortex at birth varies greatly from species to species. In marsupials, for example, the neocortex is very primitive indeed at birth, while in other animals, like the ungulates, the brain has reached an exceptionally advanced stage of development. For this reason it is not meaningful to restrict discussion of cortical development to prenatal or postnatal events alone because what is prenatal for one species is postnatal for another, and vice versa. Accordingly despite the emphasis of these volumes on prenatal ontogeny, the entire period of development of the rat cerebral cortex is covered here so that this article may have more general appeal and application.

The rat is born at a time when the cortex is quite primitive and little circuitry has been established. Proliferation, cell migration, and differentiation occur prenatally and involve the research worker in the elucidation of problems like the mechanics of nuclear and cellular movement, the meaning of specialized cell contacts, the maintenance of cell shape, and the role of germinal cells in neurogenesis *vis á vis* gliogenesis. To a large extent growth of axons and dendrites, synaptogenesis, and gliogenesis are all postnatal events, and the major problem confronting workers over this latter period is the evolution of cortical connections and the relative extents to which genetic and environmental factors are involved.

Behavior is a manifestation of central nervous function, and if some degree of orderliness within the neuropil is fundamental to this function, then behavioral maturation is contingent on the development of structural organization. In fact, it now appears that behavior may also influence the organization of structure in the later periods of development. With this in mind, it is not difficult to understand that, because the rat neocortex is structurally immature at birth, neonatal and perinatal behavior may not be influenced by this higher center but, as postnatal development proceeds, neocortical function becomes apparent with the progressive acquisition of appropriate behavioral adaptation to the environment.

II. Histogenesis of the Cerebral Cortex

The period of histogenesis of the neocortex may be divided into two stages. During the first a population of cells is established which gives rise to neurons. This stage is completed when the definitive number of nerve cells is formed and is followed by a second phase in which the same or a different population of germinal cells produces the various types of glia. There is some overlap between the end of neurogenesis and the beginning of gliogenesis.

In the rat, the former begins on about day 11 or 12 postconception and ends at birth, while the latter may begin at about birth and continue into adult life.

A. Neurogenesis

The cerebral vesicle is formed on about day 10 or 11 postconception, and at first the wall of the vesicle is only one or two cells deep (Fig. 5). The basal part of the cells is attached to a basement membrane which underlies the pia and the apical ends of adjacent cells are anchored together by terminal bars to form the lining of the lumen of the cerebral vesicle. As the cells proliferate, the wall of the vesicle increases in thickness so that a pseudostratified pallisade is formed. On about day 14 of gestation, a few cells can be seen in the subpial region which are morphologically disimilar from the rest of the population. They are rounded, having lost attachment with the pial and ventricular surfaces, and their cytoplasm is clearer than that of other cells (Fig. 5). These rounded cells are the first definitive neurons, and their appearance marks the beginning of the migratory phase. The previous stage may be called the proliferative phase.

1. The Proliferative Stage

During the proliferative stage, the wall of the cerebral vesicle (or ventricle as it may now be called) becomes a pseudostratified epithelium which increases steadily in thickness. It is now generally accepted that all the cells in the epithelium are alike (Fig. 1) and behave in the same manner. Premitotic cells are elongated and attached at their apical (inner) and basal (outer) ends along the ventricular and pial surfaces respectively. Just before mitosis the nucleus migrates into the apex of the cell, and the basal end is detached from the basement membrane and retracted so that the cell rounds up in a juxtaventricular position. Mitosis then occurs, the daughter cells separate, and the basal processes grow and become attached to the subpial basement membrane. The nucleus of each daughter cell migrates away from the ventricle into the basal part of the process, and the cycle then repeats. There are some special aspects of the proliferative stage which are worth discussing in a little more detail, namely, uniformity of cell type, nuclear movement, the mitotic cycle, cell contact, and changes in cell shape.

a. Uniformity of Cell Type. It is rather an extraordinary state of affairs that the classical theories of neurogenesis are still printed in modern text-books despite the fact that these theories were shown to be erroneous as long ago as the 1930's by the brilliant studies of F. C. Sauer. According to the classical view, the neural epithelium is stratified and contains three different cell types called germinal cells, spongioblasts, and neuroblasts (His, 1890).

Germinal cells were thought to produce spongioblasts and neuroblasts; the former develop into glia, the latter into neurons. Shortly after the formulation of this theory, slight modifications were proposed. Schaper (1897), Kölliker (1896), and Ramón y Cajal (1909) thought that the germinal (mitotic) cells and epithelial (elongated pseudostratified) cells were the mitotic and intermitotic stages of the same cell, and that spongioblasts and neuroblasts differentiated from the epithelial cells. Another less acceptable idea was that the nuclei in the epithelium of the neural tube shared a common cytoplasmic syncitium from which glia and neurons later separated (Hardesty, 1904; Sedgwick, 1895).

In 1935, F. C. Sauer (1935a, 1935b) performed a careful cytological study on the neural tube of several species and concluded that the cells did not form a syncitium but a true pseudostratified epithelium, and that a fixation artifact may have given the former impression to the earlier workers (Fig. 1). All cells in the epithelium were of the same homogeneous population, and all underwent cyclical division accompanied by changes in morphology and position within the epithelium (see later). Sauer's thesis was later substantiated by colchicine studies (Källén, 1953; Watterson, Veneziano, & Bartha, 1956; Woodard & Estes, 1944), by spectrophotometric DNA estimations (M. E. Sauer & Chittenden, 1959), by studies on the dilution of radioactive label in the DNA of neuroectoderm cells using tritiated thymidine (S. Fujita, 1960, 1962, 1963, 1964; Fujita, Shimada, & Nakamura, 1966; Sauer & Walker, 1959; Sechrist, 1969; Sidman, 1961; Sidman, Miale, & Feder, 1959), and by the use of the electron microscope (Allenspach & Roth, 1967; Bellairs, 1959; Duncan, 1957; H. Fujita & Fujita, 1963; Hinds, 1971; Hinds & Ruffett, 1971; Lyser, 1964, 1968; Meller, Breipohl, & Glees, 1966; Meller & Wechsler, 1964; Sechrist, 1969; Wechsler, 1967; Wechsler & Meller, 1967).

There is a great deal of misunderstanding among neuroembryologists about the terminology of the various layers of the neuroepithelium. The Boulder Committee (1970) recommended an unequivocal nomenclature in which the pseudostratified layer has been designated the ventricular zone. The nomenclature of the Boulder Committee is used throughout this article (Fig. 2).

b. Mitotic Cycle. S. Fujita (1960, 1962, 1963, 1964) and Fujita *et al.* (1966) have studied the cell cycle in the white leghorn chick by labeling DNA with tritiated thymidine. They found that the number of cells taking up the label increased linearly to 100%. From their graph of the percentage labeled cells plotted against time, the duration of the mitotic cycle has been calculated. Sauer and Walker (1959) found the DNA synthetic time lasted some 4 hours in the chick brain. Another estimate has been made by

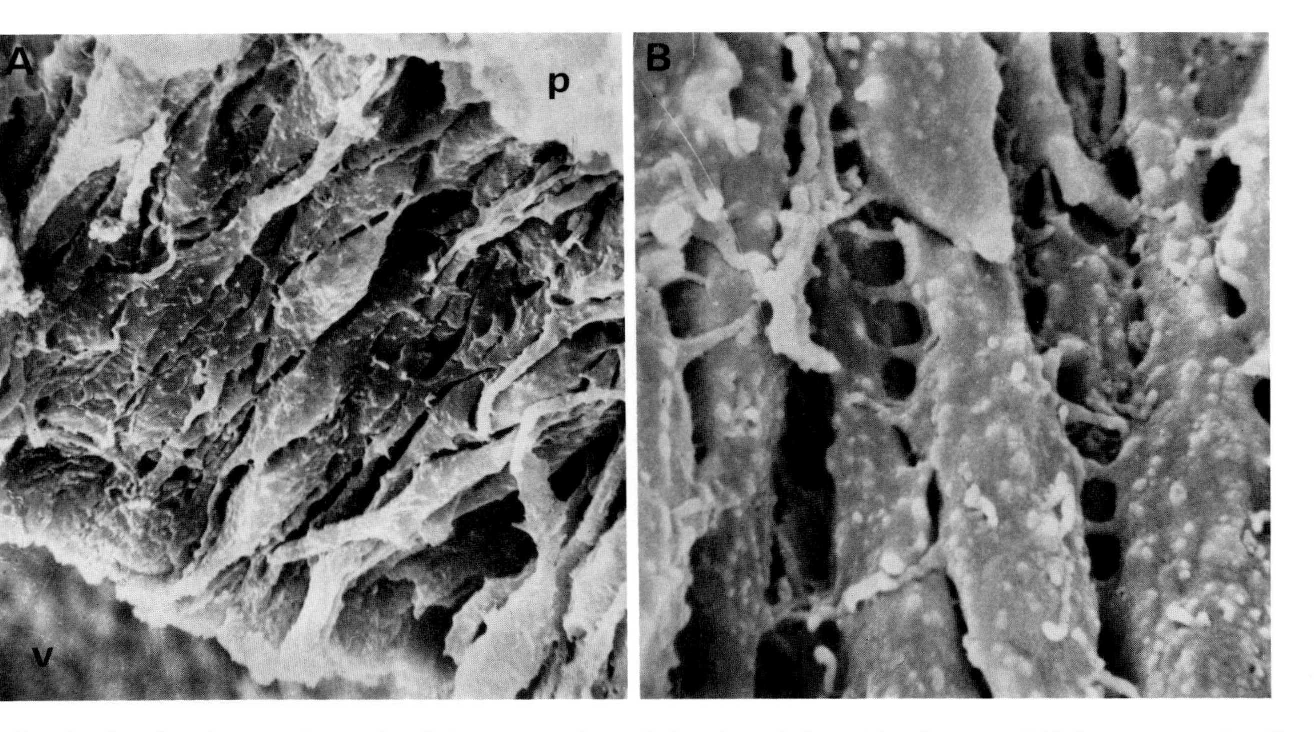

FIG. 1. Scanning electron micrographs of the neuroectoderm of the telencephalic vesicle of a rat aged 13 days *postconception*. The pseudostratified nature of the epithelium is clearly seen (A), and under higher magnification protoplasmic bridges between the processes of the cells in the epithelium are distinguishable. (A × 3.1 K; B × 7.3 K) v, ventricle; p, pial surface (from Seymore, Kemp, & Berry, 1972).

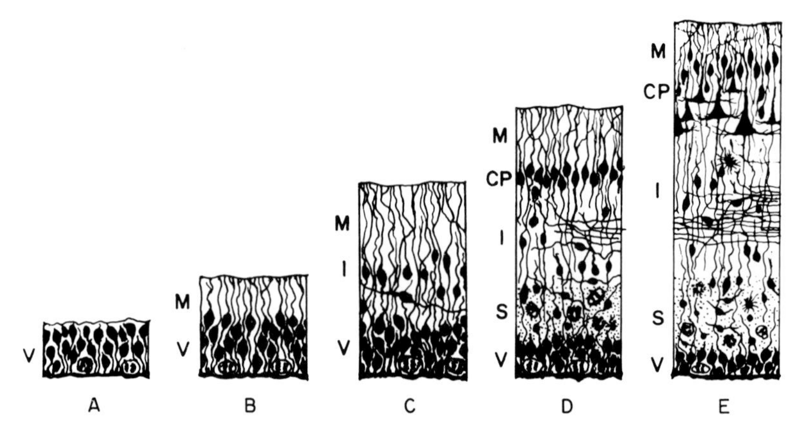

FIG. 2. A schematic drawing of five stages (A–E) in the development of the vertebrate central nervous system illustrating the nomenclature of the Boulder Committee (1970). Abbreviations: CP, cortical plate; I, intermediate zone; M, marginal zone; S, subventricular zone; V, ventricular zone (from Boulder Committee, 1970).

Langman, Guerrant, and Freeman (1966, chick cord), who obtained a DNA synthetic time of 5 hours, a postsynthetic time and prophase time of $2\frac{1}{2}$ hours, and only a brief presynthetic time (G_1). The total cycle time was 8 hours. In the mouse neural tube a generation cycle of 11 hours has been obtained (Atlas & Bond, 1965), and in the hamster the DNA synthetic phase lasts 6 hours, synthetic (G_1) and prophase some $1\frac{1}{2}$ hours, and postsynthetic $4\frac{1}{2}$ hours, giving a total generation time of 12 hours (Shimada & Langman, 1970). Any lack of agreement can be reconciled with species differences and the fact that both mitotic time and generation time vary greatly at different ages and from region to region (S. Fujita *et al.*, 1966).

c. Nuclear Migration and Cell Shape. F. C. Sauer (1935a, 1935b) deduced from his observations on the chick neural tube that during the mitotic cycle, premitotic or resting nuclei occupied the basal (or outer) process of the cell. Just before replication, the basal process became detached from the basement membrane and, as the cytoplasm rounded up, the basal process was retracted toward the lumen of the tube where the cell was firmly anchored to adjacent cells by terminal bars. Thus, the nucleus actively moved to a juxtaluminal position. The cleavage plane of divisions at this stage was such that each daughter cell maintained its attachment to its neighbors, and thus postmitotic movement away from the lumen could not occur. The basal process was seen to regrow and gain attachment to the basement membrane, while the nucleus migrated, within the process, coming to rest below the pial membrane. These movements and the accompanying changes in cell shape are repeated during each cycle. Sauer's observations have been borne out by the use of colchicine (Watterson *et al.*, 1956; Woodard & Estes, 1944) which showed that migration away from the lumen broke down under this treatment, and metaphases accumulated about the ventricle. M. E. Sauer and Chittenden (1959), using a microspectrometry technique on Feulgen stained sections, showed that the nuclei in the outer two-thirds of the wall of the chick neural tube contained approximately twice as much DNA than the telophase cells at the lumen. They concluded that premitotic cells double their DNA content in the outer wall before undergoing mitosis at the lumen. After injecting tritiated thymidine, it is possible to demonstrate premitotic cells autoradiographically and to follow their migratory movements. This has been done by many workers, and the observations of Sauer have been confirmed.

F. C. Sauer (1935a, 1935b) thought that the movement of the nucleus was a result of increased cytoplasmic turgidity and, because the cell is firmly anchored at the apex, the basal process and nucleus are pulled down to the lumen. Postmitotic cells at the lumen may no longer possess this turgidity and thus would be pushed away by simple overcrowding. This latter idea was modified (F. C. Sauer, 1936, 1937) after he noticed that postmitotic changes in cell shape were associated with the elongation of spindle fibers to produce a prominent cytoplasmic fiber which persisted through interphase into the next mitosis. He suggested that the postmitotic elongation of cells may be associated with a thrusting force generated and propagated within a cytoplasmic fiber system. Certainly one of the more prominent features of electron micrographs of the matrix cell is the presence of a large number of 60 Å microfilaments and 120 Å microtubules which are especially conspicuous in the apical and basal processes, respectively (Fig. 3) (Allenspach & Roth, 1967; Handel & Roth, 1971; Herman & Kauffman, 1966, Hinds & Ruffett, 1971; Sechrist, 1969; Tennyson, 1962).

i. Microtubules. Microtubules may be important in the development and maintenance of cell shape (Byers & Porter, 1964; Potter, Furshpan, & Lennox, 1966; de-Thé, 1964), as well as the transportation of water and ions associated with increases in nuclear volume and nuclear movement (Herman & Kauffman, 1966; Slautterback, 1963).

The functional significance of microtubules has been most closely investigated in the tiny protoplasmic processes of the heliozoans (Kitching, 1964; Roth, Pihlaja, & Shigenaka, 1970; L. G. Tilney, 1968; Tilney & Byers, 1969; Tilney, Hiramoto, & Marsland, 1966; Tilney & Porter, 1967) and in the cells of the developing lens in the eye (Arnold, 1966; Byers & Porter, 1964; Pearce & Zwaan, 1970), where it is thought that the microtubules are actively associated with the maintenance of cell shape and the active elongation of cell processes. Handel and Roth (1971) have attempted to see if the work on the heliozoans has any relevance to the nervous system. They concluded that microtubules may play a role in the development and maintenance of the shape of the proliferative cell, and that controlled dissolution of tubules may result in the passive collapse of the cell prior to mitosis. Karfunkel (1971) and Burnside (1971) came to a similar conclusion about the role of microtubules in the cells of the neural plate of two amphibians during neurulation.

Colchicine has been shown to disrupt microtubules (Brinkley, Stubblefield, & Hsu, 1967; Pearce & Zwaan, 1970; L. G. Tilney, 1968), and from the results of the colchicine studies of Källen (1953), Watterson *et al.* (1956), and Woodard and Estes (1944), it is quite clear that colchicine arrests cells in metaphase only. Cells round up normally to enter mitosis, and presumably cells completing telophase regrow basal processes, and their nuclei migrate away from the lumen in the normal way since there is no accumulation of interphase cells at the lumen. Resting cells with apical and basal processes seem quite normal. There also appears to be a controlled movement of interphase cells into mitosis, resulting in the gradual accumulation of metaphase cells at the lumen. It is difficult to equate these observations with the hypothetical role of microtubules which have been proposed.

Other workers have suggested that microtubules may be responsible for ion and water absorption and transportation (Herman & Kauffman, 1966; Slautterback, 1963). Electronmicrographs of fetal ependymal cells in the chick (Bellairs, 1959; Duncan, 1957; Meller & Wechsler, 1964), in the rat (Duckett, 1968), and in humans have shown that, in common with other absorptive cells in the body, they show evidence of intra- and intercellular pinocytosis and possess large numbers of mitochondria. By intrathecal and intraventricular injection of ^{35}S-labeled proteins (Bowsher, 1957) and ferritin (Brightman, 1965), in adult cats and rats respectively, it was possible to demonstrate the absorptive function of ependymal cells.

Microtubules may alter the shape of cells and/or initiate intracytoplasmic movements by controlling the sol/gel state of the cytoplasm from region to region. Pressman (1965) has suggested that membrane permeability may be altered by microtubules if they can induce the uptake or release of water, and L. G. Tilney and Porter (1967) favor the idea that microtubules transport and release water intracellularly, causing a local alteration from the gel to the sol state. On the other hand, Girbardt (1968) has proposed that microtubules absorb water from the cytoplasm and thus mediate the sol to gel transformation.

ii. Microfilaments. It is possible that 60 Å microfilaments may be contractile (Wessells, 1971) and function to alter the shape of cells and whole organs through local or regional contraction. Active contraction of microfilaments may occur during neurulation (Baker & Schroeder, 1967; Burnside, 1971; Karfunkel, 1971; Schroeder, 1970; Waddington & Perry, 1966), during the formation of the lens (Wren & Wessells, 1969) and the tubular glands in the wall of the thick oviduct (Wren & Wessells, 1970), and may also control morphogenesis in the salivary gland of the mouse (Spooner & Wessells, 1970). Microfilaments and microtubules have also been implicated as having important functions in the growth cones found at the growing tip of axons (see later) (Yamada, Spooner, & Wessells, 1970). Conceivably, contractile microfilaments within the apical process may actively pull down the nucleus in preparation for mitosis (Hinds & Ruffett, 1971). Wessells (1971) has suggested that Ca^{2+} may be involved in the contraction of microfilaments, and that the degrading agent cytochalasin B may counteract the effects of Ca^{2+} and inhibit microfilament contraction. It is possible to transport Ca^{2+} along electrical gradients. The fact that embryonic cells contact one another at low resistance junctions (see later), and that microfilaments appear to converge onto these junctions may also have significance with respect to their contractile function.

It is relevant to mention here that microtubules and microfilaments feature in the cytoplasm of mature neurons in great numbers and may be responsible for their characteristic argyrophilia. Accordingly, it could be argued that matrix cells exhibiting these elements are, in fact, differentiating into neurons (Sechrist, 1969).

d. Cell Contact. Junctional complexes formed between cells have been classified by Farquhar and Palade (1963). One type, the desmosome or terminal bar, as F. C. Sauer (1936, 1937) called it, has been studied in the human telencephalon (Duckett, 1968), the chick retina (Sheffield & Fischman, 1970), the rabbit telencephalon (Stensaas & Stensaas, 1968), and the rat telencephalon (Hinds & Ruffet, 1971; Holmes & Berry, 1966) (Fig. 3), and their importance in the development of the cerebral cortex has been emphasized.

It may be recalled that the apical ends of proliferative cells are anchored at the lumen of the cerebral vesicle or cord by terminal bars, and that mitosis occurs in rounded cells along this lumen. It has also been mentioned that mitotic spindles are directed in a plane at right angles to the radial axis of the lumen (S. Fujita, 1960, 1962; Fujita *et al.*, 1966; Martin & Langman, 1965; F. C. Sauer, 1935a, 1935b). F. C. Sauer (1937) suggested that the orientation of the spindle determined whether the cell remained attached at the lumen after division or migrated away. If the axis of the spindle is directed in a plane parallel with the lumen, terminal bars remain in each of the daughter cells, and attachment with neighboring cells would be maintained. If the spindle was directed in any other plane, terminal bars may be excluded from one daughter cell, and attachment with neighboring cells would be lost. Under these circumstances, daughter cells would be free to migrate away from the

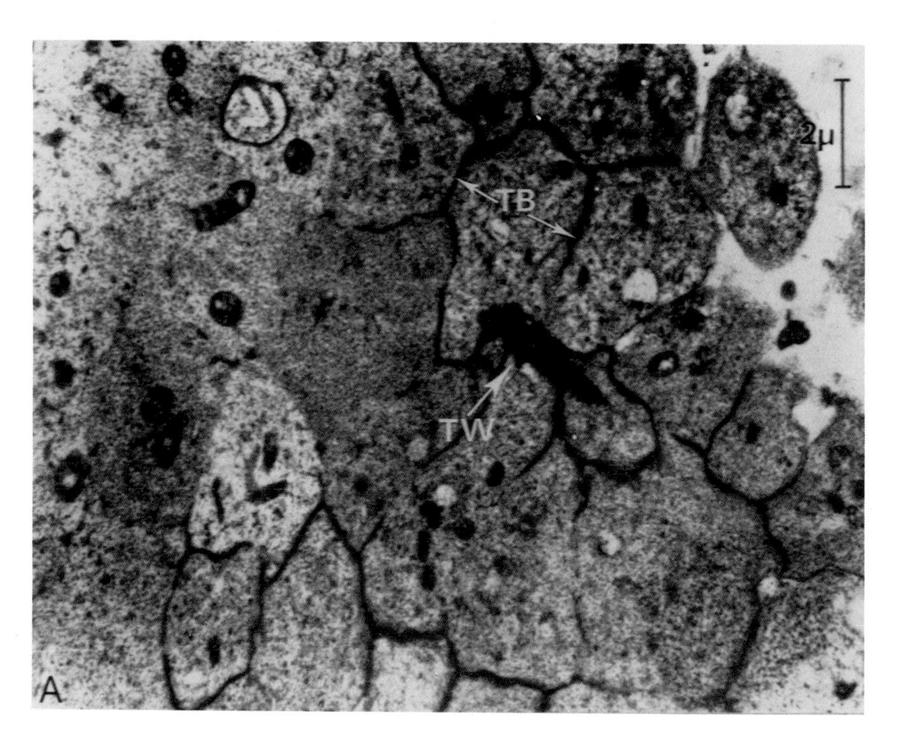
2μ
TB
TW
A

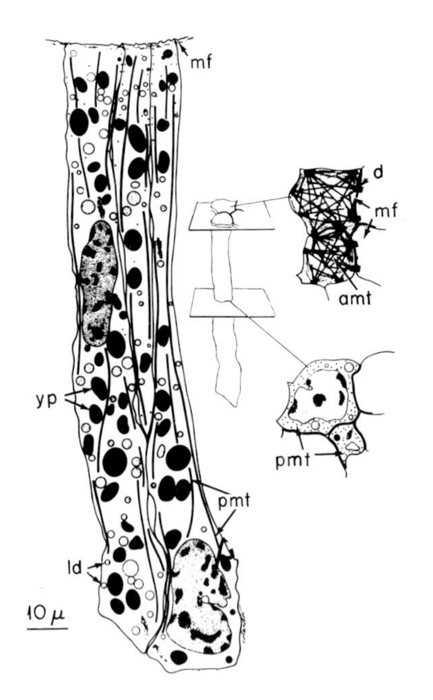
mf
d
mf
amt
yp
pmt
pmt
ld
10 μ
B

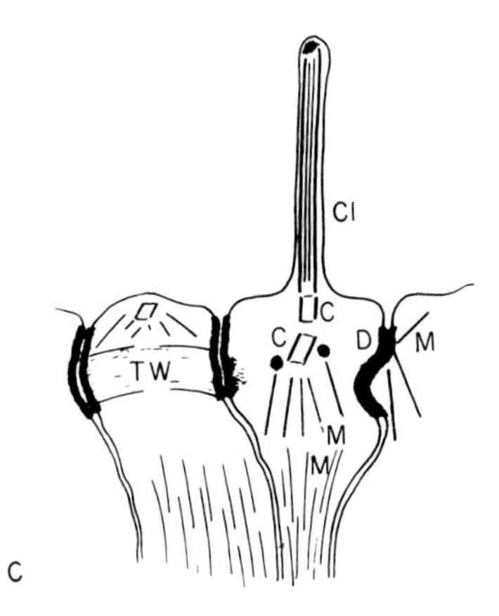
Cl
C
C
D
M
TW
M
M
C

lumen. It has been reported that during the proliferative stage, terminal bars remain intact during division (H. Fujita & Fujita, 1963; Herman & Kauffman, 1966; Wechsler, 1966) and that all spindles are parallel with the lumen (Doig & smart, 1967; Langman *et al.*, 1966; Martin, 1967; Martin & Langman, 1965). However, when migration starts and rounded cells appear under the pial membrane, mitotic spindles are found to be orientated obliquely and perpendicular to the lumen (Doig & Smart, 1967; Hinds & Ruffett, 1971; Langman *et al.*, 1966; Martin, 1967; Martin & Langman, 1965). Thus the orientation of the spindle may decide whether daughter cells remain or pass out of the ventricular zone. Later in development mitosis is no longer confined to the luminal border but may appear anywhere within the depths of the ventricular or subventricular zone (Doig & Smart, 1967) (Fig. 4). Presumably, cells undergoing division high in these zones may be unattached to the lumen, and thus both daughter cells may be free to migrate away.

Specialized cellular junctions may be more permeable to ions and large molecules than nonjunctional membranes (Payton, Bennett, & Pappas, 1969). Since the junctional complex is not accessible to the extracellular space, interchange of molecules is between cells. The flow of ions between cells means that low resistance electrical coupling can be established, and the passage of current between adjacent cells may form the basis of intercellular communication (Bennett, Pappas, Giménez, & Nakajima, 1967; Potter *et al.*, 1966; Sheridan, 1968; Trelstad, Hay, & Revel, 1967). It has also been shown that when calcium ions are removed from junctions, they become freely permeable to large molecules (Kanno & Lowenstein, 1966), and that the exchange of molecules between cells might control tissue growth (Loewenstein & Kanno, 1966). Subsequent selectivity of either synaptic contact and/or axon growth might be conferred by the interchange of macromolecules between cells. Cell contact may also be important in the execution

---

FIG. 3. (A) Horizontal section through the ependymal zone of a 14-day-old rat fetus. Terminal bars (TB) are prominent, and in one case a terminal web can be seen (TW) (from Holmes & Berry, 1966). (B) Schematic illustration of the orientation of microfilaments and microtubules in elongating neural plate cells. Numerous microtubules are aligned parallel to the long axis of the cell (paraxial microtubules, pmt). These microtubules are seen in profile in longitudinal section, in cross section and in transverse sections of the cell. Just beneath the free surface, microtubules are aligned to the free surface in a layer across the cell apex (apical microtubules, amt). In the same plane with the apical layer of microtubules, 50–70 Å microfilaments (mf) are arranged into a circumferential bundle which encircles the cell apex in pursestring fashion. yp, yolk platelet; ld, lipid droplet; d, desmosome (from Burnside, 1971). (C) Diagram of the apical surface of neural tube cells. The interrelationship of microtubules (M), desmosomes (D), terminal web (TW), and centriole (C) result in a structural specialization that seems to be important in maintaining cell relationships and therefore the morphology of the entire neural tube (cl; cilium) (from Handel & Roth, 1971).

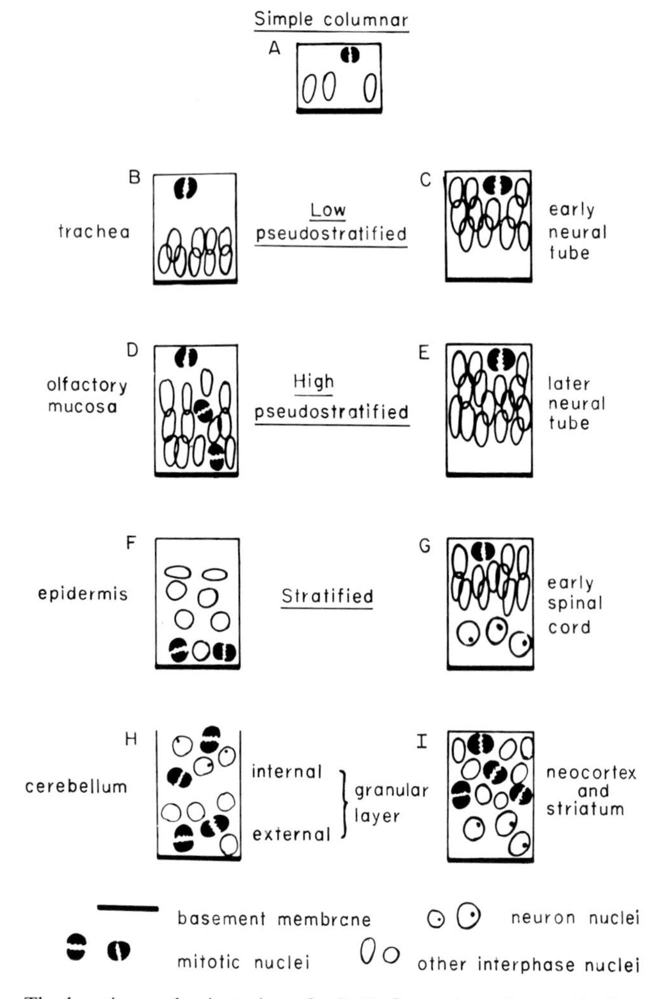

FIG. 4. The location and orientation of mitotic figures in various epithelia. Note the preponderance of apical mitotic figures in the neuroepithelium (C and E), but that this pattern breaks down later in development so that in the neocortex (I) nuclei no longer migrate and divide at the ventricular surface but lie randomly orientated in a subependymal position (from Doig & Smart, 1967).

of contact inhibition of moving cells (Abercrombie & Heaysman, 1954) and the guidance by contact of growing neuronal processes and migrating neuroblasts. The role played by tight junctions in synaptogenesis and dendritic growth will be discussed in later sections.

2. MIGRATORY PHASE

In the cerebral cortex of the rat, matrix cells become detached from their neighbors at the ventricular surface on about day 14 of gestation and move away to round up under the basement membrane (Fig. 5). These cells may be called neuroblasts because it can be shown autoradiographically that they later differentiate into neurons. The migration of neuroblasts away from the lumen accelerates, and by day 16 a definitive lamina of cells has been formed below the pial membrane (Fig. 5). The appearance of this lamina divides the cortex into five layers, or zones, called (from the pial surface inward) the marginal zone, the cortical plate, the intermediate zone, and the subventricular and ventricular zones (Fig. 2). The marginal zone later becomes layer 1 of the definitive cortex, and the cells of the cortical plate differentiate into the neurons of all the other layers. The intermediate zone becomes the white matter of the cortex. Cells dividing in the ventricular zone undergo DNA replication in the subventricular zone and not at the pial surface as before. Ultimately the cells in the ventricular and subventricular zones differentiate into ependymal and subependymal cells, respectively. To understand the migration of cells in the cerebral cortex, it is necessary to discuss two factors: the pattern and the mechanism of movement.

a. Pattern of Migration. The first research worker to study the migration of cells in the cerebral cortex was Tilney in 1933. He performed a cytological survey of Nissl stained preparations and concluded that the definitive layers of the cerebral cortex were established by three distinct and separate cellular migrations. Each was characterized by the movement of a large number of cells from the ventricular zones to the cortical plate. The first of these migrations, which he called primary migratory lamination, formed the supragranular layers II and III, the second formed the granular layer, or layer IV, and tertiary migratory lamination formed the infragranular layers, V and VI. Thus, according to F. Tilney (1933), the cerebral cortex was formed from the outside inward so that newly arriving cells took up positions below those already *in situ*. The first hint that this idea might be erroneous came from Hicks, D'Amato, and Lowe (1959), who concluded that the only acceptable way of interpreting their results of the effects of X-rays on the developing cerebral cortex was to postulate that "the major additions to the cortex in the latter days of gestation are to outer layers. Cells migrate through the cortical plate to these positions [p. 457–458]." This idea that the cerebral cortex might be formed in the reverse order to that suggested by F. Tilney (1933) was confirmed by an autoradiographic study (Angevine & Sidman, 1961) and by the further analysis of the effects of X-rays on the developing cortex (Berry & Eayrs, 1963). Berry, Rogers, and Eayrs (1964) and Berry and Rogers (1965) later worked out the sequence of migration of neuroblasts in the cerebral cortex of the rat (Fig. 6). They found that the cells formed up

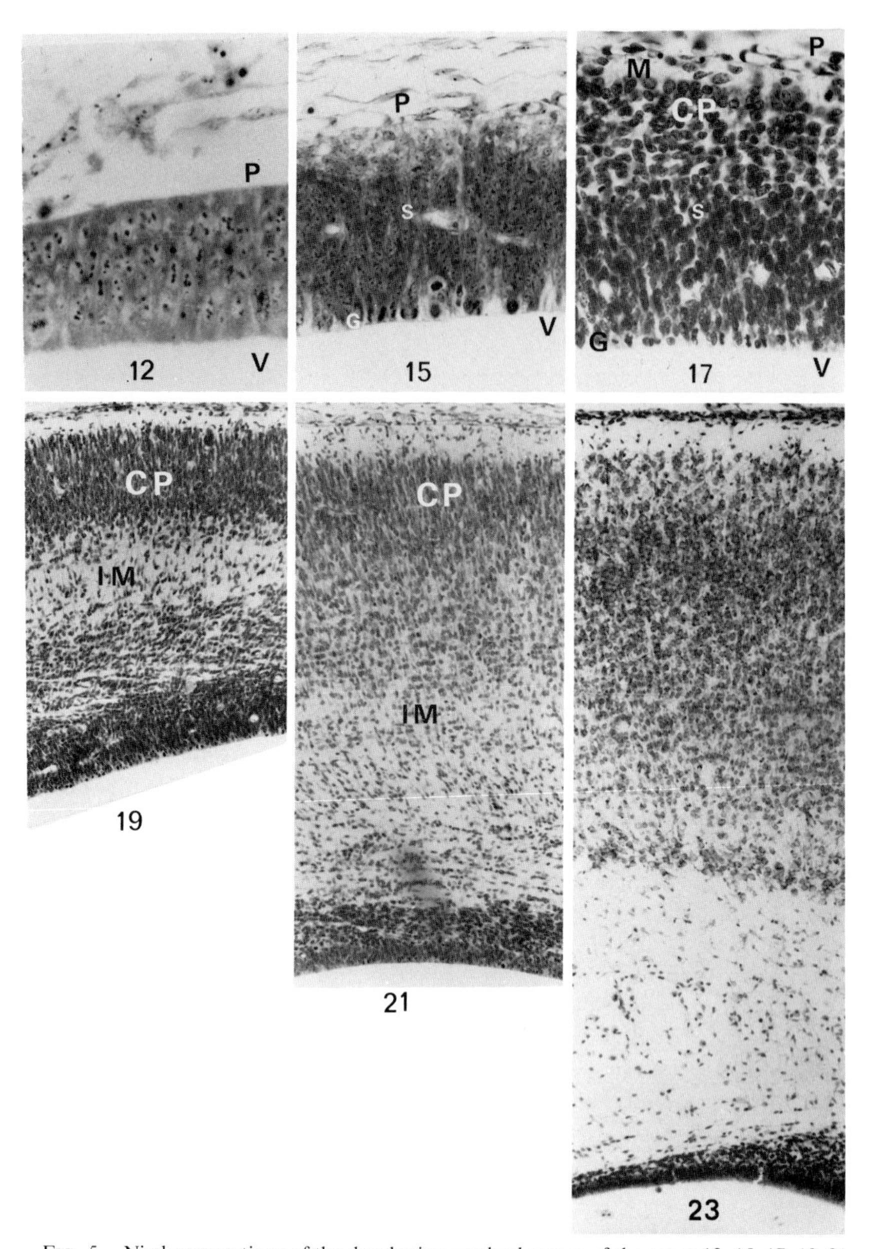

FIG. 5. Nissl preparations of the developing cerebral cortex of the rat at 12, 15, 17, 19, 21, and 23 days *postpartum*. Note that mitoses are confirmed to the ventricular zone in the 12-day specimen only, and that at all other ages cells can also be seen undergoing mitosis in the subventricular and ventricular zones. Dividing cells in these other regions may be neuroectodermal or mesodermal in origin; the latter are associated with the invasion of blood vessels. P, pial surface; V, ventricle, M, marginal zone; CP, cortical plate; IM, intermediate zone; S, subventricular zone; G, ventricular zone. (12, 15 days × 1440; 17 days × 900; 19, 21, 23 days × 360).

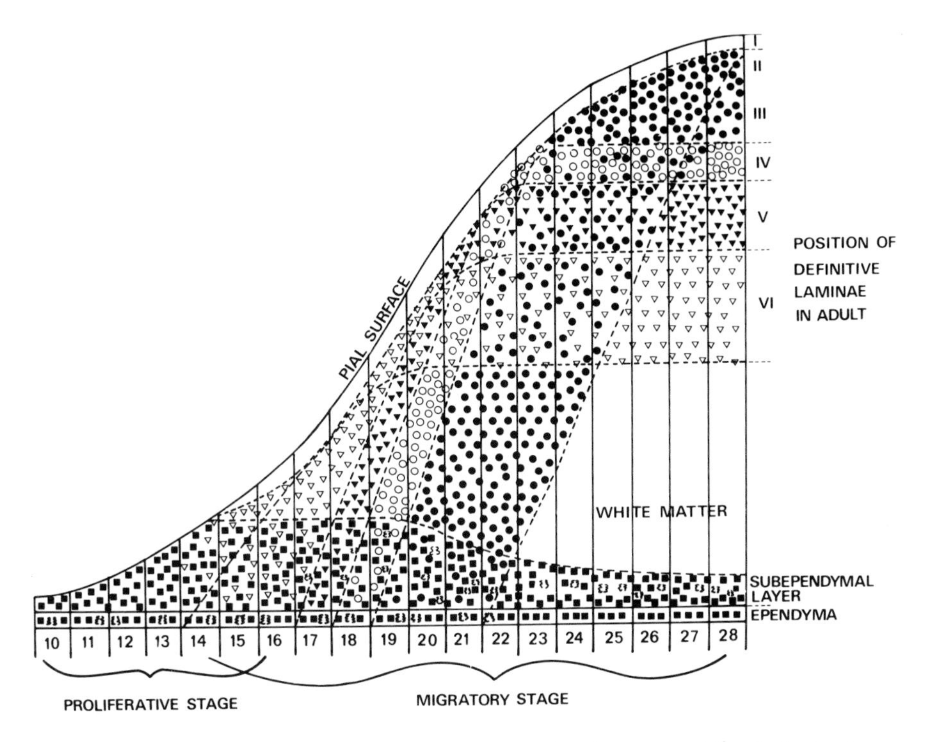

FIG. 6. Schematic representation of the pattern of migration of neuroblasts in the developing neocortex of the rat. ■, ventricular cell; ⸪, mitotic cell; ▽, ▼ infragranular cells of layers VI and V respectively; ○, granular cells; ●, supragranular cells. See text for full explanation.

to day 16 of gestation populated layer VI, those formed on about day 17 formed layer V, the cells of layer IV were formed in the ventricular zone on about the day 18, and the cells of layers II and III were formed on days 19, 20, and 21 of gestation. After their formation in the ventricular zone, migrating neuroblasts moved out into the intermediate zone and continued their migration through the cortical plate, coming to rest in a position above this lamina (Fig. 6). Thus, cellular additions to the developing cortex were not added below but above the migrated layer of cells. The first formed cells reached the cortex quite rapidly but later, as the migration path became longer, the migratory time became extended. Thus, cells formed early in the ventricular zone reached the marginal layer in about $1\frac{1}{2}$ days, but those formed later reached their definitive destination in about 6 days. These results have been confirmed in the rat (Haas, Werner, & Fliedner, 1970; Hicks & D'Amato, 1968), the mouse (Angevine & Sidman, 1961; Langman & Welch, 1967), the opossum (Morest, 1970b), and the golden hamster (Shimada & Langman,

1970). During their migration, neuroblasts must pass many obstacles before they can reach the marginal layer, for instance, developing fiber tracts, dendritic processes, and blood vessels. How do the cells do it and what starts, maintains, and terminates migration?

b. Theories on the Mechanism of Migration. 1. Morest (1970b) (Fig. 7) proposed that the nucleus rather than the whole cell migrates by moving within the cytoplasmic process of the cells in the ventricular zone. The region to which the nucleus is transported is determined by the location of the basal process. As the nucleus migrates, the apical process of the cell is retracted and the movement of the nucleus is arrested with the axon and dendrites begin to grow out from the perikaryon (Morest, 1970a, 1970b). The basal process may remain attached to the pial surface for a considerable period after the axon and dendrites have begun to differentiate. Differentiation is thought to be triggered by the arrival of afferent fibers which make contact

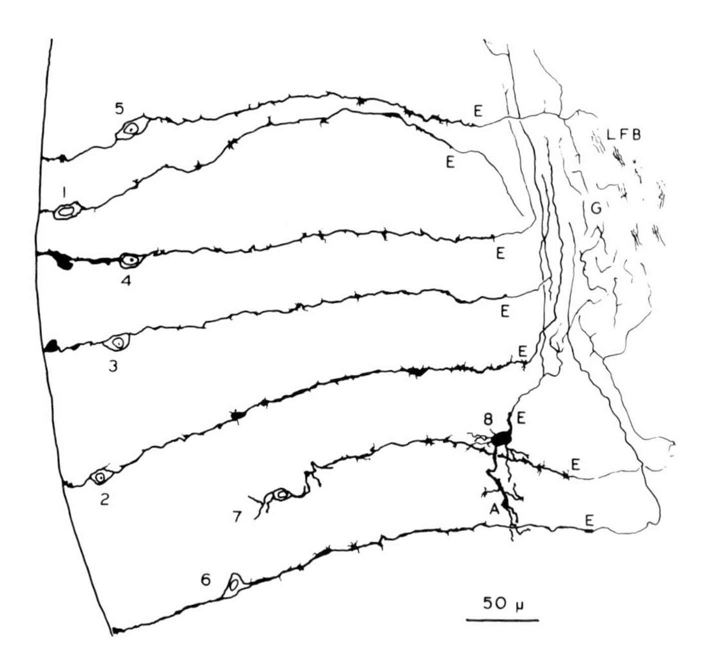

FIG. 7. Camera lucida drawings of rapid Golgi impregnated cells from the pars dorsalis of the neostriatum of the opossum. Neuroblasts (1–8) appear in progressive stages of translocation from the internal limiting layer of the matrix zone (left) to the prospective candate neuropil (G), formed by afferent branches from the incipient anterior limb of the internal capsule, or lateral forebrain bundle (LFB), and by collaterals of efferent axons (E). In cells 1–7 the impregnation was light enough that the nucleus was located. A dendritic growth cone (A) and incipient dendrites sprout from the perikaryon of cell 8 which has not quite reached its final position at the axon's origin (from Morest, 1970b).

with the primitive neuroblasts. Morest (1970b) concludes:

> the basic problem in the histogenesis of the central nervous system is to account for the growth and differentiation of the primitive epithelial process . . . [and] to determine how the afferent growth cones and other elements in the neuroepithelial mantle [subventricular zones] may relate to DNA synthesis in the germinal matrix, to the translocation of the neuroblasts and to the differentiation of its synaptogenic structure [p. 302].

2. Berry and Rogers (1965) (Fig. 8) proposed that during the migratory phase a fundamental change occurs in the mode of division of the cells in the matrix layer. As we have seen, division during the proliferative stage produces two identical cells which grow processes and establish connections at the lumen of the ventricle and at the subpial basement membrane. The theory suggests that the stage is set for migration when the nucleus migrates to the luminal surface without concomitant retraction of the basal process. The nucleus then divides, but the cytoplasm remains intact, i.e., karyokinesis without cytokinesis similar to that seen in spermatogenesis (Fawcett, Ito, & Slautterback, 1959) and oögenesis (Gondos, 1970). Thus, at this stage the two daughter nuclei are enclosed within the parent cell. One of the nuclei is thought to migrate within the basal process toward the pial surface. Cytoplasmic division occurs in the lower part of the marginal zone when the nucleus with scanty cytoplasm buds off from the parent process. The other nucleus remains in the ventricular zone to divide again, but the processes of the germinal cells never lose contact with the pial and ventricular surfaces throughout development.

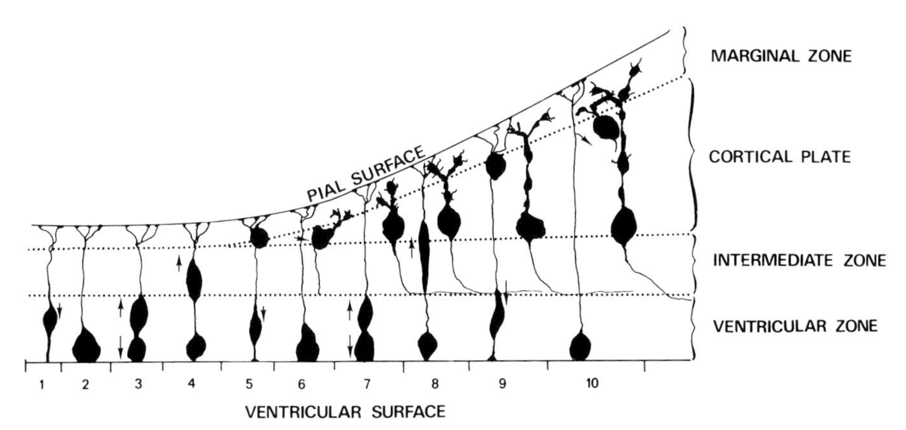

FIG. 8. Diagrammatic representation of the mechanism of migration according to Berry and Rogers (1965). Germinal cells (1–10) are depicted in various phases of the cell cycle. It can be seen that only the nucleus divides in the ventricular zone, and that one daughter nucleus migrates along the basal process and buds off under the pial membrane. (For explanation see text.)

3. Stensaas (1967b) (Fig. 9) believes that neuroblasts differentiate within the matrix layer and can be recognized in Golgi and aniline preparations (see also Sechrist, 1969). The axons of differentiating neurons grow out of the ventricular zone and may travel in a radial plane, toward the cortical surface, or horizontally within the white matter. The migratory path of the soma follows that of the axon until the trailing process, which has become detached from the ventricular surface, together with the soma itself, rotate through 180°. By this means the trailing process, or preapex as it is called, is directed at the pial surface, and dendrites grow out from it as migration continues.

4. Rakic (1971b) studied the migration of granule cells from the external granular layer to the internal granular layer in the developing cerebellum of the rhesus monkey. He concluded that cells were guided to their destination by contact with well differentiated glia cells called Bergmann glia (for fine structural details, see also Mugnaini & Forstrønen, 1967). These latter cells differentiate early and lie deep in the developing cerebellar cortex in the vicinity of the Purkinje cell bodies. Their processes run up to the pial surface and are attached to the basement membrane by end feet. The primitive germinal cells of the external granular layer lie among the end feet of the Bergmann glia. Following division, cells migrate away by sliding along the

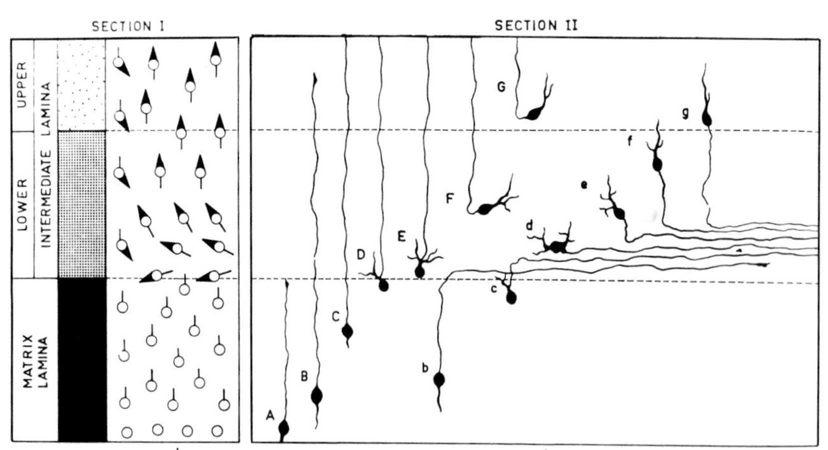

O GERMINAL CELL, NEUROBLAST WITH ASCENDING AXON, NEUROBLAST WITH ASCENDING AXON AND PREAPEX, NEUROBLAST WITH HORIZONTAL AXON AND PREAPEX, NEUROBLAST WITH DESCENDING AXON AND PREAPEX.

FIG. 9. The morphology of migrating neuroblasts is shown schematically. Section I illustrates changes in the orientation of neuroblast processes at different levels of the celebral hemisphere. Section II shows the appearance of cells impregnated with the Golgi technique. A–G depict neuroblasts with ascending axons; b–g are cells with horizontal axons in the embryonic subcortical white matter (from Stensaas, 1967b).

Bergmann glial process leading and trailing their processes. The trailing process soon develops into an axon which bifurcates within the molecular layer and becomes a parallel fiber while the granule cell is still migrating. Rakic (1971a) found a similar system to be operational in the developing parieto-occipital cortex of the macaque monkey (Fig. 10). In this situation, radially orientated glial processes appeared to guide developing neuroblasts away from the ventricular zone up through the intermediate zone and cortical plate to their definitive positions.

5. Hicks and D'Amato (1968) state that migratory cells move to the cortical plate along the curved and oblique paths of the pallial fibers, the basic plan of which is established by the early thalamocortical fibers. Migrating cells leave the fibers within the cortical plate. Neural cells may seek out and attach to fibers according to preexisting chemical affinities.

c. Possible Mechanisms of Movement during Migration. Both the theories of Berry and Rogers and of Morest imply that nuclei may be transported by some intracellular mechanism, and thus microtubules and/or microfilaments may be involved. The role played by these latter structures in the movements of nuclei during the proliferative stage has already been discussed. The ideas of Berry and Rogers are contradicted by two observations. Firstly, electron microscope investigations of developing cortex (Hinds & Ruffett, 1971; Shimada & Langman, 1970; Stensaas & Stensaas, 1968), in

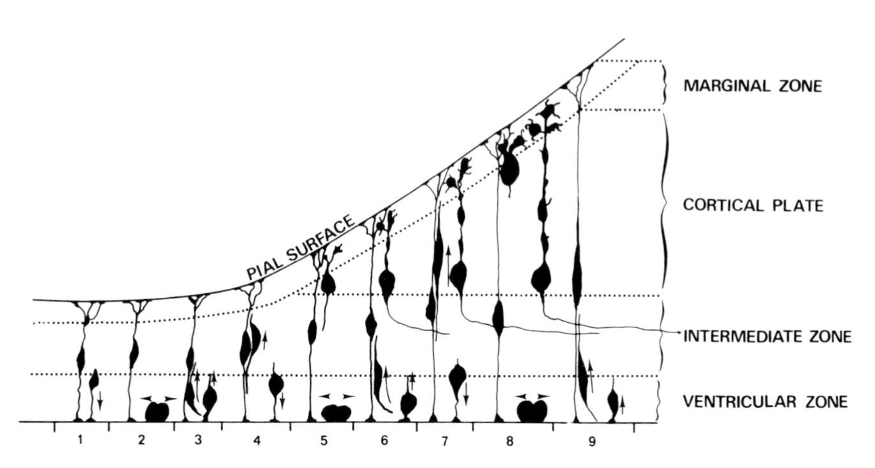

FIG. 10. Diagrammatic representation of the mechanism of migration according to Rakic (1971a, 1971b). Presumably the neuroepithelium differentiates early into two cell types: a glial cell and a germinal cell. The processes of the glial cell are attached to the pial and ventricular surfaces by long processes which form the guide wires for the migrating neuroblasts. Pairs of cells (1–9) are shown (glial cell to the left, germinal cell to the right). Differentiation of the neuroblast may occur during migration.

which serial sections were examined, have shown that mitotic cells are spherical and have no processes whatsoever, although some of these workers appear to have been examining cells in the proliferative rather than the migratory stage. Secondly, migrating neuroblasts appear to undergo considerable differentiation during their migration (Butler & Caley, 1971; Morest, 1969a, 1970a, 1970b; Rakic, 1971a, 1971b; Stensaas, 1967a, 1967b, 1967c, 1967d, 1967e, 1968; Stensaas & Stensaas, 1968).

Stensaas has suggested that the early differentiation of neuroblasts in the ventricular zone, and perhaps the initiation of migration also, may be conditioned by an inductive process mediated by the presence of the growth cones of fibers running in the ventricular zone from the cortex and extracortical centers. However, Hinds and Ruffett (1971) report that growth cones in the ventricular zone appear to belong exclusively to the basal processes of ventricular cells. Marin-Padilla (1970a, 1971) and Morest (1970a, 1970b) have both stressed the possible relationship between the presence of afferent fibers and the initiation of developmental events.

Hicks *et al.* (1959) observed thalamocortical fibers growing into the migratory zone on day 16 of gestation, and others have observed their presence in the cortex over the migratory stage (Marin-Padilla, 1970a, 1970b, 1971; Stensaas, 1967a, 1967b, 1967c, 1967d, 1967e, 1968). Berry and Hollingworth (1973) have tested the hypothesis that thalamocortical fibers might induce the migration of neuroblasts by unilateral section of the internal capsule in the embryo. They observed that in the absence of thalamocortical fibers, the migration of neuroblasts occurred normally. The observation that migration of granule cells is unimpeded in slabs of cerebellar cortex grown in tissue culture also demonstrates that migration may be under endogenous rather than exogenous control (Wolf, 1970).

The theory of Rakic (1971a, 1971b) implies that germinal cells differentiate quite early into two types: a glial cell which maintains contact with the ventricular and pial surfaces and a germinal cell which is attached at the ventricular surface only (Fig. 10). The close contact of neuroblasts with the radial glial processes may not only guide the cells to their destination but also assist the movement in some way. The phenomena of contact guidance has been discussed by Weiss (1955), and it is possible that neuroblasts may glide along glia processes by amoieboid movements. It is also possible (Mugnaini & Forstrønen, 1967) that migrating neuroblasts may actively be propelled by undulating movements in the glial membrane (Hild, 1954; Pomerat & Costero, 1956).

d. The Fate of the Germinal Cell. Following the proliferative stage, neurons, glia, and ependymal cells are formed but the relationship of germinal cells to the stem cells is unknown. Smart (1964) commented on the problem in the following passage:

> Ependymal [germinal cell] proliferation allows an exponential increase in neuron precursors, but once differentiation has begun, neuron formation follows at best an arithmetic progress. The developmental morphology of the neural tube can therefore be interpreted in terms of patterns which allow the accumulation of ependymal cells [germinal cells], e.g., (1) increase in the area of the ependymal layer [ventricular zone] by dilatation of the central canal [see also Coulombre & Coulombre, 1958]; (2) increase in the depth of the layer by mitosis-capable precursors which do not retain contact with the central canal, first by stratification as in the subependymal layer [subventricular layer] of the mammalian forebrain and secondly by migration away from the periventricular regions; (3) increase in the duration of the ependymal [germinal cell] proliferation, either relatively, by delaying differentiation or, absolutely, by continued proliferation [p. 466].

This brief statement has since been amplified in more recent work (Smart 1972a, 1972b).

During division the orientation of the spindle may be important in the postmitotic reconstitution of cell contacts. The changes in location and orientation of mitotic figures in various epithelia have been studied by Doig and Smart (1967) and Smart (1970). They found that in contrast to other epithelia, the ventricular zone of the cerebral cortex retained a pronounced apical mitotic polarity, but that as migration proceeded it was possible that the pseudostratified epithelium changed to a stratified type and, accompanying this, mitoses became more frequent away from the ventricular surface in the subventricular zone.

Thus, the germinal cell may undergo "equivalent division" (Marques-Pereira & Leblond, 1965) during the migratory stage, and the fate of the daughter cells may be decided by the presence or absence of specialized cell contacts with its neighbors. If the microenvironment of the cells is important in deciding the fate of "equivalent" daughter cells (Marques-Pereira & Leblond, 1965), it is quite easy to see how the environment of a cell attached to the ventricle is different from one which is not, especially if cerebrospinal fluid is taken up by the former via a microtubular system. Such environmental differences may induce one cell to replicate DNA and the other to differentiate.

e. The Subpial Layer. In the human cortex, a lamina of small dark cells is located below the pial surface whose nature and origin have not been determined (Rabinowicz, 1967). The layer may be similar to the external granular layer of the cerebellum and may form neurons destined to occupy layer IV and II (Brun, 1965) or deeper laminae (Rabinowicz, 1964). Others have suggested that the layer may be involved in gliogenesis (Brun, 1965; Opperman, 1929; Rabinowicz, 1964; Rauke, 1909).

B. Gliogenesis

The classical theories proposed that the stem cells of glia and neurons were demarcated early in the neural epithelium and that thereafter each developed separately. With the uncertainty about the fate of the germinal cell, however, gliogenesis has become a subject of much conjecture. Berry and Rogers (1966) studied gliogenesis autoradiographically but were unable to decide on the one hand whether germinal cells formed neurons during the first stage of their life history and glial cells subsequently (S. Fujita, 1966) or, on the other hand, if two populations of stem cells existed which gave rise to glia and neurons respectively. However, they did make the important observation that as early as day 18 of gestation, cells in the ventricular zone are destined to become glia, and thus gliogenesis begins at a time when neurogenesis is continuing in the cortex. After birth, when neurogenesis has terminated, glia cells are formed from a group of stem cells located in a subependymal region (Bryans, 1959, O. W. Jones, 1932; Kershman, 1938; Messier, Leblond, & Smart, 1958; Smart, 1961; Smart & Leblond, 1961). The cells in this layer are rounded, may have no attachment with the ventricle, and do not exhibit intermitotic nuclear migration. It is possible that one of the prerequisites of gliogenesis is that the stem cells become detached from the ventricle. The observation of Doig and Smart (1967) and Smart (1971) that mitosis is no longer confined to the ventricular region during the latter days of cortical histogenesis may suggest that stem cells are dispersed (Altman, 1966b) into the subventricular zone where they form glia. Many workers have commented on the presence of glial-like cells during the migratory phase of neurogenesis within the ventricular zone. Under the electron microscope, "gioblasts" have been recognized in the early stages of development of the olfactory bulb of the mouse (Hinds, 1968), the spinal cord and cerebral vesicle of the chick, and the fetal and neonatal mouse, rabbit, cat, and man (S. Fujita, 1965, 1966; Meller *et al.*, 1966; Ramsey, 1962; Wechsler & Meller, 1967), and the optic nerve of the cat (Vaughn, 1969). In the retina Müller cells can also be recognized early during histogenesis (Meller & Glees, 1965). In general, astrocytes appear first and oligodendroglia appear in great numbers as the tracts in the CNS become myelinated (Bensted, Dobbing, Morgan, Reid, & Payling Wright, 1957; Friede, 1961; Schonbach, Hu, & Friede, 1968).

Oligodendroglia and astrocytes may arise from a common stem cell (O. W. Jones, 1932; Penfield, 1924; Ramon-Moliner, 1958; Smart & Leblond, 1961; Stensaas, 1967a, 1967e), or one of them may be produced from a germinal precursor and differentiate into the other (Del Rio-Hortega, 1928; Farquhar & Hartman, 1957; Smart & Leblond, 1961). Smart and Leblond (1961) studied the evolution of neuroglia in the subependymal layer of the newborn mouse (Fig. 11). They identified two cell types in addition to oligondendroglia and astrocytes, which they called dark and medium dark cells on the basis of the characteristics of their nuclei after Nissl staining. By studying the distribution of tritiated thymidine in the various cells of the subependymal layer, they concluded that small dark and medium dark nuclei belonged

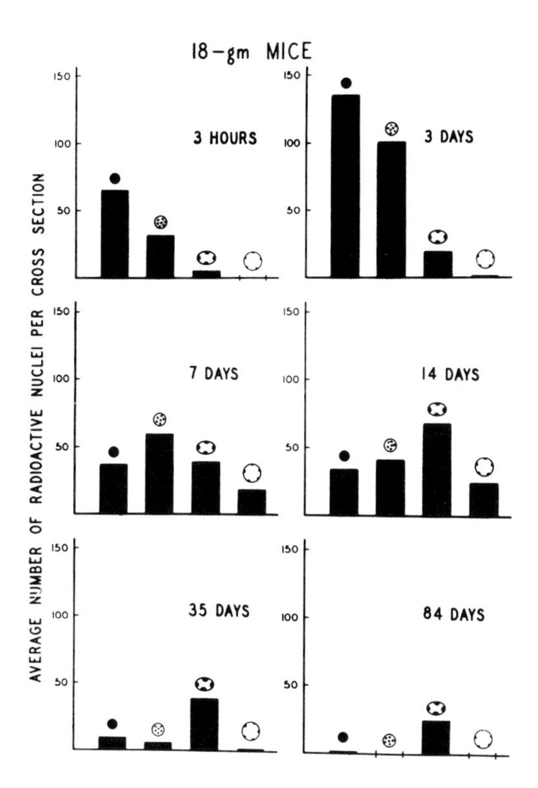

FIG. 11. Histogram showing the average numbers of different types of labelled neuroglia nuclei in cross sections of the brain of 18-gm mice. At each time interval, the first column surmounted by the solid black circle represents the number of labeled small dark nuclei; the second with lightly stippled circle represents the number of labeled medium-dark nuclei; the third with the oval containing black semicircles represents the number of labeled oligodendrocyte nuclei; the final column surmounted by the large circle with dots at the circumference represents the number of labeled astrocytes. Labeled small dark and medium dark nuclei are abundant at the early intervals but are few or absent at the late intervals. Labeled oligodendrocytes are rare and astrocytes absent at 3 hours; both reach a maximum at 14 days and slowly decrease in number thereafter (from Smart & Leblond, 1961).

to a common cell type which produced both astrocytes and oligodendroglia (Fig. 11). They postulated that astrocytes may also arise from oligodendroglia. Labeled astrocytes and oligodendroglia disappeared after some time, and this suggested to the authors that these two glial cells normally degenerated and were replaced from a stem cell pool. However, another explanation for the loss of label could be either that oligodendroglia and astrocytes may themselves divide (Altman, 1966b; Dalton, Hommes, & Leblond, 1968; Mori & Leblond, 1969, 1970; Sakla, 1965), or that metabolic DNA is present (Pelc, 1968).

Stensaas (1967a, 1967e) studied gliogenesis using the Golgi technique. Most glial cells were seen to develop from freely arborizing spongioblasts. These cells were attached at the ventricle by a long process which ended in the cortex by breaking up into fine branchlets. Young glial cells were thought to be formed from these cells as the foot process was detached from the ventricle and retracted with the nucleus toward the arbor of branching processes. These primitive glial cells can develop into astrocytes almost immediately or remain relatively unspecialized, in which case they may be capable of producing oligodendroglia and astrocytes (Ramon-Moliner, 1958).

Cammermeyer (1965) has reviewed the literature on the origin of microglia. The classical view (Del Rio-Hortega, 1928) states the microglia are of mesodermal origin and invade the CNS from blood vessels during development. An alternative hypothesis is that microglia develop directly from vascular wall cells or leucocytes. Cammermeyer (1965) presented new evidence that microglia take origin from histiocytes in the vessel walls, an hypothesis which has been supported by recent electron microscopic (EM) findings (Mori & Leblond, 1969).

III. Growth of Dendrites

A. Morphology of Growing Dentrites

The apical dentrites of pyramidal cells in the neocortex begin to grow before the basal dendrites appear (Adinolfi, 1971; Purpura, Shofer, Housepian, & Noback, 1964; Rabinowicz, 1964; Schadé, Van Backer, & Colon, 1964; Voeller, Pappas, & Purpura, 1963). After their migration, neuroblasts lie in a superficial position within or just below the zonal layer, layer I (Åström, 1967; Berry & Rogers, 1965; Berry *et al.*, 1964). A single dendrite is seen growing from one pole of the neuron and the axon stems from the other coursing into the depths. While the neuron lies within, or just below, the marginal layer, the single dendrite is directed in a random plane but, as the neuron becomes displaced by subsequent migrating cells gaining positions above them, the dendrite becomes orientated in a radial plane and can be recognized as the apical dendrite. The tip of the apical dendrite appears to remain in the marginal layer and to branch there (Berry & Rogers, 1966; Stensaas, 1968). At this stage the shaft of the dendrite does not usually possess side branches but is grossly varicose in outline. Thus, soon after migration pyramidal neurons possess an axon and apical dendrite but no basal dendrites—the same is true for the cat and rabbit (Noback & Purpura, 1961; Schadé *et al.*, 1964) and the sheep (Åström, 1967). Since the cells of layer VI are formed before other neurons in the cerebral cortex, they differentiate first, and the cells of V, IV, III, and II follow in the reverse order. It is possible, however, that although neurons in the granular and supragranular layers start to differentiate late, all cells in the cerebral cortex may mature at about the same time (Purpura, 1961).

At birth layers VI and V have migrated and occupy their definitive positions, but layers, IV, III, and II are actively migrating, and the six laminae of the neocortex do not become fully established until some 7–10 days after birth (Berry & Rogers, 1965; Haas *et al.*, 1970) (Fig. 6). In Golgi preparations (Fig. 12) basal dendrites are poorly developed at birth, and it is not until 30 days postpartum that the parameters of their dendritic fields approach adult dimensions (Eayrs & Goodhead, 1959). It is interesting that the mean number of dendrites arising from the perikaryon has reached an adult figure as early at 12 days postpartum, and that subsequent development of the dendritic field is marked by a peripheral extension of dendrites and by an increased amount of branching (Eayrs & Goodhead, 1959). Schadé *et al.* (1964) obtained similar results in their quantitative study on the growth of dendrites in the developing neocortex of the rabbit.

Morest (1969a, 1969b) and Scheibel and Scheibel (1971), using the rapid Golgi and Golgi-Cox techniques, identified the points of growth of dendrites as local irregular swellings, often as large or larger than the cell body itself. These enlargements were called growth cones and were located at the tip, anywhere along the shaft, or at the base of the dendrites. Exactly similar structures are found in growing axons. Radiating from the growth cones, from all parts of the primitive dendrites, and from the soma are numerous filopodia (see also Scheibel & Scheibel, 1971). Growth of the dendrite may occur at the tip of the growth cone, and the vesicles accumulating there (Bodian, 1966; Del Cerro & Snider, 1968) may be a source of membrane for the growing tip (Morest, 1969b). Another source of membrane may be the filopodia (Morest, 1969b). They may be viewed as acting much like the bellows of a concertina and thus, as the dendrite grows, filopodia are retracted and their membrane is applied to the main shaft.

Although Morest (1969a) has suggested that dendrites may grow at their tips, at their bases, or along their trunks, Hollingworth, Berry, and Anderson (1973) and Berry and Hollingworth (1972) have devised a quantitative method which shows that dendrites *branch* at their terminal segments only. Hollingworth *et al.* (1973), studied the topology of mature dendritic trees of pyramidal cells in the cerebral cortex and Purkinje cells in the vermis of the cerebellum. They showed that in both sites the distribution of topological branching types within the dendritic trees followed a pattern which could only be obtained if branches originated from terminal segments. Network analysis of the dendritic tree showed that the frequency of the different orders of dendritic segments formed an inverse geometric series, and that the ratio between adjacent numbers in the series always approxi-

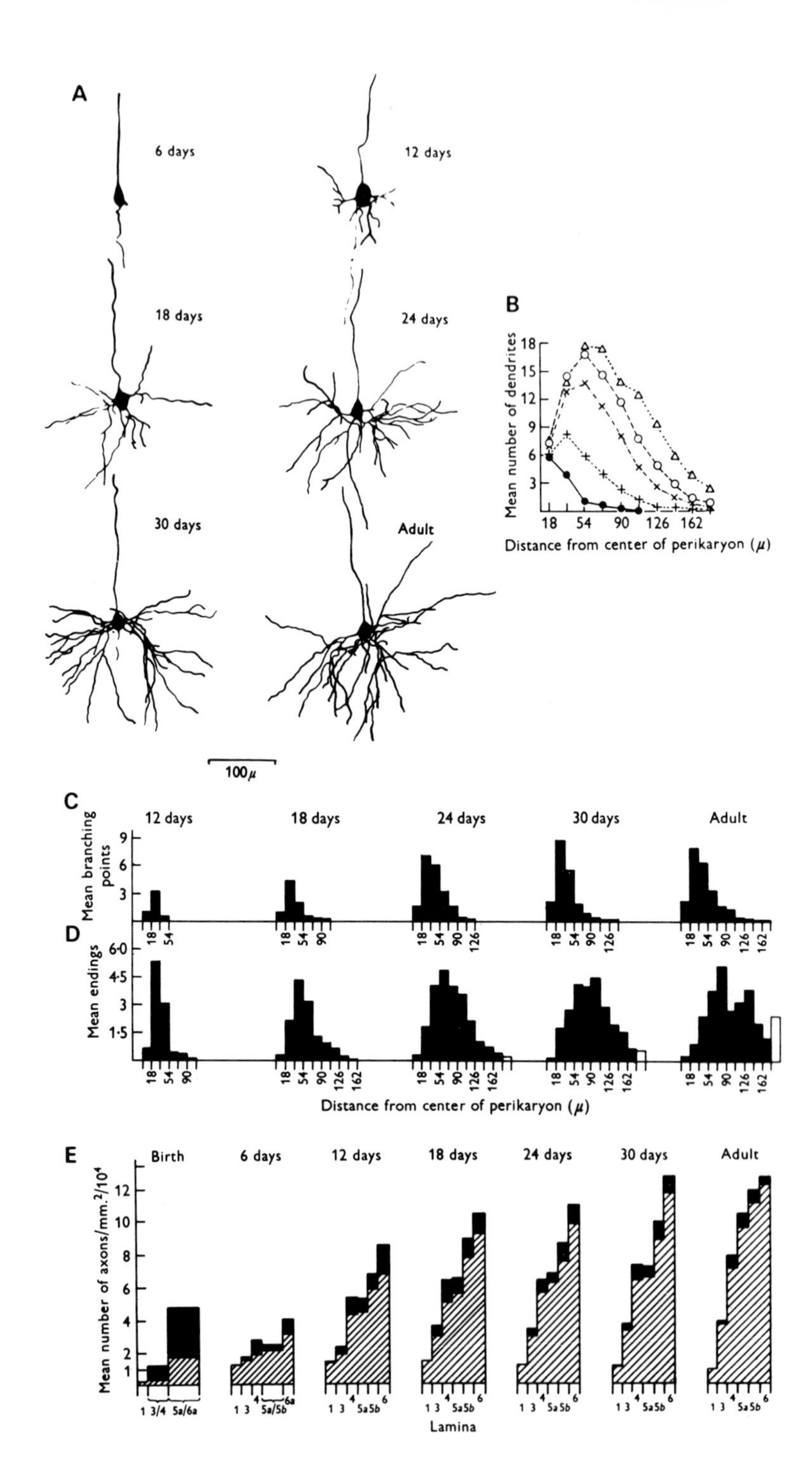
A
6 days
12 days
18 days
24 days
30 days
Adult
100μ
B
Mean number of dendrites
Distance from center of perikaryon (μ)
C
12 days
18 days
24 days
30 days
Adult
Mean branching points
D
Mean endings
Distance from center of perikaryon (μ)
E
Birth
6 days
12 days
18 days
24 days
30 days
Adult
Mean number of axons/mm.²/10⁴
Lamina

mated to 3. This number is called the bifurcation ratio. It was shown that exactly the same geometric series could be obtained by computer growth simulation of a network using a random terminal growth model and, further, that the probability of occurrence of distinct topological types obtained in a random terminal network gave a frequency distribution of orders which fitted exactly an inverse geometric series with a bifurcation ratio of 3. It was concluded that dendrites branch at their terminal segments in a random manner. These results are supported by the findings of Bray (1970) and Bray and Bunge (1973).

Bray (1970) has perfected a method of observing the growing dendrites of embryonic chick sympathetic neurons in tissue culture by marking discrete parts of the cell membrane of growing dendrites with glass or carmine particles. He observed that although the particles on the membrane exhibited continual small jerky movements, they did not show any overall distal progression away from the soma, but the growth cones at the tips of the dendrites were freely mobile and covered considerable distances during the periods of observation. Bray concluded that membrane was added at the tip, and thus growth was taking place at growth cones and not along the shafts of dendrites. Bray and Bunge (1973) made additional observations on the branching patterns of sympathetic neurons in culture and concluded that the growth cones generate most of the branch points by their bifurcation, and that the frequency with which they divide is the same at all parts of the cell and throughout the period of growth.

B. Factors Affecting Dendritic Growth—Genetic vis á vis *Environment*

Hollingworth and Berry's results also showed that branching per se does not determine the architecture of the dendritic tree. For example, in the cerebellum and cerebral cortex the dendritic trees of Purkinje and pyramidal cells respectively are quite different and yet they branch in exactly the same manner. Clearly, additional important factors in determining the character-

---

FIG. 12. (A) Characteristic changes in appearance of pyramidal cells of layer V in the neocortex of the rat from 6 days old to maturity. Note the precocious development of the apical relative to the basal dendritic system. (B) Basal dendritic density at successive distances from the perikaryon at 12 days, ●——●; 18 days, + ... + ; 24 days, × -.-.-. × , and 30 days *post-partum*, ○ --- ○ , and in the adult, △ .... △ .) (C) and (D) Distribution of branching and ending points (respectively) of basal dendrites in relation to the center of the perikaryon. The white areas of the histogram in (D) represent the increasing number of dendrites extending beyond 180 μ. (E) Density of axons by laminae at successive ages. The hatched portion of each histogram gives the density in the cortex taken as a whole; the solid portion is the increment resulting from correction for the presence of formed elements other than axons, the total giving the axonal density within the neuropil (from Eayrs & Goodhead, 1959).

istics of the tree are the length of segments and their solid angles at the nodes. The observations of Van der Loos (1965) strongly suggests that both these parameters may be controlled by genetic factors, and that the environment in which neurons find themselves may have little influence on the final pattern of the dendritic array. Van der Loos (1965) observed that no matter what the orientation of the cell body within the cerebral cortex (i.e., whether inverted or tilted to one side of the radial plane), the dendritic tree maintained an orientation referable to the long axis of the soma and not to the neuropil (Fig. 13). These observations shed new light on the results of a study by Berry and Eayrs (1966) on the effects of X-rays on the differentiation of dendrites.

After irradiation of the fetal rat cortex on day 19 of gestation, layers II, III, and IV do not develop at all, and after irradiation on day 21 of gestation these layers are present but are represented by a small band of cells. The environment in which layer V and VI neurons differentiate in cortex irradiated on day 19 of gestation is more hypoplastic and the cells themselves are more disorientated than is the case in cortex irradiated on day 21. But the dendritic fields of 19-day irradiated neurons were less affected than 21-day neurons. In fact, 19-day neurons were in many respects quite normal. This result may be explained by assuming that the environment has a limited effect on the ultimate organization of dendrites, and that the effects of irradiation are only manifest as a direct effect at a time when basal dendrites are starting to grow—on day 21 of gestation in the rat.

It is an old axiom of neuroembryology that neuronal processes grow by contact guidance within the neuropil (Barron, 1943; Weiss, 1955). The importance of this factor in the growth of dendrites must be small, however, since the architecture of the dendritic tree is not affected when neurons are variously orientated in the predominantly undirectional neuropil of the neocortex (Berry & Eayrs, 1966; Van der Loos, 1965), nor is there any gross difference in dendritic trees between the neurons in one center which are developing at different times in a rapidly changing neuropil (Morest, 1969a).

A possible prerequisite to dendritic differentiation in the amphibian spinal cord is that the axons of the motor neuron should firstly innervate muscle (Barron, 1944) or, as seems more likely, simply gain access to and invade the primordial limb bud (Hamburger & Keefe, 1944). Once this is accomplished, these motor neurons may begin to grow dendrites and as the latter ramify among neighboring neuroblasts, their presence will promote differentiation. At first sight it seems unlikely that such a mechanism has any relevance to the development of neocortical dendrites, since the axons of cortical cells remain inside the central nervous system and innervate multiple targets via a complex collateral system (Morest, 1969b). In any event, the apical dendrites of neocortical cells appear to grow out from the cell body at the same

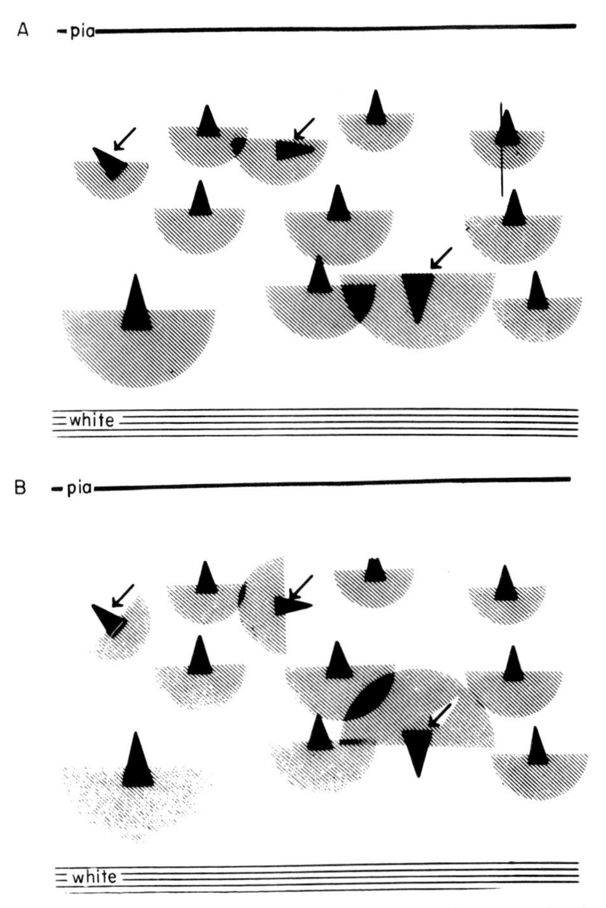

FIG. 13. Schematic summary of the argument that not only emanation but also further growth of dendrites in governed by factors intrinsic to the maturing neuron. (A) Depicts the morphological condition that would ensue if extrinsic directive factors governed the growth of basal dendrites, i.e., disoriented perikaryon bear dendritic systems whose orientation is similar to that of properly oriented cells. In fact this condition is never encountered. In (B) basal dendrite systems have developed under the influence of factors residing in the neurons. Orientation of all dendritic domains is in accordance with orientation of the corresponding cell bodies (from Van der Loos, 1965).

time as the axon. Furthermore, if dendrodendritic induction were taking place, the contacts between dendrites necessary for the mediation of induction should be observable in the developing cortex. But no such relationships have been found (Morest, 1969b), although dendrodendritic synapses are formed in various sites in the adult CNS (Ralston, 1971). However, the recent discovery by Kristensson, Olsson, and Sjöstrand (1971) that hypoglossal nerves can take up proteins at their terminals and transport these macromolecules to the soma has demonstrated a substrate by which the end organ could exert a trophic influence on the cell body.

C. The Importance of Synaptic Activity in the Growth and Maintenance of the Dendritic Tree

Deafferentation of developing neurons has a remarkable effect on the subsequent growth and differentiation of dendrites (Chase, 1945; DeLong & Sidman, 1962; Hess, 1957; Levi-Montalcini, 1967; Moskowitz & Noback, 1962; Mugnaini & Forstrønen, 1967). Dendritic maturation appears to be causally related to synaptic formation, and functioning synapses may exert a trophic influence on dendritic growth. Conversely, dendritic maturity may be a prerequisite for synaptic formation (Molliver & Van der Loos, 1970; Morest, 1968, 1969a, 1969b). Deafferentation alone can cause dramatic changes in the developing mouse superior colliculus, where proliferation is reduced, maturation is arrested and cells are lost, the size of cell bodies is reduced, and a reduction in the volume of the neuropil occurs (DeLong & Sidman, 1962). Similar effects are seen in the cochlear centers in the absence of the VIIIth nerve root (Levi-Montalcini, 1949). In the visual cortex of animals with hereditary anophthalmia, the line of Gennari is absent, the striate cortex reduced in thickness, and the packing density of cells increased (Chase, 1945; Duckworth & Cooper, 1966; Hess, 1958). Marin-Padilla (1970a, 1971) and Poliakov (1961) have observed in human and cat fetal cortex that the differentiation and maturation of neurons is related to the arrival of afferent fibers in the cortex, and Morest (1969b) has stated that the differentiation of the dendritic branches coincides in time and place with the differentiation of the afferent axonal end branches that form synaptic contacts with the dendrites. Morest (1969a) has attached special significance to the filopodia and proposed that they may function to secure contact with growing afferent axons. Once contact is made it is possible that either the subsequent growth of both the axon and the definitive dendrite along the surface of the filopodia will result in the formation of a synapse, or that actual retraction of the filopodia (Nakai & Kawasaki, 1959) may pull axon and dendrite together and effect a synaptic contact. But whatever the mechanisms are which guide axons and dendrites to establish their synaptic interrelationships, there now seems little doubt that the dendritic trees of neurons are stimulated to grow and are maintained by afferent input.

It is now established that, on the one hand, deafferentation causes a reduction in the volume and thickness of the neocortex and an increase in the packing density of cells (Fifková, 1967, 1968, 1970a; Gyllensten, Malfors, & Norrlin, 1965; Krech, Rosenzweig, & Bennett, 1963; Tsang, 1937) and, on the other, rearing animals in complex environments increases neocortical weight and depth, but decreases neuron density (Bennett, Diamond, Krech, & Rosenzweig, 1964; Diamond, Krech, & Rosenzweig, 1964; Krech *et al.*, 1963; Rosenzweig, Bennett, Diamond, Wu, Slagle, & Saffran, 1969; Rosenzweig, Krech, Bennett, & Diamond, 1962; Rosenzweig, Love, & Bennett, 1968). These findings may be explained by the hypothesis that dendritic branching is reduced by deafferentation and is made more extensive by the increased afferent input contingent on environmental complexity—although the effects of a gliosis in the latter case also needs evaluation. So far quantitative estimates of the dendritic field of neurons in the cortex of deafferented animals or of animals placed in complex environments have yielded conflicting results. Globus and Scheibel (1967d) found no quantitative difference in the dendritic fields of stellate and pyramidal cells in the striate cortex in normal and dark reared rats other than an increased variance of all parameters in the treated group. This result contrasted with the findings of Coleman and Riesen (1968) who studied the effect of rearing in the dark on the dendritic fields of stellate cells in layer IV of the striate cortex and pyramidal cells in the posterior cingulate gyrus. They showed that although dendritic length was unaffected, the probability of branching, and thus dendritic density, was reduced in both types of cell. Some explanation for the disagreement between the results of Globus and Scheibel (1967d) and Coleman and Riesen (1968) may be found in the work of Ruiz-Marcos and Valverde (1969) and Valverde (1971). These workers were able to show that unilateral enucleation of mice at birth may not have any effect on the total basal dendritic density of pyramidal cells but can specifically reduce density in an inferior sector of the field while the remainder undergoes compensatory hypertrophy. Valverde (1968) also noted that the orientation of the dendrites of stellate cells in layer IV in the striate area of mice unilaterally enucleated at birth was grossly abnormal. Dendrites appeared to grow out of layer IV into layer III and Va rather than ramify within this layer as is normally the case (Fig. 14).

There has been one preliminary study on the effects of "enriched" environment on the growth of dendritic fields (Holloway, 1966), and this very tentatively suggested that dendritic branching may occur more frequently in the neurons of these animals.

Once established, the normal architecture of the dendritic field may be maintained by sustained afferent input. If this factor is lacking, then dendrites partly atrophy. The dendrites of cells in the medial superior olive undergo shrinkage in 2 weeks after ablation of the anteroventral cochlear nucleus, and by 6 weeks dendritic diameters are reduced by a factor of 3 (Liu & Liu, 1971). In the prepyriform cortex, the dendrites of pyramidal cells atrophy after interruption of the olfactory tract (Jones & Thomas, 1962).

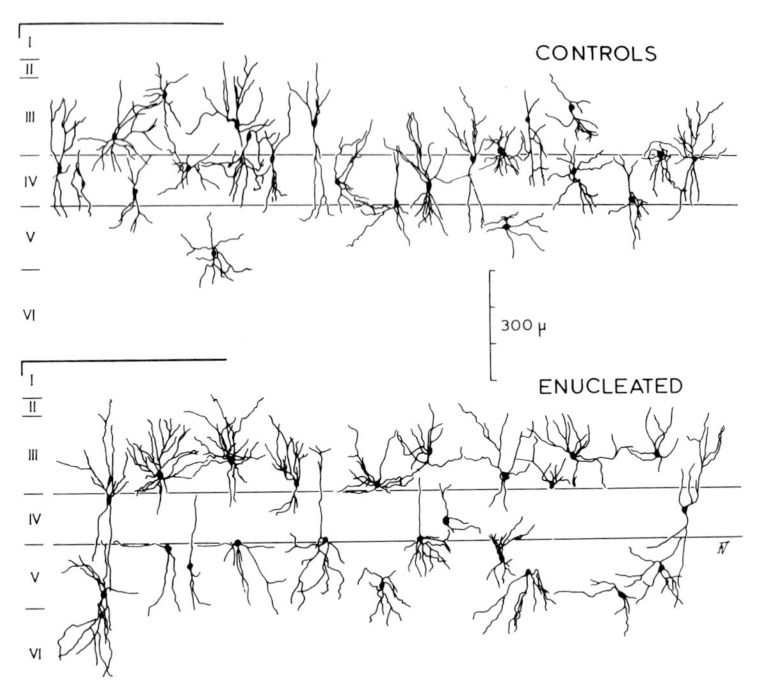

FIG. 14. Composite camera lucida drawing of Golgi triple impregnations of stellate cells with ascending axons in the area striata from mice 48 days old. Stellate cells in normal mice appear with bodies and dendrites distributed randomly through layers V, IV, and III (Controls). In mice enucleated at birth, the orientation of dendrites outside layer IV is evident (Enucleated) (from Valverde, 1968).

Schadé and Baxter (1960) and Schadé *et al.* (1964) have devised methods of direct measurement of the surface area and volume of soma and dendrites, and they have been able to show how these parameters are interrelated during the development of cortical cells in the rabbit. Several computations can be made which give an indirect measure of the rate of growth of dendrites. The cell/gray coefficient is the ratio of the volume of cortex occupied by cells to the volume occupied by everything else (Brizzee, Vogt, & Kharetchko, 1964; Haug, 1956; Shariff, 1953). In developing cortex, the volume of gray matter unoccupied by cells (stained nuclei) is filled with neuronal and glial processes and blood vessels. If the vascular volume is measured, a very crude estimate of dendritic growth can be made. Changes in the packing density of cells (i.e., cell/mm^3 of brain, Brizzee & Jacobs, 1959) is another crude measure which can be used to monitor the rate of dendritic growth during development. Eayrs and Goodhead (1959) showed that the cell/gray coefficient changed little after the day 18 postpartum in all layers of the rat cerebral cortex. Electron microscope studies have given the opportunity of illustrating this change in the cell/gray coefficient as the cortex develops. Figure 15 is taken from a paper by Caley and Maxwell (1971) and clearly shows how the cells nuclei are separated from one another by increasingly large amounts of internuclear material as the cortex matures.

IV. Growth of Axons

A. Growth Cones

The terminals of growing axons are expanded into structures called growth cones. Their morphology has been studied in the rat cerebellum (Del Cerro & Snider, 1968), in dorsal root neuroblasts of rabbit embryos (Tennyson, 1970), in monkey spinal cord (Bodian, 1966), and in tissue culture (Yamada *et al.*, 1970). In the cerebellum growth cones are devoid of any organelles except vesicles which are usually oval in section but may also appear round or even tubular. Their largest diameter may be as much as 1100 Å. Microfilaments and microtubules are also present in large numbers (Yamada *et al.*, 1970).

The biological significance of the growth cone is not understood, although judging from observations on dendritic (Bray, 1970) and axonal (Pomerat, 1961; Speidel, 1942; Yamada *et al.*, 1970) growth cones in tissue culture, they are the sites of active movement and branching. The vesicles within the cone have been assigned several functions. Morest (1969a, 1969b) suggested that they may be a source of membrane for the growing tip and also that the growth cone, like the filopodium, may have some vital role to play in synaptogenesis. Another idea is that the vesicles may be encapsulated particles pinocytosed at the growing tip (Tennyson, 1970) and destined for transportation proximally, along the axon, to the cell body (Hughes, 1953). Tissue culture studies have confirmed that the tips of neurites can ingest substances which can be transported to the soma in cytoplasmic vacuoles. Recently, Kristensson *et al.* (1971) have shown that nerve terminals can take up macromolecules at their tips and transport them to the soma, where they accumulate. The terminals of young animals are more proficient at this than those of older animals. Thus, one can speculate that the vesicles in the growth cone may represent some inductive substance destined for the perikaryon or for release at another terminal. The role of trophic stimuli in the induction of neuronal differentiation is discussed in Section III, C.

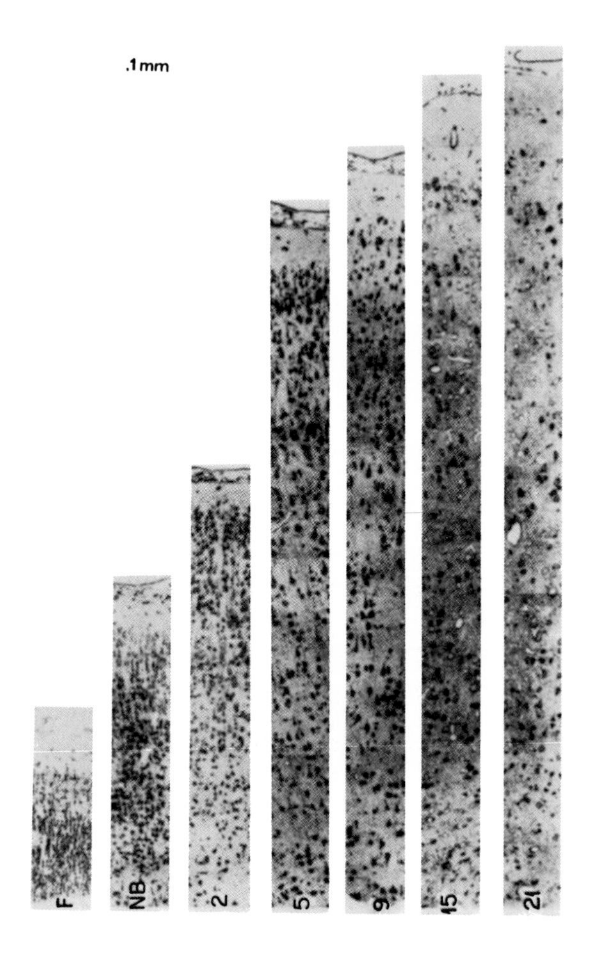

FIG. 15. Composite photomicrographs of sensorimotor cortex of rats aged 2 weeks fetal and newborn, 2, 5, 9, 15, and 21 days old. Each micrograph extends from the surface to the white matter. Comparison can be made of cortical thickness, cell packing density, and cell size (from Caley & Maxwell, 1971).

B. *Myelination*

S. Jacobson (1963) has studied the myelination of the cerebral axons of the rat and observed that the process is initiated on about the day 10 postpartum in the primary motor, somesthetic, auditory, limbic, and pyriform cortex and spreads to adjacent regions as development proceeds. Detailed studies of myelination in the corpus callosum and pyramidal tracts of rats (Schonbach *et al.*, 1968; Seggie & Berry, 1972) have shown that there is a wave of production of glial cells just prior to myelination which has been called "myelination gliosis" and associated with this there is the concomitant appearance of large numbers of glia processes among the axons (Seggie & Berry, 1972). The glial process may engage the axon at a discrete point and the first few turns of the process may be localized by allowing growth to occur at the mesoaxon only (Gaze & Peters, 1961; Maturana, 1960; Peters, 1960; Wechsler, 1967). Myelination may subsequently proceed by the addition of lamellae and the longitudinal growth of the myelin sheath over the segment of the axon. Glial processes do not appear to engage axons unless their diameter is more than .3 mμ (Matthews, 1968; Seggie & Berry, 1972). The number of turns made by the mesoaxon is determined by the diameter of the axon by some unknown mechanism. Correlation between axon diameter and number of lamellae is, at first, poor, but good correlation is established within a few days (Matthews & Duncan, 1971; Samorajski & Friede, 1968; Seggie & Berry, 1972). The initial lack of a relationship may be associated with the presence of a large number of varicosities along immature axons, but as the axon diameter become more uniform, correlation with the number of lamellae becomes constant. When growth of the myelin sheath is complete, the inner and outer tongues of the mesoaxon tend to lie opposite one another.

Myelination of axons of the corpus callosum begins on day 10 postpartum, reaches a peak by day 26, but does not appear to be complete even at 300 days. Unlike unmyelinated fibers in peripheral nerves, those in the CNS are completely denuded of sheath cell cytoplasm.

The old idea that a causal relationship exists between myelination and the acquisition of function can no longer be upheld since it is now established that fetal and neonatal behavior develop before myelination has begun. Both the interhemispheric and callosal responses can be elicited before the corpus callosum is myelinated (Grafstein, 1963; Meyerson, 1968; Seggie & Berry, 1972; Ulett, Dow, & Larsell, 1955), and stimulation of the unmyelinated optic nerve evokes a response in the visual cortex of neonatal kittens (Hunt & Goldring, 1951). Thus, the limiting factor as far as the functional integrity of the developing nervous system is concerned seems to be the ontogeny of the synapse and possibly the maturation of peripheral sensory receptors, since a high level of function can be achieved in the presence of incomplete maturation of other structures (see Introduction to Volume 1 by Gottlieb).

C. Specificity of Axon Growth

The mechanisms by which axons are guided to their destinations and specific synaptic connections are made is unknown. Many theories have been put forward to explain the phenomenon, and for a more detailed review of the subject the reader is referred to Gottlieb (Introduction to Volume 1 and Gaze (1970).

Ramón y Cajal (1928, 1960) suggested that specific neural connections might be formed by chemotropism. Individual nerves were thought to grow to their destinations along chemical gradients and effect connections by specific chemical affinities between pre- and postsynaptic membranes. Ariëns Kappers,Huber and Crosby (1936) proposed that:

> If several centers of stimulation are present in the nervous system, the outgrowth of the chief dendrites and eventually the shifting of the cells takes place in the direction whence the greatest number of stimulations reach the cell. This outgrowth or shifting, however, only takes place between stimulatively correlated centers. Temporarily correlated excitation plays a part also in establishing the connections of the neuraxis [Pp. 78–79].

Ariëns Kapper's ideas were backed by two experimental findings. In the first, Ingvar (1920) showed that weak galvanic current has an orientating influence on cell and fiber outgrowth in tissue culture which occurred almost along the lines of forces of the galvanic current. In the second, Marsh and Beams (1946) found that nerve fibers in tissue culture were orientated toward the cathode, and no fibers at all grew toward the anode. Bok (1915) introduced his theory of stimulogenous fibrillation, which considered that stimulation currents generated in fiber tracts induced neighboring cells to differentiate. Their axons grow away from and their dendrites grow toward the source of stimulation.

The contact guidance theory of Weiss (1955) proposed that, given a correct timing and sequence in developmental events, mechanical guidance of nerve fibers, initially along tension lines in the intercellular matrix and later along existing fiber tracts, could explain how the CNS was wired. Specificity of function was believed to be achieved by impulse specificity based on a resonance principle.

The current theory, which is backed by considerable indirect experimental evidence (Sperry, 1965), maintains that each neuron possesses a chemical specificity all of its own. Axons find their way along chemically coded paths to establish connections with specific cells according to a genetic blueprint. The chemistry of such nerve growth is little understood, however. Sperry himself (1958) has suggested that the entire surface of the neuron is coated with chemically individual molecules. If a series of molecules is arranged from one end of a neuron to the other in a reciprocal graded fashion, then a mechanism is available for identifying any locus on the neuron surface according to the "unit ratio" of molecules in the two graded series at that locus. Another possible mechanism for chemical specificity is selective cell adhesion where specificity of growth path and eventual innervation are dictated by the relative adhesiveness of the neuropil during the growth of the axon (Steinberg, 1964). Specific molecules likely to fill the bill for both roles are the brain specific mucoids, the almost infinite variety of which has already suggested that they could be involved in the chemistry of memory (Bogoch, 1968).

The observation that regenerating axons produce many sprouts at their tips and along their shafts, but that only one of these neurites reinnervates the end organ does suggest that nerve connections may be formed by natural selection among a number of axons in which only the fittest survives. M. Jacobson (1970) has endorsed this idea, believing that axons branch randomly and find their targets, during growth, by trial and error. In this respect it is interesting to recall that dendrites grow by random terminal branching (Berry & Hollingworth, 1972; Bray & Bunge, 1973).

To explain the mechanisms of connectivity by chemical specificity alone appears too rigid because it is clear that environment, behavior, experience, etc., also play a part. Following Altman (1967), M. Jacobson (1970) has allowed for this contingency by postulating the existence of two types of neuron in the CNS (see Jacobson, this volume). Class I neurons are said to be highly specified early in development, after which their connectivity is tightly constrained and unmodified—all long-axoned neurons may be of this type. Class II neurons are said to remain unspecified until late in ontogeny when the connections may be modified or maintained by function and experience of an appropriate type. Short-axoned microneurons may be of this type.

D. *Afferent Input to the Cortex*

Afferent fibers invade the rat cortex on about day 16 of gestation (Hicks *et al.*, 1959), and by birth the internal capsule is well developed and corticofugal fibers, as well as the recurrent collaterals of intrinsic pyramidal cells, are undoubtedly present. Eayrs and Goodhead (1959) noted that both specific and nonspecific afferents were present in the cortex at birth, and that the corpus callosum had formed. All fibers run predominantly in a tangential plane. The adult radial orientation of afferent fibers (Lorente de Nó, 1946) was not attained until about day 6 after birth. Scheibel and Scheibel (1971) and Adinolfi (1971) have noted in the cat that both specific and nonspecific afferents invade the cortex early but do not exhibit their normal arborizations until 60–90 days.

In their quantitative study on the postnatal development of the cerebral cortex of the rat, Eayrs and Goodhead (1959) noted that the density of axons increased markedly over the period from day 6–18 to about half the adult value. By 30 days postpartum, this figure was only some 15% below the adult figure. The growth of axons was not uniform in each cortical lamina. In layer I the axon density increased rapidly to reach a peak by day 12 and to remain constant thereafter. In layer III, IV, Vb, and VI, the rate of growth was greatest over the period from day 6–18, but layer Va lagged behind all the others some 30% appearing after the age of 30 days (Fig. 12E).

One method of monitoring the maturation of cortical projection systems is to study the development of the appropriate evoked cortical response. The interhemispheric and callosal evoked responses are present at 10 days postpartum (Seggie & Berry, 1972). The first response to light flash in the visual cortex occurs at 11 days postpartum (Rose, 1968). Bradley, Eayrs, and Schmalbach (1960) have noted that the EEG is readily blocked by sensory stimuli at 15 days postpartum. There appears to be a definitive sequence of maturation of projection fibers. The nonspecific thalamocortical system matures first, since the recruiting potential is elicited before any other thalamocortical response (Bernhard, Kolmodin, & Meyerson, 1967; Do Carmo, 1960). The somesthetic evoked response appears before both visual and auditory evoked potentials (Bernhard *et al.*, 1967; Marty & Scherrer, 1964). It is to be appreciated that the appearance of cortically evoked responses does not reflect developmental changes in the neocortex alone because these potentials are a manifestation of the integrity of the entire projection path from the level of stimulation to the cerebral cortex. For the details of the development of somesthetic evoked cortical responses in fetal sheep, see the Myerson and Persson, this volume. For a general discussion of the ontogeny of sensory and perceptual processes, see Introduction to Section I by Gottlieb, this volume.

E. Microneurons

Short-axoned neurons, also called stellate cells, granule cells, or microneurons appear late in ontogeny. In some regions of the brain these cells develop after birth (Altman, 1962a, 1962b, 1963, 1966a, 1966b, 1967; Altman & Das, 1965a,b, 1966). In the cerebral cortex of the rat the granular and supragranular cells do develop late and migrate to their definitive positions postnatally, but details of the time of origin of stellate cells in the deep lamina have not been worked out. However, many workers have observed that in other species, certain stellate (Golgi type II) neurons are slow to mature, and thus their processes form new neuropil at a late ontogenetic stage (Åström, 1967; Noback & Purpura, 1961; Scheibel & Scheibel, 1963). Marin-Padilla (1970b) observed that the development and subsequent maturation of the interneurons in human fetal cortex paralleled the growth and differentiation of efferent neurons, and that the two systems became interconnected via intracortical neuronal chains. The thesis that microneurons have some special significance in the evolution of the higher integrative functions of the nervous system has been discussed by Altman (1967). In the case of the rat cerebral cortex, the differentiation of microneurons coincides with the acquisition of a more sophisticated behavioral repertoire and the maturation of both spontaneous and evoked electrocortical activity and they may be associated with the acquisition of inhibitory mechanisms (see Crain, this volume).

F. Horizontal Cells of Retzius-Cajal

An exceptionally well-developed cell can be found in layer I of the cerebral cortex of most mammals at birth which is called the horizontal cell of Retzius-Cajal (Meller, Breipohl, & Glees, 1968; Molliver & Van der Loos, 1970; Purpura, 1961; Ramón y Cajal, 1960). Ramón y Cajal (1960) described the cell as having a diverse configuration, but that despite this "all possessed one or more peripheral dendrons which terminate beneath the pia mater as well as two or more voluminous and very long, polar branches. The latter travel horizontally describing small curves and emit enumerable perpendicular, ascending branches which always terminate in spherules beneath the pia mater [p. 343]." Fig. 16. It is quite possible that this cell has no axon and thus may be classed as a unique neuron (Stensaas, 1967c), but it is also possible that the cell is some form of glial element. In the human cortex it is the first cell to differentiate (Brun, 1965; Opperman, 1929; Poliakov, 1961; Rabinowicz, 1964, 1967), and in all species it disappears after birth. Some workers have suggested that tangentially running fibers make synaptic contact with these cells, and that the characteristic propogation times and negativity of the direct cortical response in fetal cortex is a manifestation of the genesis and conduction of excitatory postsynaptic potentials in the dendrites of Retzius-Cajal cells (Purpura, 1961; Purpura *et al.*, 1964).

V. Synaptogenesis

A. Morphological Changes in Synapses during Development

In fine structural studies of the development of the rat neocortex (Caley & Maxwell, 1971; Sarkisov, Popova, & Bogolepov, 1966; Seggie & Berry, 1973), it has been observed that at birth there were few synapses and that the majority were axodendritic contacts. Axodendritic synapses were immature and exhibited a small area of contact, few synaptic vesicles, and relatively little thickening of the opposing membranes, giving the junctions a symmetrical character (Type I, Gray, 1959) (Fig. 17). As the neuropil matured, axodendritic synapses gradually showed increased thickening of the postsynaptic membrane, synaptic vesicles became more numerous, there was greater area of contact, more distinct subsynaptic thickening, and more uni-

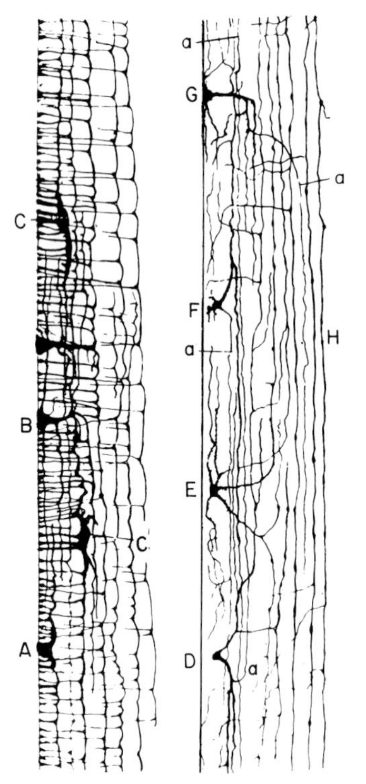

Fig. 16. Golgi preparations of Retzius-Cajal cells in layer I of an infant. A, B, and C are from the visual cortex of a neonate, and D, E, F, and G are similar cells from the visual cortex of a 20 day-old infant; H, elongated tangential fibers; a, possibly the axons of Retzius-Cajal cells (from Ramón y Cajal, 1960).

formity of width of the synaptic cleft. By some 22 days postpartum, axosomatic synapses became more frequent and, on qualitative judgment, appeared to reach adult frequencies by 30 days postpartum. During this latter period dendritic spines had formed. All axospinous synapses were asymmetrical (Type II, Gray, 1959), while those formed on dendritic shafts and the soma were both symmetrical and asymmetrical. These results bear out those of many former studies in other species (Adinolfi, 1971; Noback & Purpura, 1961; Scheibel & Scheibel, 1971; Voeller *et al.*, 1963).

In the kitten exactly the same sequence of events characterizes the development of synapses, although additional features have also been recorded (Adinolfi, 1971). Before birth, desmosomal junctions are present between cell bodies and processes in the neuropil. Presumptive symmetrical axodendritic contacts are present, but few vesicles can be seen in the presynaptic terminal. In the newborn, desmosomal junctions disappear, and recogniz-

cuplike protuberances along the surfaces of apical shafts and later along basal dendrites but do not acquire a mature configuration until between week 3 and 6. These axospinous synapses are always asymmetrical (Adinolfi, 1971).

Spines disappear, or are not impregnated, when the presynaptic bouton is lost or following prolonged sensory deprivation. In the striate cortex, after visual deprivation (usually effected by lid closure, enucleation, or dark rearing), spines are lost on the part of the apical shaft of layer V neurons which courses through layers III and IV (Fifková,1970a; Globus & Scheibel, 1967a, 1967b, 1967c, 1967d; Valverde, 1967, 1968). The effects of lid closure from birth can be reversed if the eyes are opened at 10–30 days, but beyond 2 months there is no recovery after opening of the lids (Fifková, 1970b). In fact, there appears to be several distinct populations of spines which react differently to sensory deprivation and exhibit differing recovery patterns. For example, the growth of some spines in the visual cortex of the mouse is not dependent on the presence or absence of visual stimuli, since they are formed before the eyes are opened and may continue to grow in dark-reared animals after the period when the eyelids would normally open. The growth of a second group of dendritic spines is contingent on the normal arrival of visual impulses after spontaneous opening of the eyes (Valverde, 1971). When animals are removed from darkness at the time of eye opening and allowed to survive for up to 30 days in normal conditions, some apical dendrites recover their full quota of spines while others maintain a permanent deficit.

Hubel and Wiesel (1963) and Wiesel and Hubel (1963) suggested that the effects of visual deprivation on neurons in the visual cortex were those of disuse atrophy, since their neurophysiological findings suggested that all connections were present at birth but became defective with disuse. However, the results of Valverde (1971) strongly imply that normal visual "experience" triggers the growth of spines.

Spines are distributed over the surface of dendrites in a precise pattern which can be defined by a mathmatical equation (Valverde & Ruiz-Marcos, 1969). The number of apical spines in the striate cortex of mice increases constantly over the period from 10 to 180 days (practically the average lifespan of the mouse), but the largest increment occurs at a time when the eyes are opening. It has been proposed that the distribution of spines is determined by the density of afferent fibers in a given area of cortex (Marin-Padilla & Stibitz, 1968). However, there is some evidence to suggest that this may not be true, since the distribution is not altered over the apical dendrites of inverted pyramidal cells when compared with normally orientated cells, nor is it altered following sensory deprivation although, in this latter case, there is an overall reduction in number (Ruiz-Marcos & Valverde, 1969). These findings have led Valverde and Ruiz-Marcos (1969) to postulate that the distribution of spines is determined by a "soma-dendrite" factor, while the quantity is related to function.

D. Ontogeny of Cortical Synaptology

Globus and Scheibel (1967b, 1967c) and Valverde (1968) present evidence that specific afferents may primarily contact the spines over the central three-fifths of apical dendrites of deep pyramids as they pass through layer IV and also engage stellate cells in layer IV of the striate cortex (Coleman & Riesen, 1968). This view is supported by the EM studies of Jones and Powell (1970) and Garey and Powell (1971) on the degenerating terminals of specific afferents. They have presented evidence that these fibers may engage stellate cells and apical dendrites in layer IV and the bordering regions of layer V and III. They also speculated that the axosomatic synapses on pyramidal cells, which exhibit the same morphological characteristics as junctions elsewhere in the CNS which have been assigned an inhibitory role (Uchizono, 1965; Walberg, 1968), may be formed by stellate cells. These findings are of great interest because they are entirely in accord with those of Marin-Padilla (1970b) who described the ontogeny of Golgi type II neurons and pyramidal cells in the human neocortex. In layer IV stellate cell axons ramify over a large area and are seen to form dense arborizations about the soma of pyramidal cells in other layers similar to the basket cell networks about Purkinje cells in the cerebellum.

Thus the late development of stellate cells in the neocortex may be correlated with the delayed development of axosomatic synapses relative to axodendritic synapses. The equally late development of axospinous synapses may be correlated with the morphological and functional maturation of specific afferent networks in layer IV. This later quantity presumably has a multivariate dependence on the maturation of sensory and behavioral processes as a whole.

It must be mentioned that the idea that pyramidal and stellate cells are connected in parallel has not been generally accepted. Valverde and Ruiz-Marcos (1969) support the classical viewpoint that these cell types are arranged in series, the stellate cell being the interneuron between afferent terminal and pyramidal dendrite. Many neurophysiologists believe that the primary somatosensory volleys activate pyramidal cells secondary to at least one internuncial neuron (Amassian, Walter, & Macy, 1964; Li, Cullen, & Jasper, 1956; Mountcastle, Davies, & Berman, 1957).

V. Summary

Before birth and during the neonatal period the development of the cerebral cortex is characterized by the formation of the full complement of neurons and their organization into six layers. The laminae are formed in a phylogenetic sequence which has allowed new additions to accumulate on the pial aspect of the older laminae. Thus, it appears that the neocortex has evolved from the primitive pyriform type through archicortex to neocortex by a genetic/environmental change which prolongs mitosis in the ventricular zone and permits the guidance system to persist so that neuroblasts are able to move to their destinations above the older laminae. The factors which control mitosis in the ventricular zone are unknown, and thus the mechanisms involved in stopping or switching off division at about birth remain an enigma. Further advance in the evolution of the mammalian neocortex will occur if the switching mechanism fails and mitosis is allowed to continue in the ventricular zone so that new cellular laminae can be formed.

The appearance of the EEG at some 10 days after birth (Crain, 1952) presumably means that nerve networks are bioelectrically active. The substrate for the mediation of this activity is certainly present at this time, since both dendrites and synapses are seen in increasing numbers. We should now ask ourselves if this activity has any functional significance to the behavior of the animal? If it does, what is it? If it does not, then how does the part of the developing CNS, which is working properly, protect itself from the jamming effect of disorganized activity? The structural development of the nervous system appears to proceed in a cumulative manner, and presumably the physiology follows *pari passu*. The first activity is thus likely to be haphazard and functionally meaningless, but the other parts of the CNS may remain insulated by the development of inhibitory mechanisms or by the delayed maturation of one link in the network until a late stage. In the latter respect the late ontogeny of microneurons (interneurons) may have significance, and in the former respect it is interesting to record that a preponderance of inhibitory mechanisms in early development has been a finding of many works (see Crain, Meyerson and Persson,and Bergström, this volume; and Corner, Bakhuis and van Wingerden, Volume 1, and others in this book).

At present there is little understanding of how axons and dendrites are organized into the circuits which subserve behavior. Genetic factors may be primarily involved in the growth of axons and dendrites, but much of their synaptology appears to be influenced by the environment. The sensory experience of the animal, which to a large extent is dependent on behavior, is an important factor, and if animals suffer sensory deprivation, connections in the CNS are lost or are not formed since dendritic and axonal arborizations atrophy. Similar effects occur in the adult in the absence of afferent input, which suggests that mature connections are maintained by what may be called sensory tone.

References

Abercrombie, M., & Heaysman, J. E. M. Observations on the social behaviour of cells in tissue culture. II. "Monolayering" of fibroblasts. *Experimental Cell Research*, 1954, **6**, 293–306.

Adinolfi, A. M. The postnatal development of synaptic contacts in the cerebral cortex. In M. B. Sterman, D. J. McGinty, & A. M. Adinolfi (Eds.), *Brain development and behavior*. New York: Academic Press, 1971. Pp. 71–89.

Aghajanian, G. K., & Bloom, F. E. The formation of synaptic junctions in developing rat brain: a quantitative electron microscopic study. *Brain Research*, 1967, **6**, 716–727.

Allenspach, A. L., & Roth, L. E. Structural variations during mitosis in the chick embryo. *Journal of Cell Biology*, 1967, **33**, 179–196.

Altman, J. Are new neurons formed in the brains of adult mammals; *Science*, 1962, **135**, 1127–1128. (a)

Altman, J. Autoradiographic study of degenerative and regenerative proliferation of neuroglia cells with tritiated thymidine. *Experimental Neurology*, 1962, **5**, 302–318. (b)

Altman, J. Autoradiographic investigation of cell proliferation in the brains of rats and cats. *Anatomical Record*, 1963, **145**, 573–591.

Altman, J. Autoradiographic and histological studies of postnatal neurogenesis. II. A longitudinal investigation of the kinetics, migration and transformation of cells incorporating tritiated thymidine in infant rats, with special reference to postnatal neurogenesis in some brain regions. *Journal of Comparative Neurology*, 1966, **128**, 431–473. (a)

Altman, J. Proliferation and migration of undifferentiated precursor cells in the rat during postnatal gliogenesis. *Experimental Neurology*, 1966, **16**, 263–278. (b)

Altman, J. Postnatal growth and differentiation of the mammalian brain, with implications for a morphological theory of memory. In G. C. Quarton, T. Melnechuk, & F. O. Schmitt, (Eds.), *The neurosciences: A study program.* New York: Rockefeller University Press, 1967. Pp. 723–743.

Altman, J. and Das, G. D. Autoradiographic and histological evidence of postnatal hippocampal neurogenesis in rats. *Journal of Comparative Neurology*, 1965, **124**, 319–335. (a)

Altman, J., & Das, G. D. Post-natal origin of microneurones in the rat brain. *Nature* (*London*), 1965, **207**, 953–956. (b)

Altman, J., & Das, G. D. Autoradiographic and histological studies of postnatal neurogenesis. I. A longitudinal investigation of the kinetics, migration and transformation of cells incorporating tritiated thymidine in neonate rats, with special reference to postnatal neurogenesis in some brain regions. *Journal of Comparative Neurology*, 1966, **126**, 337–390.

Amassian, V. E., Walter, H. J., & Macy, J., Jr. Neural mechanism of the primary somatosensory evoked potential. *Annals of the New York Academy of Sciences*, 1964, **112**, 5–32.

Angevine, J. B., Jr., & Sidman, R. L. Autoradiographic study of cell migration during histogenesis of cerebral cortex in the mouse. *Nature* (*London*), 1961, **192**, 766–768.

Ariëns Kappers, C. U., Huber, G. C., & Crosby, E. C. *The comparative anatomy of the nervous system including man.* Vol. 1. New York: Macmillan, 1936. (Republished: New York, Hafner, 1960.)

Arnold, J. M. On the occurrence of microtubules in the developing lens of the squid *Loligo pealii*. *Journal of Ultrastructure Research*, 1966, **14**, 534–539.

Åström, K. E. On the early development of the isocortex in fetal sheep. *Progress in Brain Research*, 1967, **26**, 1–59.

Atlas, M., & Bond, V. P. The cell generation cycle of the eleven-day mouse embryo. *Journal of Cell Biology*, 1965, **26**, 19–24.

Baker, P. C., & Schroeder, T. E. Cytoplasmic filaments and morphogenetic movement in the amphibian neural tube. *Developmental Biology*, 1967, **14**, 432–450.

Barron, D. H. The early development of the motor cells and columns in the spinal cord of the sheep. *Journal of Comparative Neurology*, 1943, **78**, 1–27.

Barron, D. H. The early development of the sensory and internuncial cells in the spinal cord of the sheep. *Journal of Comparative Neurology*, 1944, **81**, 193–225.

Bellairs, R. The development of the nervous system in chick embryos, studied by electron microscopy. *Journal of Embryology and Experimental Morphology*, 1959, **7**, 94–115.

Bennett, E. L., Diamond, M. C., Krech, D., & Rosenzweig, M. R. Chemical and anatomical plasticity of the brain. *Science*, 1964, **146**, 610–619.

Bennett, M. V. L., Pappas, G. D., Giménez, M., & Nakajima, Y. Physiology and ultrastructure of electronic junctions. IV. Medullary electromotor nuclei in gymnotid fish. *Journal of Neurophysiology*, 1967, **30**, 236–300.

Bensted, J. P. M., Dobbing, J., Morgan, R. S., Reid, R. T. W., & Payling Wright, G. Neurological development and myelination in the spinal cord of the chick embryo. *Journal of Embryology and Experimental Morphology*, 1957, **5**, 428–437.

Bernhard, C. G., Kolmodin, G. M., & Meyerson, B. A. On the prenatal development of function and structure in the somesthetic cortex of the sheep. *Progress in Brain Research*, 1967, **26**, 60–77.

Berry, M., & Eayrs, J. T. Histogenesis of the cerebral cortex. *Nature (London)*, 1963, **197**, 984–985.

Berry, M., & Eayrs, J. T. The effects of x-irradiation on the development of the cerebral cortex. *Journal of Anatomy*, 1966, **100**, 707–722.

Berry, M., & Hollingworth, T. Growth of dendrites of the Purkinje cells in the rat cerebellum. *Journal of Anatomy*, 1972, **111**, 491–492.

Berry, M., & Hollingworth, T. Development of isolated neocortex. *Experientia*, 1973, **29**, 204–207. (a)

Berry, M., & Rogers, A. W. The migration of neuroblasts in the developing cerebral cortex. *Journal of Anatomy*, 1965, **99**, 691–709.

Berry, M., & Rogers, A. W. Histogenesis of mammalian neocortex. In R. Hassler & H. Stephan (Eds.), *Evolution of the forebrain*. Stuttgart: Thieme, 1966. Pp. 197–205.

Berry, M., Rogers, A. W., & Eayrs, J. T. Pattern of cell migration during cortical histogenesis. *Nature (London)*, 1964, **203**, 591–593.

Bodian, D. Development of fine structure of spinal cord in monkey fetuses. I. The motoneuron neuropil at the time of onset of reflex activity. *Bulletin of the Johns Hopkins Hospital*, 1966, **119**, 129–149.

Bogoch, S. *The biochemistry of memory*. London & New York: Oxford University Press, 1968.

Bok, S. T. Die Entwicklung der Hirnnerven und ihrer zentralen Bahnen. Die stimulogene Fibrillation. *Folia Neuro-Biologicum*, 1915, **9**, 475–565.

Boulder Committee. Embryonic vertebrate central nervous system: Revised terminology. *Anatomical Record*, 1970, **166**, 257–262.

Bowsher, D. Pathways of absorption of protein from the cerebrospinal fluid: An autoradiographic study in the cat. *Anatomical Record*, 1957, **128**, 23–39.

Bradley, P. B., Eayrs, J. T., & Schmalbach, K. The electroencephalogram of normal and hypothyroid rats. *Electroencephalography and Clinical Neurophysiology*, 1960, **12**, 467–477.

Bray, D. Surface movements during the growth of single explanted neurons. *Proceedings of the National Academy of Sciences, U.S.*, 1970, **65**, 905–910.

Bray, D., & Bunge, M. B. Branching patterns of sympathetic neurons in culture. (In press).

Brightman, M. W. Distribution within the brain of ferritin injected into cerebrospinal fluid compartments by ependymal distribution. *Journal of Cell Biology*, 1965, **26**, 99–121.

Brinkley, B. R., Stubblefield, E., & Hsu. T. C. The effect of colcemid inhibition and reversal of the fine structure of the mitotic apparatus of Chinese hamster cells *in vitro*. *Journal of Ultrastructure Research*, 1967, **19**, 1–18.

Brizzee, K. R., & Jacobs, L. A. Early post-natal changes in neuron packing density and volumetric relationships in the cerebral cortex of the white rat. *Growth*, 1959, **23**, 337–347.

Brizzee, K. R., Vogt, J., & Kharetchko, X. Postnatal changes in glia/neuron index with a comparison of methods of cell enumeration in the white rat. *Progress in Brain Research*, 1964, **4**, 136–149.

Brun, A. The subpial granular layer of the foetal cerebral cortex in man. *Acta Pathologica et Microbiologica Scandinavica, Supplement 1965*, **179**, 1–98.

Bryans, W. A. Mitotic activity in the brain of the adult rat. *Anatomical Record*, 1959, **133**, 65–71.

Burnside, B. Microtubules and microfilaments in Newt neuralation. *Developmental Biology*, 1971, **26**, 416–441.

Butler, A. B., & Caley, D. W. The migrating neuroblast: an ultrastructural study in hamster cortex. *Anatomical Record*, 1971, **169**, 287.

Byers, B., & Porter, K. R. Oriented microtubules in elongating cells of the developing lens rudiment after induction. *Proceedings of the National Academy of Sciences U.S.*, 1964, **52**, 1091–1099.

Caley, D. W., & Maxwell, D. S. Ultrastructure of the developing cerebral cortex in the rat. In M. B. Sterman, D. J. McGinty, & A. M. Adinolfi (Eds.), *Brain development and behavior*. New York: Academic Press 1971. Pp. 91–107.

Cammermeyer, J. Juxtavascular karyokinesis and microglia cell proliferation during retrograde reaction in the mouse facial nucleus. *Ergebnisse der Anatomie und Entwicklungsgeschichte*, 1965, **38**, 1–22.

Chase, H. B. Studies on an anophthalmic strain of mice. V. Associated cranial nerves and brain centers. *Journal of Comparative Neurology*, 1945, **83**, 121–139.

Coleman, P. D., & Riesen, A. H. Environmental effects on cortical dendritic fields. I. Rearing in the dark. *Journal of Anatomy*, 1968, **102**, 363–374.

Coulombre, A. J., & Coulombre, J. L. The role of mechanical factors in brain morphogenesis. *Anatomical Record*, 1958, **130**, 289–290.

Crain, S. M. Development of electrical activity in the cerebral cortex of the albino rat. *Proceedings of the Society for Experimental Biology and Medicine*, 1952, **81**, 49–51.

Dalton, M. M., Hommes, O. R., & Leblond, C. P. Correlation of glial proliferation with age in the mouse brain. *Journal of Comparative Neurology*, 1968, **134**, 397–399.

Del Cerro, M. P., & Snider, R. S. Studies on the developing cerebellum. Ultrastructure of growth cones. *Journal of Comparative Neurology*, 1968, **133**, 341–362.

DeLong, G. R., & Sidman, R. L. Effects of eye removal at birth on histogenesis of mouse superior colliculus. An autoradiographic analysis with tritiated thymidine. *Journal of Comparative Neurology*, 1962, **118**, 205–224.

Del Rio-Hortega, P. Tercera aportación al conocimento morfologico e interpretación functional de la oligodendrendroglia. *Memorias de la Real Sociedad Español de Historia Natural*, 1928, **14**, 5–122.

de-Thé, G. Cytoplasmic microtubules in different animal cells. *Journal of Cell Biology*, 1964, **23**, 265–275.

Diamond, M. C., Krech, D., & Rosenzweig, M. R. The effects of an enriched environment on the histology of the rat cerebral cortex. *Journal of Comparative Neurology*, 1964, **123**, 111–120.

Do Carmo, R. J. Direct cortical and recruiting responses in postnatal rabbit. *Journal of Neurophysiology*, 1960, **23**, 496–504.

Doig, C. M., & Smart, I. H. M. The location and orientation of mitotic figures in various epithelia. *Journal of Anatomy*, 1967, **101**, 634–636.

Duckett, S. The germinal layer of the growing human brain during early foetal life. *Anatomical Record*, 1968, **161**, 231–246.

Duckworth, T., & Cooper, E. R. A. A study of anophthalmia in an adult. *Acta Anatomica*, 1966, **63**, 509–522.

Duncan, D. Electron microscope study of the embryonic neural tube and notochord. *Texas Reports on Biology and Medicine*, 1957, **15**, 367–377.

Eayrs, J. T., & Goodhead, B. Postnatal development of the cerebral cortex of the rat. *Journal of Anatomy*, 1959, **93**, 385–402.

Farquhar, M. G., & Hartman, J. F. Neurological structure and relationships as revealed by electron microscopy. *Journal of Neuropathology and Experimental Neurology*, 1957, **16**, 18–39.

Farquhar, M. G., & Palade, G. E. Junctional complexes in various epithelia. *Journal of Cell Biology*, 1963, **17**, 375–412.

Fawcett, D. W., Ito, S. & Slautterback, D. The occurrence of intercellular bridges in groups of cells exhibiting synchronous differentation. *Journal of Biophysical and Biochemical Cytology*, 1959, **5**, 453–460.

Fifková, E. The influence of unilateral visual deprivation on optic centers. *Brain Research*, 1967, **6**, 763–766.

Fifková, E. Changes in the visual cortex of rats after unilateral deprivation. *Nature (London)*, 1968. **220**, 379–381.

Fifková, E. The effects of monocular deprivation on the synaptic contacts of the visual cortex. *Journal of Neurobiology*, 1970, **1**, 285–294. (a)

Fifková, E. The effects of unilateral deprivation of visual centers in rats. *Journal of Comparative Neurology*, 1970, **140**, 431–438. (b)

Friede, R. L. A histochemical study of DPN-diaphorase in human white matter with some notes on myelination. *Journal of Neurochemistry*, 1961, **8**, 17–30.

Fujita, H., & Fujita, S. Electron microscope studies on the neuroblast differentiation in the central nervous system of domestic fowl. *Zeitschrift für Zellforschung und Mikroskopische Anatomie, Abteilung Histochemie*, 1963, **60**, 463–478.

Fujita, S. Mitotic pattern and histogenesis of the central nervous system. *Nature (London)*, 1960, **185**, 702–703.

Fujita, S. Kinetics of cellular proliferation. *Experimental Cell Research*, 1962, **28**, 52–60.

Fujita, S. The matrix cell and cytogenesis in the developing central nervous system. *Journal of Comparative Neurology*, 1963, **120**, 37–42.

Fujita, S. Analysis of neuron differentiation in the central nervous system by tritiated thymidine autoradiography. *Journal of Comparative Neurology*, 1964, **122**, 311–328.

Fujita, S. An autoradiographic study on the origin and fate of the subpial glioblast in the embryonic chick spinal cord. *Journal of Comparative Neurology*, 1965, **124**, 51–60.

Fujita, S. Application of light and electron microscopic autoradiography to the study of cytogenesis of the forebrain. In R. Hassler & H. Stephan (Eds.), *Evolution of the forebrain.* Stuttgart: Thieme, 1966, Pp. 180–196.

Fujita, S., Shimada, M., & Nakamura, T. H^3-thymidine autoradiographic studies on the cell proliferation and differentiation in the external and internal granular layers of the mouse cerebellum. *Journal of Comparative Neurology*, 1966, **128**, 191–208.

Garey, L. J. & Powell, T. P. S. An experimental study of the termination of the lateral geniculo-cortical pathway in the cat and monkey. *Proceedings of the Royal Society London, ser. B.*, 1971, 179, 41–63.

Gaze, R. M. *Formation of nerve connections.* London: Academic Press, 1970.

Gaze, R. M. & Peters, A. The development, structure and composition of the optic nerve of *Xenopus laevis (Daudin). Quarterly Journal of Experimental Physiology and Cognate Medical Sciences*, 1961, **46**, 299–309.

Girbardt, M. Ultrastructure and dynamics of the moving nucleus. *Symposia of the Society for Experimental Biology*, 1968, **22**, 249–260.

Globus, A., & Scheibel, A. B. Dendritic branching in visually deprived rats. *Experimental Neurology*, 1967, **19**, 331–345. (a)

Globus, A., & Scheibel, A. B. The effects of visual deprivation on cortical neurons. A Golgi study. *Experimental Neurology*, 1967, **19**, 331–345. (b)

Globus, A., & Scheibel, A. B. Effects of visual deprivation on neurons of the visual cortex. *Anatomical Record*, 1967, **157**, 248. (c)

Globus, A., & Scheibel, A. B. Synaptic loci in cortical neurons of rabbit: the specific afferent radiation. *Experimental Neurology* 1967, **18**, 116–131. (d)

Gondos, B. Germ cell relationships in the developing ovary. In W. R. Butt, A. L. Crooke, & M. Ryle (Eds.), *Gonadotrophins and ovarian development.* Edinburgh: Livingstone, 1970.

Grafstein, B. Postnatal development of the transcallosal evoked response in the cerebral cortex of the cat. *Journal of Neurophysiology*, 1963, **26**, 79–99.

Gray, E. G. Axo-somatic and axo-dendritic synapses of the cerebral cortex: an electron microscope study. *Journal of Anatomy*, 1959, **93**, 420–433.

Gray, E. G., & Guillery, R. W. Synaptic morphology in the normal and degenerating nervous system. *International Review of Cytology*, 1966, **19**, 111–182.

Gyllensten, L., Malfors, T., & Norrlin, M-L., Effects of visual deprivation in optic centers of growing and adult mice. *Journal of Comparative Neurology*, 1965, **124**, 149–160.

Haas, R. J., Werner, J., & Fliedner, T. M. Cytokinetics of neonatal brain cell development in rats as studied by the 'complete ^{3}H-thymidine labelling' method. *Journal of Anatomy*, 1970, **107**, 421–437.

Hamburger, V., & Keefe, E. L. 1944. The effects of peripheral factors on the proliferation and differentiation in the spinal cord of chick embryos. *Journal of Experimental Zoology*, 1944, **96**, 223–242.

Handel, M. A., & Roth, L. E. Cell shape and morphology of the neural tube: implications for microtubule function. *Developmental Biology*, 1971, **25**, 78–95.

Hardesty, I. On the development and nature of the neuroglia. *American Journal of Anatomy*, 1904, **3**, 229–268.

Haug, H. Remarks on the determination and significance of the gray cell coefficient. *Journal of Comparative Neurology*, 1956, **104**, 473–492.

Herman, L., & Kauffman, S. L. The fine structure of the embryonic mouse neural tube with special reference to cytoplasmic microtubules. *Developmental Biology*, 1966, **13**, 145–162.

Hess, A. The experimental embryology of the foetal nervous system. *Biological Reviews of the Cambridge Philosophical Society*, 1957, **32**, 231–260.

Hess, A. Optic centers and pathways after eye removal in fetal guinea pigs. *Journal of Comparative Neurology*, 1958, **109**, 91–116.

Hicks, S. P., & D'Amato, C. J. Cell migration to the isocortex in the rat. *Anatomical Record*, 1968, **160**, 619–634.

Hicks, S. P., D'Amato, C. J., & Lowe, M. J. The development of the mammalian nervous system. I. Malformations of the brain, especially the cerebral cortex, induced in rats by radiation. II.

Some mechanisms of the malformations of the cortex. *Journal of Comparative Neurology*, 1959, **113**, 435–470.

Hild, W. Das Morphologische, kinetische und endokrinologische Verhalten von hypothalamischen und neurohypophysäran geweb in vitro. *Zeitschrift für Zellforschung und Mikroskopische Anatomie*, 1954, **40**, 257–312.

Hinds, J. W. Autoradiographic study of histogenesis in the mouse olfactory bulb. I. Time of origin of neurons and neuroglia. *Journal of Comparative Neurology*, 1968, **134**, 287–304.

Hinds, J. W. Early neuroblast differentiation in the mouse olfactory bulb. *Anatomical Record*, 1971, **169**, 340–341.

Hinds, J. W., & Ruffett, T. L. Cell proliferation in the neural tube: an electron microscopic and Golgi analysis in the mouse cerebral vesicle. *Zeitschrift für Zellforschung und Mikroskopische Anatomie*, 1971, **115**, 226–264.

His, W. Histogenese und zusammenhaug der Nervenelemente. *Archiv für Anatomie und Physiolgie, Anatomie Arbitung, Supplement Band*, 1890, **5**, 95–117.

Hollingworth, T., Berry, M., & Anderson, E. M. Network analysis of dendritic fields of pyramidal cells in neocortex and Purkinje cells in the cerebellum of the rat. *Journal of Anatomy* (in press).

Holloway, R. L., Jr. Dendritic branching: some preliminary results of training and complexity in rat visual cortex. *Brain Research*, 1966, **2**, 393–396.

Holmes, R. L., & Berry, M. Electron-microscopic studies of developing foetal cerebral cortex of the rat. In R. Hassler & H. Stephan (Eds.), *Evolution of the forebrain.* Stuttgart: Thieme, 1966. Pp. 206–212.

Hubel, D. H., & Wiesel, T. N. Receptive fields of cells in striate cortex of very young, visually inexperienced kittens. *Journal of Neurophysiology*, 1963, **26**, 994–1002.

Hughes, A. The growth of embryonic neurites. A study on cultures of chick neural tissues. *Journal of Anatomy*, 1953, **87**, 150–162.

Hunt, W. E., & Goldring, S. Maturation of evoked response of the visual cortex in the postnatal rabbit. *Electroencephalography and Clinical Neurophysiology*, 1951, **3**, 465–471.

Ingvar, S. Reaction of cells to the galvanic current in tissue culture. *Proceedings of the Society for Experimental Biology and Medicine*, 1920, **17**, 198–199.

Jacobson, M. Development, specification, and diversification of neuronal connections. In G. C. Quarton, T. Melnechuk, & G. Adelenen (Eds.), *The neurosciences: Second study program.* New York: Rockefeller University Press, 1970. Pp. 116–129.

Jacobson, S. Sequence of myelinization in the brain of the albino rat. A cerebral cortex, thalamus and related structures. *Journal of Comparative Neurology*, 1963, **121**, 5–29.

Jones, E. G., & Powell, T. P. S. An electron microscopic study of the laminar pattern and mode of termination of afferent fibre pathways in the somatic sensory cortex of the cat. *Philosophical Transactions of the Royal Society of London, Series B*, 1970, **257**, 45–62.

Jones, H. G., & Thomas, D. B. Changes in the dendritic organization of neurons in the cerebral cortex following deafferentation. *Journal of Anatomy*, 1962, **96**, 375–381.

Jones, O. W., Jr. Cytogenesis of oligodendroglia and astrocytes. *Archives of Neurology and Psychiatry*, 1932, **28**, 1030–1045.

Källen, B. On the significance of the neuromeres and similar structures in vertebrate embryos. *Journal of Embryology and Experimental Morphology*, 1953, **1**, 387–392.

Kanno, Y. & Loewenstein, W. R. Cell-to-cell passage of large molecules. *Nature* (*London*), 1966, **212**, 629–630.

Karfunkel, P. The role of microtubules and microfilaments in neurulation in *Xenopus*. *Developmental Biology*, 1971, **25**, 30–56.

Kershman, J. The medulloblast and the medulloblastoma. A study on human embryos. *Archives of Neurology and Psychiatry*, 1938, **40**, 937–967.

Kitching, J. A. The axopods of the sun animalicule Actinophrys Sol (Heliozoa). In R. R. Allen & N. Kamiya (Eds.), *Primitive motile systems in cell biology*. New York: Academic Press, 1964. Pp. 445–456.

Kolliker, A. *Handbuch der Gewebelehre des Menschen. (6th ed.)* Leipzig: W. Engelmann, 1896.

Krech, D., Rosenzweig, M. R., & Bennett, E. L. Effects of complex environment and blindness on rat brain. *Archives of Neurology*, 1963, **8**, 403–412.

Kristensson, K., Olsson, Y., & Sjöstrand, J. Axonal uptake and retrograde transport of exogenous proteins in the hypoglossal nerve. *Brain Research*, 1971, 32, 399–406.

Langman, J., Guerrant, R. L., & Freeman, B. G. Behavior of neuro-epithelial cells during closure of the neural tube. *Journal of Comparative Neurology*, 1966, **127**, 399–412.

Langman, J., & Welch, G. W. Excess vitamin A and development of the cerebral cortex. *Journal of Comparative Neurology*, 1967, **131**, 15–26.

Levi-Montalcini, R. The development of the acoustico-vestibular centers in the chick embryo in the absence of the afferent root fibers and of descending fiber tracts. *Journal of Comparative Neurology*, 1949, **91**, 209–241.

Levi-Montalcini, R. Differentiation and growth control mechanisms in the nervous system. *Experimental Biology and Medicine*, 1967, **1**, 170–182.

Li, C. L., Cullen, C., & Jasper, H. H. Laminar microelectrode studies of specific somatosensory cortical potentials. *Journal of Neurophysiology*, 1956, **19**, 111–130.

Liu, C. N., & Liu, C. Y. Role of afferents in maintenance of dendritic morphology. *Anatomical Record*, 1971, **169**, 369.

Loewenstein, W. R., & Kanno, Y. Intercellular communication and the control of tissue growth: lack of communication between cancer cells. *Nature* (*London*), 1966, **209**, 1248–1249.

Lorente de Nó, R. Cerebral cortex: architecture, intracortical connections, motor projections. Cortical afferents. In J. F. Fulton (Ed.), *Physiology of the nervous system*. London & New York: Oxford University Press, 1946. Pp. 300–301.

Lyser, K. M. Early differentiation of motor neuroblasts in the chick embryo as studied by electron microscopy. I. General aspects. *Developmental Biology*, 1964, **10**, 433–466.

Lyser, K. M. Early differentiation of motor neuroblasts in the chick embryo as studied by electron microscopy. II. Microtubules and neurofilaments. *Developmental Biology*, 1968, **17**, 117–142.

Marin-Padilla, M. Prenatal and early postnatal ontogenesis of the human motor cortex: a Golgi study. I. The sequential development of the cortical layers. *Brain Research*, 1970, **23**, 167–183. (a)

Marin-Padilla, M. Prenatal and early postnatal ontogenesis of the human motor cortex: a Golgi study. II. The basket-pyramidal system. *Brain Research*, 1970, **23**, 185–191. (b)

Marin-Padilla, M. Early ontogenesis of the cerebral cortex (neocortex) of the cat (Felis domestica). A Golgi study. I. The primordial neocortical organisation. *Zeitschrift für Anatomie und Entwicklungsgeschichte*, 1971, **134**, 117–145.

Marin-Padilla, M., & Stibitz, G. R. Distribution of the apical dendritic spines of layer V pyramidal cells of the hamster neocortex. *Brain Research*, 1968, **11**, 580–592.

Marques-Pereira, J. P., & Leblond, C. P. Mitosis and differentiation in the stratified squamous epithelium of the rat esophagus. *American Journal of Anatomy*, 1965, **117**, 73–90.

Marsh, G., & Beams, H. W. Orientation of chick nerve fibers by direct electric currents. *Anatomical Record*, 1946, **94**, 370.

Martin, A. H. Significance of mitotic spindle fibre orientation in the neural tube. Nature (*London*), 1967, **216**, 1133–1134.

Martin, A., & Langman, J. The development of the spinal cord examined by autoradiography. *Journal of Emrbyology and Experimental Morphology*, 1965, **14**, 25–35.

Marty, R., & Scherrer, J. Critères de maturation des systèmes afférents corticaux. *Progress in Brain Research*, 1964, **4**, 222–236.

Matthews, M. A. An electron microscopic study of the relationship between axon diameter and the initiation of myelin production in the peripheral nervous system. *Anatomical Record*, 1968, **161**, 337–352.

Matthews, M. A., & Duncan, D. A quantitative study of morphological changes accompanying the initiation and progress of myelin production in the dorsal funiculus of the rat spinal cord. *Journal of Comparative Neurology*, 1971, **142**, 1–22.

Maturana, H. R. The fine anatomy of the optic nerve of anurans–An electron microscope study. *Journal of Biophysical and Biochemical Cytology*, 1960, **7**, 107–119.

Meller, K., Breipohl, W., & Glees, P. Early cytological differentiation in the cerebral hemisphere of mice. An electronmicroscopical study. *Zeitschrift für Zellforschung und Mikroskopische Anatomie*, 1966, **72**, 525–533.

Meller, K., Breipohl, W., & Glees, P. The cytology of the developing molecular layer of mouse. motor cortex. An electron microscopical and a Golgi impregnation study. *Zeitschrift für Zellforschung und Mikroskopische Anatomie*, 1968, **86**, 171–183.

Meller, K., & Glees, P. The differentiation of neuroglia-Müller-cells in the retina of the chick. *Zeitschrift für Zellforschung und Mikroskopische Anatomie*, 1965, **66**, 321–332.

Meller, K., & Wechsler, W. Electron microscope findings in the ependymal lining of the developing brain of the chick embryo. *Acta Neuropathologica*, 1964, **3**, 609–626.

Messier, B., Leblond, C. P., & Smart, I. Presence of DNA synthesis and mitosis in the brain of young adult mice. *Experimental Cell Research*, 1958, **14**, 224–226.

Meyerson, B. A. Electrophysiological signs of interhemispheric functions during development. In L. Jílek & S. Trojan (Eds.), *Ontogenesis of the brain*. Prague: Charles University, 1968. Pp. 61–71.

Molliver, M. E., & Van der Loos, H. The ontogenesis of cortical circuitry: The spatial distribution of synapses in somesthetic cortex of newborn dog. *Ergebnisse der Anatomie und Entwicklungsgeschichte*, 1970, **42**, 7–53.

Morest, D. K. The growth of synaptic endings in the mammalian brain: a study of the calyses of the trapezoid body. *Zeitschrift für Anatomie und Entwicklungsgeschichte*, 1968, **127**, 201–220.

Morest, D. K. The differentiation of cerebral dendrites: a study of the post-migratory neuroblast in the medial nucleus of the trapezoid body. *Zeitschrift für Anatomie und Entwicklungsgeschichte*, 1969, **128**, 271–289. (a)

Morest, D. K. The growth of dendrites in the mammalian brain. *Zeitschrift für Anatomie und Entwicklungsgeschichte*, 1969, **128**, 290–317. (b)

Morest, D. K. The pattern of neurogenesis in the retina of the rat. *Zeitschrift für Anatomie und Entwicklungsgeschichte*, 1970, **131**, 45–67. (a)

Morest, D. K. A study of neurogenesis in the forebrain of opossum pouch young. *Zeitschrift für Anatomie und Entwicklungsgeschichte*, 1970, **130**, 265–305. (b)

Mori, S., & Leblond, C. P. Electron microscopic features and proliferation of astrocytes in the corpus callosum of the rat. *Journal of Comparative Neurology*, 1969, **137**, 197–226.

Mori, S., & Leblond, C. P. Electron microscopic identification of three classes of oligodendrocytes and a preliminary study of their proliferative activity in the corpus callosum of young rats. *Journal of Comparative Neurology*, 1970, **139**, 1–30.

Moskowitz, N., & Noback, C. R. The human lateral geniculate body in normal development and congenital unilateral anophthalmia. *Journal of Neuropathology and Experimental Neurology*, 1962, **21**, 377–382.

Mountcastle, V. B., Davies, P. W., & Berman, A. L. Response properties of neurons of cat's somatosensory cortex to peripheral stimuli. *Journal of Neurophysiology*, 1957, **20**, 374–407.

Mugnaini, E. The relation between cytogenesis and the formation of different types of synaptic contact. *Brain Research*, 1970, **17**, 169–179.

Mugnaini, E., & Forstrønen, P. F. Ultrastructural studies on the cerebellar histogenesis. I.

Differentiation of granule cells and development of glomeruli in the chick embryo. *Zeitschrift für Zellforschung und Mikroskopische Anatomie*, 1967, **77**, 115–143.

Nakai, J., & Kawasaki, Y. Studies on the mechanism determining the course of nerve fibres in tissue culture. I. The reaction of the growth cone to various obstructions. *Zeitschrift für Zellforschung und Mikroskopische Anatomie*, 1959, **51**, 108–122.

Noback, C. R. & Purpura, D. P. Postnatal ontogenesis of neurons in cat neocortex. *Journal of Comparative Neurology*, 1961, **117**, 291–307.

Opperman, K. Cajalische Horizontalzellen und ganglienzellen des Marks. *Zeitschrift für die gesamte Neurologie Psychiatrie*, 1929, **120**, 121.

Palay, S. L. Synapses in the central nervous system. *Journal of Biophysical and Biochemical Cytology Supplement*, 1956, **2**, 193–202.

Payton, B. W., Bennett, M. V. L., & Pappas, G. D. Permeability and structure of junctional membranes at an electronic synapse. *Science*, 1969, **166**, 1641–1643.

Pearce, T. L., & Zwaan, J. A light and electron microscopic study of cell behaviour and microtubules in the embryonic chicken lens using Colcemid. *Journal of Embryology and Experimental Morphology*, 1970, **23**, 491–507.

Pelc, S. R. Turnover of DNA and function. *Nature* (*London*), 1968, **219**, 162–163.

Penfield, W. Oligodendroglia and its relation to classical neuroglia. *Brain*, 1924, **47**, 430–452.

Peters, A. The structure of myelin sheaths in the central nervous system of *Xenopus laevis* (Davidson) *Journal of Biophysical and Biochemical Cytology*, 1960, **7**, 121–126.

Pick, J., Gerdin, C., & Delemos, C. An electron microscopic study of developing sympathetic neurons in man. *Zeitschrift für Zellforschung und Mikroskopische Anatòmie*, 1964, **62**, 402–415.

Poliakov, G. I. Some results of research into the development of the neuronal structure of the cortical ends of the analysers in man. *Journal of Comparative Neurology*, 1961, **117**, 197–212.

Pomerat, C. M. Cinematology, indispensable tool for cytology. *International Review of Cytology*, 1961, **11**, 307–334.

Pomerat, C. M., & Costero, I., Tissue culture of cat cerebellum. *American Journal of Anatomy*, 1956, **99**, 211–241.

Potter, D. D., Furshpan, E. J., & Lennox, E. S. Connection between cells of the developing squid as revealed by electrophysiological methods. *Proceedings of the National Academy of Sciences, U.S.*, 1966, **55**, 328–336.

Pressman, B. C. Induced active transport of ions in mitochondria. *Proceedings of the National Academy of Sciences, U.S.*, 1965, **53**, 1076–1083.

Purpura, D. P. Analysis of axodendritic synaptic organizations in immature cerebral cortex. *Annals of the New York Academy of Sciences*, 1961, **94**, 604–654.

Purpura, D. P., Shofer, R. J., Housepian, E. M., & Noback, C. R. Comparative ontogenesis of structure-function relations in cerebral and cerebellar cortex. *Progress in Brain Research*, 1964, **4**, 187–221.

Rabinowicz, Th., The cerebral cortex of the premature infant of the 8th month. *Progress in Brain Research*, 1964, **4**, 39–92.

Rabinowicz. Th., Quantitative appraisal of the cerebral cortex of the premature infant of 8 months. In A. Minkowski (Ed.), *Regional development of the brain in early life*. London: Blackwell, 1967.

Rakic, P. Guidance of neurons migrating to the fetal monkey neocortex. *Brain Research*, 1971, **33**, 471–476. (a)

Rakic, P. Neuron-glia relationship during granule cell migration in developing cerebellar cortex. A Golgi and electronmicroscopic study in *Macacus rhesus*. *Journal of Comparative Neurology*, 1971, **141**, 283–312. (b)

Ralston, H. J. III. Evidence for presynaptic dendrites and a proposal for their mechanism of action. *Nature* (*London*), 1971, **230**, 585–587.

Ramon-Moliner, E. A study on neuroglia. The problem of transitional forms. *Journal of*

Comparative Neurology, 1958, **110**, 157–171.

Ramón y Cajal, S. *Histologie du système nerveux de l'homme et des vertébrés.* (Française révue et mise à jour par l'auteur. Traduite de l'espagnol par L. Azoulay.) Paris: 1909.

Ramón y Cajal, S. *Degeneration and regeneration of the nervous system.* London: Oxford University Press, 1928.

Ramón y Cajal, S. *Studies on vertebrates neurogenesis.* (Translated by L. Guth.) Springfield, Ill.: Thomas, 1960.

Ramsey, H. Differentiation of oligodendroglia from migratory spongioblasts. In S. S. Breese (Ed.), *Fifth international congress for electron microscopy.* Vol. 2. New York: Academic Press, 1962. pp. N–3.

Rauke, O. Beiträge zur Kenntnis der normalen und pathologischen Hirnrindenbildung. *Beiträge zur Pathologischen Anatomie*, 1909, **45**, 51.

Robertson, J. D., Dodenheimer, T. S., & Stage, D. E. The ultrastructure of Mauthner cell synapses and nodes in goldfish brains. *Journal of Cell Biology*, 1963, **19**, 159–199.

Rose, G. H. The comparative ontogenesis of visually evoked responses in rat and cat. In L. Jílek & S. Trojan (Eds.), *Ontogenesis of the brain.* Prague: Charles University, 1968. Pp. 347–358.

Rosenzweig, M. R., Bennett, E. L., Diamond, M. C., Wu, S-Y., Slagle, R. W., & Saffran, E. Influence of environmental complexity and visual stimulation on development of occipital cortex in the rat. *Brain Research*, 1969, **14**, 427–445.

Rosenzweig, M. R., Krech, D., Bennett, E. L., & Diamond, M. C. Effects of environmental complexity and training on brain chemistry and anatomy: a replication and extension. *Journal of Comparative Physiology and Psychology*, 1962, **55**, 529–437.

Rosenzweig, M. R., Love, W., & Bennett, E. L. Effects of a few hours a day of enriched experience on brain chemistry and brain weights. *Physiology & Behavior*, 1968, **3**, 819–825.

Roth, L. E., Pihlaja, D. J., & Shigenaka, Y. Microtubules in the heliozoan axopodium. I. The gradion hypothesis of allosterism in structural proteins. *Journal of Ultrastructure Research*, 1970, **30**, 7–37.

Ruiz-Marcos, A., & Valverde, F. The temporal evolution of the distribution of dendritic spines in the visual cortex of normal and dark raised mice. *Experimental Brain Research*, 1969, **8**, 284–294.

Sakla, B. F. Post-natal growth of neuroglia cells and blood vessels of the cervical spinal cord of the albino mouse. *Journal of Comparative Neurology*, 1965, **124**, 189–202.

Samorajski, T., & Friede, R. L. A quantitative electron microscopic study of myelination in the pyramidal tract of rat. *Journal of Comparative Neurology*, 1968, **134**, 323–328.

Sarkisov, S. A., Popova, E. N., & Bogolepov, N. N. Structure of synapses in evolutionary aspect (optic and electron-microscopic studies). In R. Hassler & H. Stephan (Eds.), *Evolution of the forebrain.* Stuttgart: Thieme, 1966. Pp. 225–236.

Sauer, F. C. The cellular structure of the neural tube. *Journal of Comparative Neurology*, 1935, **63**, 13–23. (a)

Sauer, F. C. Mitosis in the neural tube. *Journal of Comparative Neurology*, 1935, **62**, 337–405. (b)

Sauer, F. C. The interkinetic migration of embryonic epithelial nuclei. *Journal of Morphology*, 1936, **60**, 1–11.

Sauer, F. C. Some factors in the morphogenesis of vertebrate embryonic epithelia. *Journal of Morphology*, 1937, **61**, 563–579.

Sauer, M. E., & Chittenden, A. C. Deoxyribonucleic acid content of cell nuclei in the neural tube of the chick embryo: evidence for intermitotic migration of nuclei. *Experimental Cell Research*, 1959, **16**, 1–6.

Sauer, M. E., & Walker, B. E. Radioautographic study of interkinetic nuclear migration in the neural tube. *Proceedings of the Society for Experimental Biology and Medicine*, 1959, **101**, 557–560.

Schadé, J. P., & Baxter, C. F. Changes during growth in the volume and surface area of cortical neurons in the rabbit. *Experimental Neurology*, 1960, **2**, 158–178.

Schadé, J. P., Van Backer, H., & Colon, E. Quantitative analysis of neuronal parameters in the maturing cerebral cortex. *Progress in Brain Research*, 1964, **4**, 150–175.

Schaper, A. Die Frühesten Differenzirungsvorgange in Centralnervensystem. *Archiv für Entwicklungsmechanik*, 1897, **5**, 81–132.

Scheibel, M. E., & Scheibel, A. B. Some structuro-functional correlates of development in young cats. *Electroencephalography and Clinical Neurophysiology*, 1963, Suppl. **24**, 235–246.

Scheibel, M. E., & Scheibel, A. B. Selected structural-functional correlations in postnatal brain. In M. B. Sterman, D. J. McGinty, & A. M. Adinolfi (Eds.), *Brain development and behavior*. New York: Academic Press, 1971. Pp. 1–21.

Schonbach, J., Hu, K. H., & Friede, R. L. Cellular and chemical changes during myelination: Histologic, autoradiographic, histochemical and biochemical data on myelination in the pyramidal tract and corpus callosum of rat. *Journal of Comparative Neurology*, 1968, **134**, 21–38.

Schroeder, T. E. Neurulation in *Xenopus laevis*. An analysis and model based upon light and electron microscopy. *Journal of Embryology and Experimental Morphology*, 1970, **23**, 427–462.

Sechrist, J. W. Neurocytogenesis I. Neurofibrils, neurofilaments and the terminal mitotic cycle. *American Journal of Anatomy*, 1969, **124**, 117–134.

Sedgwick, A. On the inadequacy of the cellular theory of development and on the early development of nerves, particularly of the third nerve and of the sympathetic ganglion in Elasmobranchii. *Quarterly Journal of Microscopical Science of New York*, 1895, **37**, 87–101.

Seggie, J. & Berry, M. Ontogeny of interhemispheric evoked potentials in the rat: significance of myelination of the corpus callosum. *Experimental Neurology*, 1972, **35**, 215–232.

Seggie, J., & Berry, M. Synaptogenesis in the cortex of the rat. In preparation, 1973.

Seymore, R. M., Kemp, J. M., & Berry, M. Scanning and transmission electron microscope studies on the neuroectoderm of the telencephalic vesicle. *Journal of Anatomy*, 1972, **111**, 508–509.

Shariff, G. A. Cell counts in the primate cerebral cortex. *Journal of Comparative Neurology*, 1953, **98**, 381–400.

Sheffield, J. B., & Fischman, D. A. Intercellular junctions in the developing neural retina of the chick embryo. *Zeitschrift für Zellforschung und Mikroskopische Anatomie*, 1970, **104**, 405–418.

Sheridan, J. D. Electrophysiological evidence for low-resistance intercellular junctions in the early chick embryo. *Journal of Cell Biology*, 1968, **37**, 650–659.

Shimada, M., & Langman, J. Cell proliferation, migration and differentiation in the cerebral cortex of the golden hamster. *Journal of Comparative Neurology*, 1970, **139**, 227–244.

Sidman, R. L. Histogenesis of mouse retina studied with thymidine-H^3. In G. K. Smelser (Ed.), *The structure of the eye*. New York: Academic Press, 1961. pp. 487–506.

Sidman, R. L., Miale, I. L., & Feder, N. Cell proliferation and migration in the primitive ependymal zone; An autoradiographic study of histogenesis in the nervous system. *Experimental Neurology*, 1959, **1**, 322–333.

Slautterback, D. B. Cytoplasmic microtubules. I. Hydra. *Journal of Cell Biology*, 1963, **18**, 367–388.

Smart, I. The subependymal layer of the mouse brain and its cell production as shown by radioautography after thymidine-H^3 injection. *Journal of Comparative Neurology*, 1961, **116**, 325–348.

Smart, I. The evolution of neurone production in the vertebrate central nervous system. *Journal of Anatomy*, 1964, **98**, 466–467.

Smart, I. H. M. Changes in location and orientation of mitotic figures in mouse oesophageal epithelium during the development of stratification. *Journal of Anatomy*, 1970, **106**, 15–21.

Smart, I. H. M. Location and orientation of mitotic figures in the developing mouse olfactory epithelium. *Journal of Anatomy*, 1971, **109**, 243–251.

Smart, I. H. M. Proliferative characteristics of the ependymal layer during the early development of the spinal cord in the mouse. *Journal of Anatomy*, 1972, **111**, 365–380. (a)

Smart, I. H. M. Proliferative characteristics of the ependymal layer during early development of the mouse diencephalon, as revealed by recording the number, location, and plane of cleavage of mitotic figures, *Journal of Anatomy*, 1972, **113**, 109–129. (b)

Smart, I., & Leblond, C. P. Evidence for division and transformations of neuroglia cells in the mouse brain, as derived from radioautography after injection of thymidine-H^3. *Journal of Comparative Neurology*, 1961, **116**, 349–367.

Speidel, C. C. Studies on living nerves. VII. Growth adjustments of cutaneous terminal arborizations. *Journal of Comparative Neurology*. 1942, **76**, 57–73.

Sperry, R. W. Developmental basis of behavior. In A. Roe & G. T. Simpson (Eds.), *Behavior and evolution.* New Haven: Yale University Press, 1958, Pp. 128–139.

Sperry, R. W. Chemoaffinity in the orderly growth of nerve fiber patterns and connections. *Proceedings of the National Academy of Sciences, U.S.*, 1963 **50**, 703–710.

Sperry, R. W. Embryogenesis of behavioral nerve nets. In R. L. De Haan & H. Ursprung (Eds.), *Organogenesis.* New York: Holt Rinehart and Winston, 1965. Pp. 161–186.

Spooner, B. S., & Wessells, N. K. Effects of cytochalasin B upon microfilaments involved in morphogenesis of salivary epithelium. *Proceedings of the National Academy of Sciences, U.S.*, 1970, **66**, 360–364.

Steinberg, M. S. The problem of adhesive selectivity in cellular interactions. In M. Locke (Ed.), *Cellular membranes in development.* New York: Academic Press, 1964. Pp. 321–366.

Stensaas, L. J. The development of hippocampal and dorsolateral pallial regions of the cerebral hemisphere of fetal rabbits. I. Fifteen millimeter stage spongioblast morphology. *Journal of Comparative Neurology*, 1967, **129**, 59–70. (a)

Stensaas, L. J. The development of hippocampal and dorsolateral pallial regions of the cerebral hemisphere in fetal rabbits. II. Twenty millimeter stage, neuroblast morphology. *Journal of Comparative Neurology*, 1967, **129**, 71–84. (b)

Stensaas, L. J. The development of hippocampal and dorsolateral pallial regions of the cerebral hemisphere in fetal rabbits. III. Twenty-nine millimeter stage, marginal lamina. *Journal of Comparative Neurology*, 1967, **130**, 149–162. (c)

Stensaas, L. J. The development of hippocampal and dorsolateral pallial regions of the cerebral hemispheres in fetal rabbits. IV. Forty-one millimeter stage, intermediate lamina. *Journal of Comparative Neurology*, 1967, **131**, 409–422. (d)

Stensaas, L. J. The development of hippocampal and dorsolateral pallial region of the cerebral hemisphere in fetal rabbits. V. Sixty-millimeter stage, glial cell morphology. *Journal of Comparative Neurology*, 1967, **131**, 423–436. (e)

Stensaas, L. J. The development of hippocampal and dorsolateral pallial regions of the cerebral hemispheres in fetal rabbits. VI. Ninety-millimeter stage, cortical differentiation. *Journal of Comparative Neurology*, 1968, **132**, 93–108.

Stensaas, L. J., & Stensaas, S. S. An electron microscope study of cells in the matrix and intermediate laminae of the cerebral hemisphere of the 45 mm. rabbit embryo. *Zeitschrift für Zellforschung und Mikroskopische Anatomie*, 1968, **91**, 341–365.

Tennyson, V. M. Electron microscope observations of the development of the neuroblast in the rabbit embryo. In S. S. Breese (Ed.), *Fifth international congress for electron microscopy.* Vol. 2, New York: Academic Press, 1962. pp. 4–8.

Tennyson, V. M. The fine structure of the axon and growth cone of the dorsal root neuroblasts of the rabbit embryo. *Journal of Cell Biology*, 1970, **44**, 62–79.

Tilney, F. Behavior in its relation to the development of the brain. Part II. Correlation between the development of the brain and behavior in the albino rat from embryonic states to matùrity. *Bulletin of the Neurological Institute of New York*, 1933, **3**, 252–358.

Tilney, L. G. Studies on microtubules in Heliozoa. IV. The effect of colchicine on the formation and maintenance of axopodia and the redevelopment of pattern in *Actinosphaerium nucleofilium* (Barrett). *Journal of Cell Science*, 1968, **3**, 549–562.

Tilney, L. G., & Byers, B. Studies on the microtubules in Heliozoa. V. Factors controlling the organization of microtubules in the axonemal pattern in Echinosphaerium (*Actinosphaerium nucleofilum*). *Journal of Cell Biology*, 1969, **43**, 148–165.

Tilney, L. G., Hiramoto, Y., & Marsland, D. Studies on the microtubules in Heliozoa. III. A pressure analysis of the role of these structures in the formation and maintenance of the axopodia of *Actinosphaerium nucleofilum* (*Barrett*). *Journal of Cell Biology*, 1966, **29**, 77–95.

Tilney, L. G., & Porter, K. R. Studies on microtubules in Heliozoa. II. The effect of low temperature on these structures in the formation and maintenance of the axopodia. *Journal of Cell Biology*, 1967, **34**, 327–343.

Trelstad, R. L., Hay, E. D., & Revel, J-P. Cell contact during early morphogenesis in the chick embryo. *Developmental Biology*, 1967, **16**, 78–106.

Tsang, Y.-C. Visual centers in blinded rats. *Journal of Comparative Neurology*, 1937, **66**, 211–261.

Uchizono, K. Characteristics of excitatory and inhibitory synapses in the central nervous system of the cat. *Nature* (*London*), 1965, **207**, 642–643.

Ulett, G.,Jr., Dow, R. S., & Larsell, O. The inception of conductivity in the corpus callosum and the cortico-ponto-cerebellar pathway in young rabbits with reference to myelinization. *Journal of Comparative Neurology*, 1955, **80**, 1–10.

Valverde, F. Apical dendritic spines of the visual cortex and light deprivation in the mouse. *Experimental Brain Research*, 1967, **3**, 337–352.

Valverde, F. Structural changes in the area striata of the mouse after enucleation. *Experimental Brain Research*, 1968, **5**, 274–292.

Valverde, F. Rate and extent of recovery from dark rearing in the visual cortex of the mouse. *Brain Research*, 1971, **33**, 1–11.

Valverde, F., & Ruiz-Marcos, A. Dendritic spines in the visual cortex of the mouse: Introduction to a mathematical model. *Experimental Brain Research*, 1969, **8**, 269–283.

Van der Loos, H. The "improperly" orientated pyramidal cell in the cerebral cortex and its possible bearing on problems of neuronal growth and cell orientation. *Bulletin of the Johns Hopkins Hospital*, 1965, **117**, 228–250.

Vaughn, J. E. An electron microscopic analysis of gliogenesis in rat optic nerves. *Zeitschrift für Zellforschung und Mikroskopische Anatomie*, 1969, **94**, 293–324.

Voeller, K., Pappas, G. D., & Purpura, D. P. Electron microscope study of development of cat superficial neocortex. *Experimental Neurology*, 1963, **7**, 107–130.

Waddington, C. H., & Perry, M. M. A note on the mechanism of cell deformation in the neural folds in the amphibian. *Experimental Cell Research*, 1966, **41**, 691–693.

Walberg, F. Morphological correlates of postsynaptic inhibitory processes. In C. von Euler, S. Skoglund, & V. Soderberg (Eds.), *Structure and function of inhibitory neural mechanisms.* Oxford: Pergamon, 1968, Pp. 7–14.

Watterson, R. L., Veneziano, P., & Bartha, A. Absence of a true germinal zone in neural tubes of young chick embryos as demonstrated by the colchicine technique. *Anatomical Record*, 1956, **124**, 379.

Wechsler, W. Electron-microscopy of the cytodifferentiation in the developing brain of chick embryos. In R. Hassler & H. Stephan (Eds.), *Evolution of the forebrain.* Stuttgart: Thieme, 1966. Pp. 213–224.

Wechsler, W. Developmental analysis of the fine structure of different nerve cell types. *Experimental Biology and Medicine*, 1967, **1**, 153–169.

Wechsler, W., & Meller, K. Electron microscopy of neuronal and glial differentiation in developing brain of chick. *Progress in Brain Research*, 1967, **26**, 93–144.

Weiss, P. Special vertebrate organogenesis. Nervous system. In B. H. Willier, P. A. Weiss, & V. Hamburger (Eds.), *Analysis of development*. Philadelphia: Saunders, 1955.

Wessells, N. K. How living cells change shape. *Scientific American*, 1971, **225**, 77–82.

Wiesel, T. N., & Hubel, D. H. Single-cell responses in striate cortex of kittens deprived of vision in one eye. *Journal of Neurophysiology*, 1963, **26**, 1003–1017.

Wolf, M. Anatomy of cultured mouse cerebellum. II. Organotypic migration of granule cells demonstrated by silver impregnation of normal and mutant cultures. *Journal of Comparative Neurology*, 1970, **140**, 281–298.

Woodard, T. M., Jr., & Estes, S. B. Effect of colchicine on mitosis in the neural tube of the forty-eight hour chick embryo. *Anatomical Record*, 1944, **90**, 51–54.

Wren, J. T., & Wessells, N. K. An ultrastructural study of lens invagination in the mouse. *Journal of Experimental Zoology*, 1969, **171**, 359–368.

Wren, J. T., & Wessells, N. K. Cytochalasin. B: Effects upon microfilaments involved in morphogenesis of estrogen-induced glands of oviduct. *Proceedings of the National Academy of Sciences, U.S.*, 1970, **66**, 904–908.

Yamada, K. M., Spooner, B. S., & Wessells, N. K. Axon growth: roles of microfilaments and microtubules. *Proceedings of the National Academy of Sciences, U.S.*, 1970, **66**, 1206–1212.

Zwaan, J., Bryan, P. R., & Pearce, T. L. Intermitotic nuclear migration during the early stages of lens formation in the chicken embryo. *Journal of Embryology and Experimental Morphology*, 1969, **21**, 71–83.

TISSUE CULTURE MODELS OF DEVELOPING BRAIN FUNCTIONS

*STANLEY M. CRAIN**

Department of Physiology
Albert Einstein College of Medicine
Bronx, New York

I. Introduction

Cultures of immature central nervous tissues provide a powerful model system for studies of developing brain functions. Arrays of CNS neurons growing in a culture chamber on a thin coverglass offer a remarkable

*Kennedy Scholar at the Rose F. Kennedy Center for Research in Mental Retardation and Human Development.

"window" to facilitate not only direct observation but also flexible experimental manipulation of the intricate cellular networks of the *mammalian* brain. The feasibility of this model system is based upon demonstrations, during the past decade, that small groups of embryonic mammalian CNS neurons possess intrinsic "self-organizing" properties even after isolation in culture (Crain, 1970c). Microelectrode recordings in explants of fetal mammalian CNS tissues have shown that these neurons can still develop *in vitro* the capacity to generate complex patterned bioelectric discharges resembling the activity of synaptic networks of the central nervous system (Crain, 1966). The relevance of these tissue culture models to studies of mechanisms underlying early development of the central nervous system and behavior has been noted in recent reviews (Gottlieb, 1971, see also Introduction to Section I, this Volume; Hamburger, 1968; Jacobson, 1970; Skoglund, 1969). The present report summarizes the major evidence in support of this model system and points out many of the limitations and pitfalls involved in extrapolating data obtained from these tiny neuronally isolated bits of CNS tissues in culture back to problems of CNS development in the intact organism.

II. Synaptogenesis in Embryonic CNS Cultures

Demonstration that synaptogenesis and development of functional synaptic networks can occur in isolated CNS explants sharply reduces the number of factors which must be considered in analyzing the mechanisms underlying these complex phenomena. Systematic experiments have, therefore, been carried out to clarify the degree to which groups of immature CNS neurons, explanted prior to formation of synaptic junctions *in situ*, could proceed to develop such interrelationships in culture. It was, furthermore, of great interest to determine whether such *de novo* synapses could function *in vitro*, and also whether organotypic patterns could be detected in the structure or function of any groups of these synapses which might form within the explanted tissue. Experiments along these lines were, indeed, successful, utilizing fetal mammalian CNS explants, and the basic techniques will be briefly outlined before proceeding to applications of this model system to various problems in neural and behavioral development.

A. *Within Individual Explants*

1. Methods

The culture technique which has produced the most highly differentiated CNS tissues *in vitro* involves explantation of 1 mm^3 fragments (Fig. 1), at embryonic stages, onto collagen-coated coverglasses, and incubation at

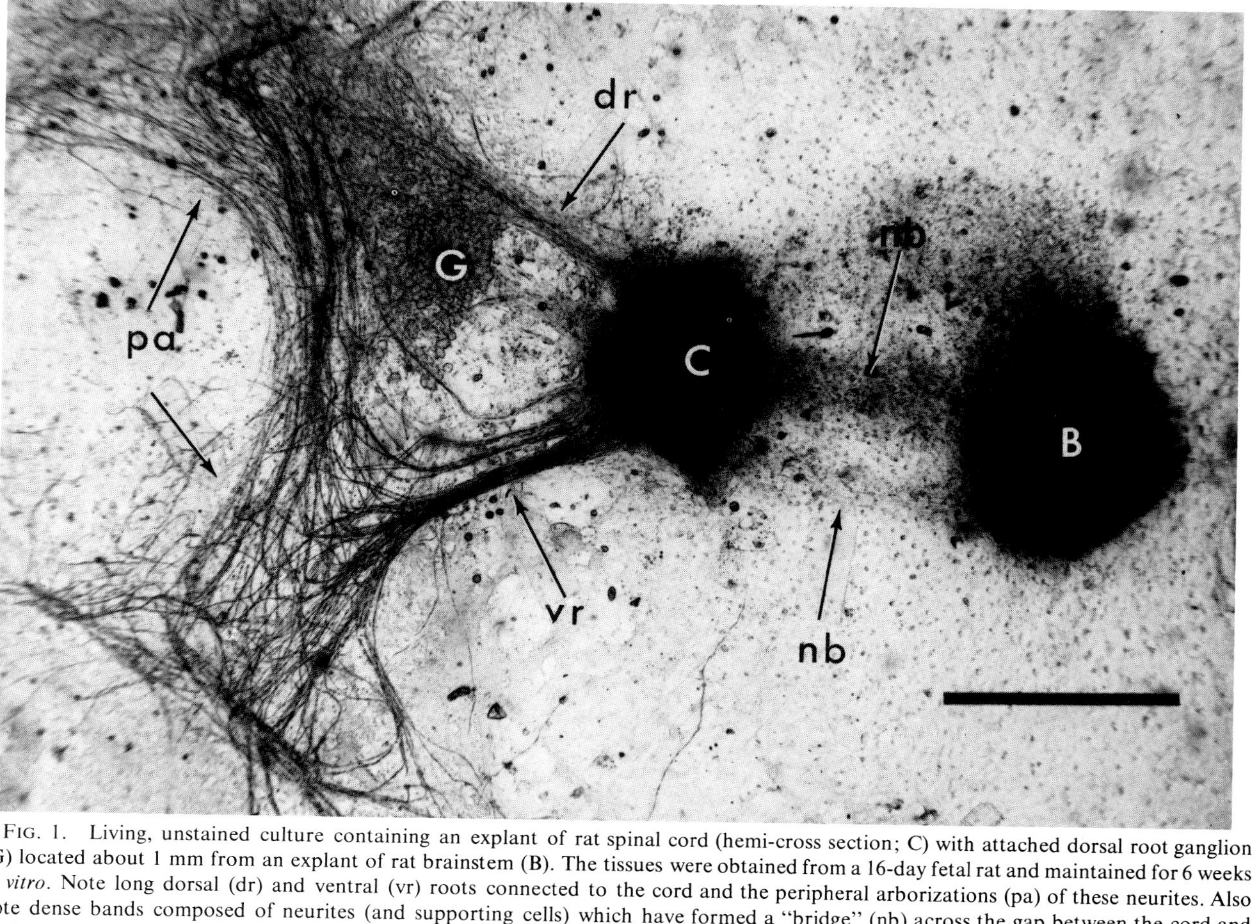

FIG. 1. Living, unstained culture containing an explant of rat spinal cord (hemi-cross section; C) with attached dorsal root ganglion (G) located about 1 mm from an explant of rat brainstem (B). The tissues were obtained from a 16-day fetal rat and maintained for 6 weeks *in vitro*. Note long dorsal (dr) and ventral (vr) roots connected to the cord and the peripheral arborizations (pa) of these neurites. Also note dense bands composed of neurites (and supporting cells) which have formed a "bridge" (nb) across the gap between the cord and brainstem explants. (Neurites in "bridge" could be clearly seen at higher magnification.) Scale: 1 mm. (from Crain *et al.*, 1968b).

35°C in Maximow depression-slide chambers, as "lying-drop" preparations (Murray, 1965; Peterson, Crain, & Murray, 1965). The explants are generally cut so that one dimension is well under 1 mm, to facilitate diffusion of metabolites to and from the cells within the central region of the tissue. The culture medium is changed twice a week, and generally contains human placental serum in a balanced salt solution, with chick embryo extract or other special nutrients. The total volume of medium is about .1 ml and the overlying airspace about 2 ml. Coordinated electrophysiologic and electron microscopic studies have been carried out on explants of spinal cord from 14- to 15-day fetal rats, a stage shortly before the first ultrastructural evidence of synapse formation has been detected (M. B. Bunge, Bunge, & Peterson, 1967; Crain & Peterson, 1967). Cultures selected after serial microscopic examinations during days or weeks of incubation in Maximow slides are transferred to a micrurgical chamber for bioelectric study. Openings in the chamber walls permit micromanipulation of microelectrodes, under direct visual control at high magnification, for focal recording and stimulation within an explant (Crain, 1970a). Extracellular microelectrode recordings are made with chloridized silver electrodes via saline-filled pipettes with tip diameters of 1–5 μ, and electric stimuli (.1 to .5-msec duration) are applied through pairs of similar pipettes with 10-μ tips. In some cases, chloridized silver-core pipettes with 25-μ tips are used as recording electrodes. Recently developed miniaturized, magnetically coupled micromanipulators (Baer & Crain, 1971; Crain, 1973) now permit incorporation of an entire array of microelectrodes and micromanipulators within a *sealed* micrurgical chamber, using magnetic controls *external* to the chamber for positioning each electrode into the tissue (Fig. 2; see also Fig. 11). This sealed chamber array permits far more rigorous control of the physicochemical environment of the culture during electrophysiologic studies, and sterilized assemblies are now being developed for longitudinal bioelectric recordings over days or weeks, instead of the usual limit of less than 1 day (Crain, 1970b, 1973).

2. Spinal Cord

During the first 2 to 3 days after explantation of rat spinal cord at "presynaptic" stages, only simple spike potentials can be elicited by either single or tetanic electric stimuli applied to these immature cord explants. The spikes (Fig. 3) are similar to those observed in neurons of cultured dorsal root ganglia (Crain, 1956, 1965), where impulses can propagate along the conductile portions of the neurons, but no bioelectric evidence of transmission from one neuron to another has been detected.

By 3 to 4 days *in vitro*, on the other hand, facilitation effects can be demonstrated in the cord explants with paired stimuli at long test intervals (Fig. $3C_{1,2}$), and long-lasting spike barrages and "slow waves" may be evoked with

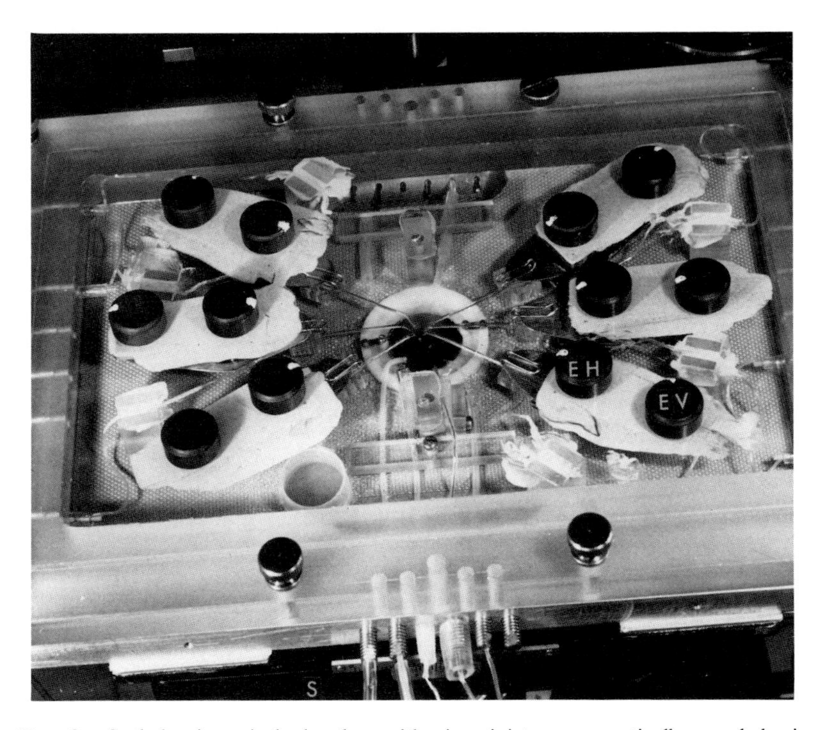

FIG. 2. Sealed micrurgical chamber with six miniature magnetically coupled micromanipulators suspended from greased glass roof. Note pairs of external manually operated control magnets (EH and EV), resting on glass roof, which are used to position micropipette electrodes (bent at right angle near tip) into central glass-bottomed culture dish. Entire array is mounted on mechanical stage (S) of inverted microscope (stage is positioned in three dimensions by standard rack and pinion controls). Microscope condenser lens and illuminator are normally located above central region of chamber (removed for clarity), and microscope objective lens is located below culture dish. Flexible insulated silver wires connect electrodes with sockets sealed into chamber wall. External couplings can then be readily made from these sockets to electronic recording and stimulating apparatus. Teflon tubes for perfusion of the culture dish, leads for bath electrodes, temperature probes, etc., are all sealed into the floor of the chamber (entering through gasketed holes in front edge of metal baseplate), and they are mounted so as to contact the fluid in the peripheral region of the culture dish (from Crain, 1972c; see also Baer & Crain, 1971).

brief tetanic stimulation at critical thresholds (Fig. $3C_{3-5}$). The appearance of these complex bioelectric activities indicates that polysynaptic networks are beginning to function in the cultured cord tissue. The responses in 4-day and older cultures can often be enhanced with strychnine (Fig. $3C_{2-5}$), whereas no significant effects are produced by the application of this drug during the first 2 to 3 days *in vitro*. Furthermore, all of the complex bioelectric discharges can be rapidly blocked by raising the Mg^{2+} concentration of the

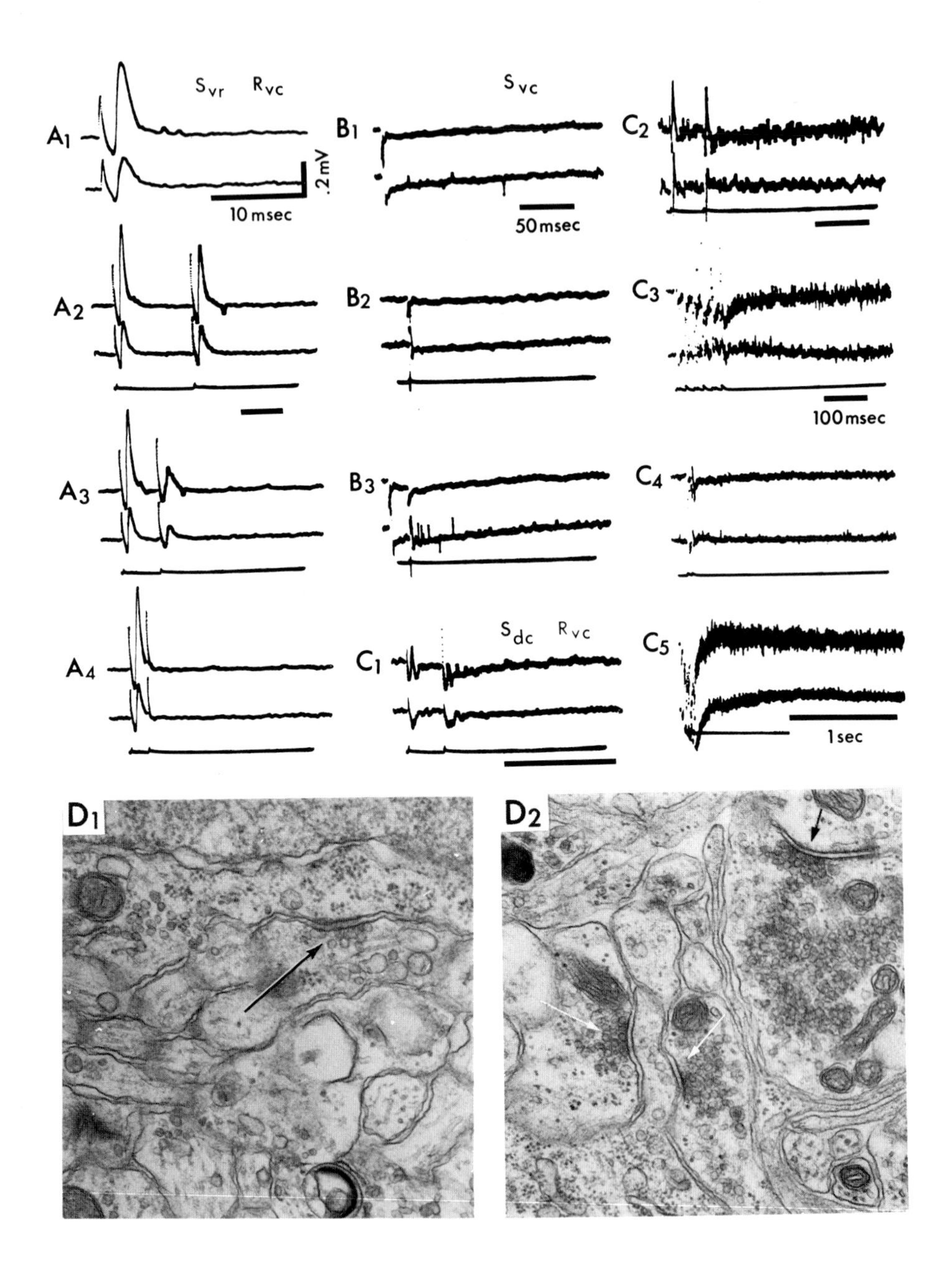
A1
A2
A3
A4
B1
B2
B3
C1
C2
C3
C4
C5
D1
D2
Svr
Rvc
Svc
Sdc
Rvc
.2 mV
10 msec
50 msec
100 msec
1 sec

medium from 1 to 5m*M* (Crain, Bornstein, & Peterson, 1968a), although short-latency spike potentials can still be evoked (see also Section III, Part B and Fig. 8C). Although intracellularly recorded postsynaptic potentials have not yet been obtained from these cultured CNS explants (see the first addendum, p. 114) electrophysiologic analyses of extracellular data provide excellent, although less elegant, evidence of activities mediated through synaptic pathways (Crain & Peterson, 1963, 1964). Recent intracellular recordings of excitatory and inhibitory postsynaptic potentials (EPSPs and IPSPs) in cultures of dissociated chick and mouse spinal cord neurons (Dichter & Fischbach, 1971; Fischbach, 1970; Peacock, Nelson & Goldstone, 1973) add further support to this interpretation (see also Section III B). The marked sensitivity of the cord explant to strychnine at 4 days *in vitro* suggests, moreover, that inhibitory circuits may already be functioning quite early during CNS synaptogenesis (see Section V). During the next few days of culture beyond the critical 4-day period, the afterdischarges increase in amplitude and complexity, and they can be elicited at lower thresholds with fewer stimuli (Table I). Still more elaborate repetitive dis-

---

FIG. 3. Transition from simple to complex bioelectric responses in spinal cord tissue cultured for 2–4 days after explantation from 14-day fetal rat. (A and B) 2 days *in vitro*. (A_1) Simultaneous recordings of simple spike potentials evoked in two sites of ventral cord (300 μ apart) by stimulus applied to ventral root (400 μ from edge of explant). Application of paired stimuli demonstrates relative ($A_{2,3}$) and absolute (A_4) refractoriness to test stimulus. (Responses to dorsal cord, or root, stimulus were much smaller in amplitude, both in dorsal and ventral cord.) ($B_{1,2}$) Similar simple spike potentials evoked in another region of ventral cord by stimulus applied nearby, within cord explant. (B_3) Paired stimuli, at 15-msec test interval, elicit multiple spike burst, of small amplitude, lasting more than 35 msec (barely detectable in most explants at 2 days *in vitro*, even with tetanic stimuli and strychnine). (C) 4 days *in vitro*. (C_1) Longer lasting afterdischarge (small amplitude) in ventral cord evoked by paired stimuli to dorsal cord. (C_2) Strychnine (10 μg/ml) now enhances barrage response even at test intervals of 30 msec. (C_{3-5}) Brief tetanic stimulation (20 per second) produces further increase in duration and amplitude of afterdischarges. Note: In this and all subsequent figures, time and amplitude calibrations, and specification of recording and stimulating sites, *apply to all succeeding records, until otherwise noted.* Upward deflection indicates negativity at active recording electrode, and onset of stimuli is indicated, where necessary, by sharp pulse (or arrow) or break in baseline of third sweep. (D_1) Electron micrograph of cultured spinal cord tissue about 70 hours after explantation as a "synapse-free" slice from $14\frac{1}{2}$-day fetal rat. Note typical newly formed synapse (at arrow), with moderate synaptic membrane density and intervening cleft substance. A few synaptic vesicles are clustered on the presynaptic side of this axosomatic junction (near arrowhead) (× 32,500). (D_2) Similarly prepared electron micrograph of fetal rat cord explant after 10 weeks *in vitro*. Synaptic membrane density and cleft substance are more pronounced at the two axosomatic synapses (white arrows) and the axodendritic one (black arrow). Many more synaptic vesicles have accumulated at the presynaptic side of all three junctions (× 28, 500) (A to C: from Crain & Peterson, 1967; D: from M. B. Bunge *et al.*, 1967).

TABLE I
DEVELOPMENT OF ORGANIZED BIOELECTRIC ACTIVITIES IN CULTURES OF SPINAL CORD WITH ATTACHED DORSAL ROOT GANGLIA (DRG)

Cord activity	Days after explantation of 14- to 15-day fetal rat spinal cord					
	0–2	3	4	6	12	21
Only simple spike responses with cord or DRG stimuli	+					
Weak barrages of spikes with tetanic cord stimuli	0	+[a]				
Weak barrages with single cord stimuli; facilitation with paired stimuli; marked enhancement with strychnine	0	0	+			
Long lasting afterdischarges (spikes and slow waves) with tetanic DRG stimuli	0	0	0	+[b]		
Complex afterdischarges with paired DRG stimuli or tetanic VR stimuli[c]	0	0	0	0	+	
Complex afterdischarges with single DRG or VR stimuli	0	0	0	0	0	+

[a]Earliest stage at which synapses are regularly seen in electron micrographs; this degree of function reached within 1 day after explantation of 18-day fetal rat cord.
[b]This stage reached within 3 days after explantation of 18-day fetal rat cord.
[c]VR, ventral root (from Crain & Peterson, 1967).

charges often occur in older explants, e.g., long-lasting rhythmic (7–15 per second) oscillatory afterdischarges (Fig. 4). The bioelectric responses evoked in 4-day cultures of 14-day fetal rat spinal cord tissue already include, however, the *basic* organotypic properties characteristic of mature explants of cord and other CNS tissues (Crain, 1966).

The onset of complex bioelectric activity in 14- to 15-day fetal rat spinal cord explants at about 3 days *in vitro* correlates closely with the earliest time at which clear-cut synaptic profiles, mainly axodendritic, are regularly seen in electron micrographs (M. B. Bunge *et al.*, 1967) of these cultured tissues (Fig. $3D_1$). The marked increase in quantity of synapses as the explants mature in culture and the concomitant developments in synaptic membrane density, cleft substances, and presynaptic vesicle accumulation (Fig. $3D_2$) provide important morphologic parameters which may underlie the sequential developments in bioelectric activities seen during the first few weeks *in vitro.* Functional connections also develop between dorsal root ganglion cells and cord neurons in these cultures during the second week *in vitro* (Table I).

3. Cerebral Cortex

Explants of late fetal or newborn mouse cerebral cortex appear to undergo a similar sequence of developmental changes in bioelectric properties as occurs in rat spinal cord cultures during the first week after explantation

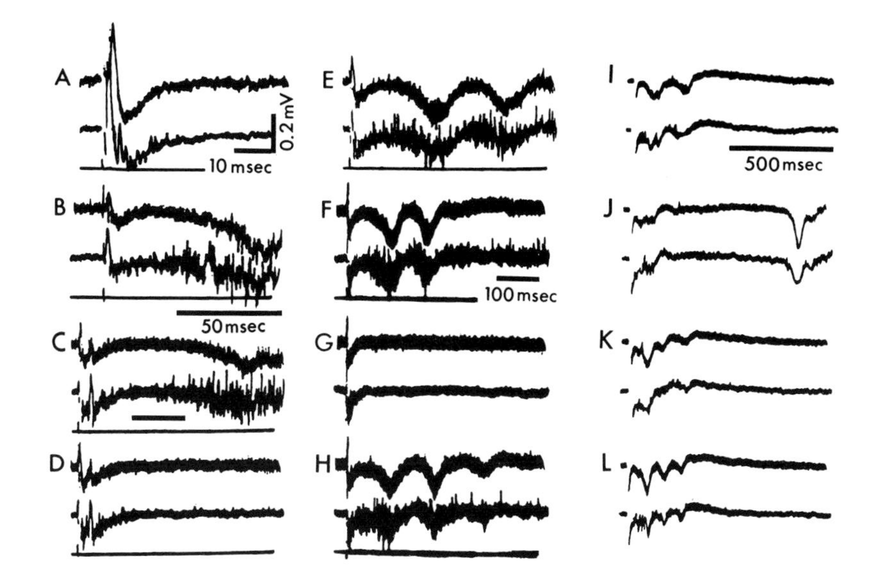

FIG. 4. Oscillatory afterdischarges evoked by single brief, electric stimuli in long-term culture of rat spinal cord (3 months *in vitro*). (A–C) Simultaneous recordings of typical repetitive, spike barrage responses evoked in two regions of the explant, 400 μ apart, by stimulus applied 500 μ from both recording sites. (D) Short-duration response when stimulus was applied 1 second after spike barrage in (C). (E, F, H) Longlasting oscillatory sequences (up to 400 msec) evoked shortly after records (A–D). Note regularity of pattern of these 7–15 per second, diphasic potentials, and synchronization of the responses between the two recording sites. (G): Control record (subthreshold stimulus).) (I–L) Similar oscillatory afterdischarges at slower sweep rate. Note second sequence in J, appearing after silent period of 500 msec (from Crain & Peterson, 1964).

(Crain, 1964; Crain & Bornstein, 1964; morphological correlates in Bornstein, 1964). For the first 2 or 3 days *in vitro*, only simple spike responses (Fig. 5A) can be evoked with electric stimuli (as in cord cultures, Fig. 3A). By 4 days in culture, however, evoked potentials with durations of the order of 400 msec (Fig. 5B) may occur, with latencies of as much as 100 msec following the early spike response to a single electric stimulus. Repetitive spike barrages often appear concomitant with these long-duration potentials. The latter increase in amplitude and regularity during the following week in culture, and their duration generally decreases below 100 msec (Fig. 5C). They can generally be greatly enhanced with picrotoxin, strychnine and caffeine, and they probably represent extracellular recordings of summated postsynaptic potentials (Crain, 1966, 1973b). They resemble responses evoked by local electric stimuli in neonatal rat cerebral cortex *in situ*

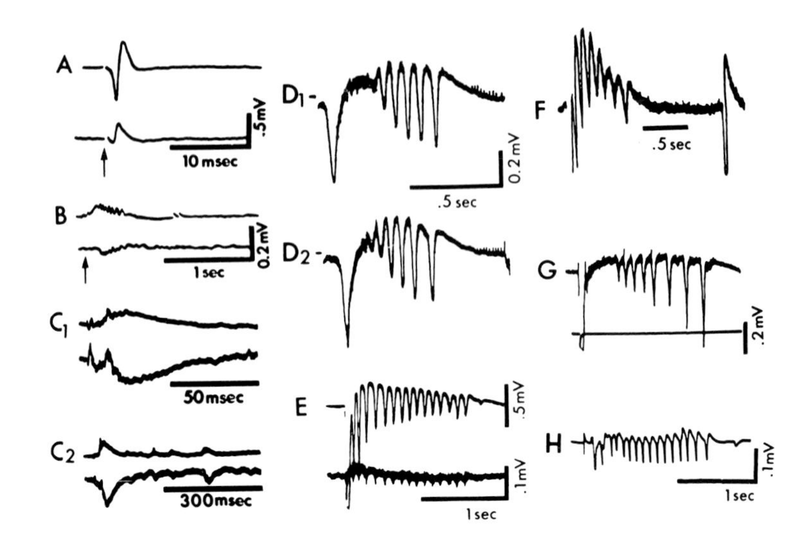

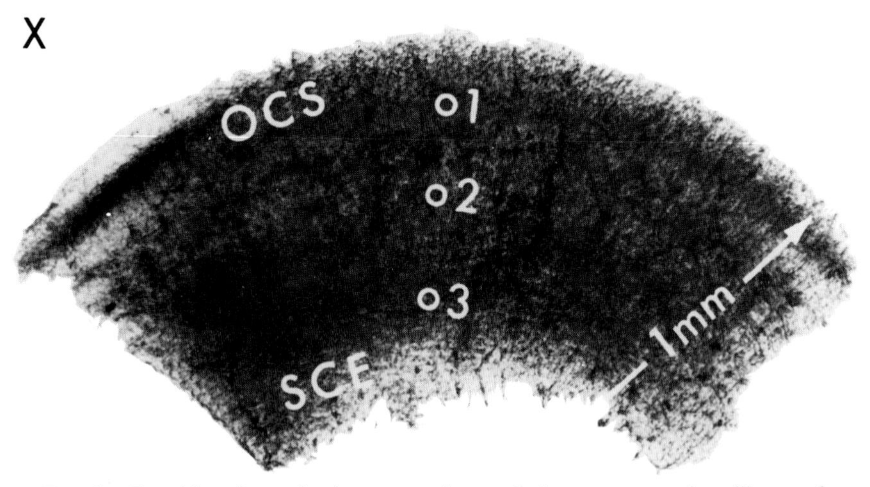

FIG. 5. Transition from simple to complex evoked responses and oscillatory after-discharges in cultured cerebral cortex tissue, during first 2 weeks after explantation from 1-day-old mouse. (A) three days *in vitro*. Simultaneous records showing simple spikes evoked, at "cortical depths" (see X) of 200 μ (upper sweep) and 400 μ, by stimulus applied near subcortical edge of explant (about 800 μ from original cortical surface). (B) Early signs of complex response patterns recorded, at much slower sweep rate, in same culture and at same electrode loci as in A. Long-duration negativity arises gradually with a latency of about 100 msec after the early superficial spike (upper sweep); also note long-duration positivity which develops with a still longer latency after early deep spike (lower sweep). Arrow indicates onset of dual stimuli spaced 50 msec apart. Note that the second pair of stimuli, applied 1 second after first pair, is ineffective. (C_1) Ten days *in vitro*.

(Armstrong-James & Williams, 1963) and, under similar conditions, in the neonatal cat (Purpura, Carmichael, & Housepian, 1960).

The onset of complex bioelectric activity in these mouse cerebral explants after 4 days *in vitro* is consonant with the paucity of synaptic junctions detectable in electron micrographs of the tissues at explantation and their abundance in 10-day cultures (Model, Bornstein, Crain, & Pappas, 1971), but close correlations of ultrastructure and function have not yet been carried out during the critical 3- to 5-day period.

B. Between Separate Explants

Functional synaptic networks can, therefore, develop *in vitro* even after explantation of immature "presynaptic" CNS tissues. However, since the general topography of the neurons and glial cells within these tissues are not radically disturbed by the explantation procedure, the patterns of cellular interrelationships may already be sufficiently developed so that synaptogenesis after explantation is automatically determined. If, on the other hand, the neurons were *completely* separated at explantation, could functional synaptic relations still develop in culture? This problem was first approached experimentally by explanting pairs or groups of fetal rodent spinal cord

---

(FIG. 5 *continued*)
Simultaneous records of characteristic evoked potentials at "cortical depths" of 250 μ (upper sweep) and 650 μ following single stimulus applied at depth of 700 μ (but 300 μ from deep recording site). Note 60-msec negative evoked response in superficial region and positive response in deep zone which is similar, but of longer duration and greater latency. (C_2) Same as C_1, but at slower sweep rate. Note that small-amplitude repetitive potentials at 10–20 per second follow primary responses at both sites and are also of opposite polarities. (D–G) From 2 to 6 weeks *in vitro*. Repetitive oscillatory afterdischarges evoked in four mouse cerebral explants by single stimulus applied several hundred micra from recording site. Lower record in E shows simultaneous recording from another region of explant (800 μ away). Note variation in latency of onset of repetitive discharge following initial, positive evoked potential ($D_{1,2}$). (H) Characteristic repetitive afterdischarge evoked in cerebral cortical slab in 5-day-old kitten, 3 days after neuronal isolation, *in situ*. Note similarity between this response pattern and those obtained from cerebral explants. (X) Photomicrograph of freshly prepared explant of neonatal mouse cerebral cortex (about 0.5 mm thick). OCS, original cortical surface; SCE, subcortical edge. The tissue has assumed the characteristic crescent shape which it generally maintains for months *in vitro* (Bornstein, 1964). Focal recording electrodes were often positioned, in contact with the tissue, at 1 and 2, and a cathodal stimulating lead placed at 3. Indifferent electrodes were located near each active electrode, in fluid, just below the tissue. Distance of locus from OCS is referred to as "cortical depth" (see text). A–G and X from Crain, 1964; H from Purpura & Housepian, 1961.

ganglia, brainstem, and cerebral fragments onto collagen-coated coverglasses (Fig. 1), separated by gaps up to 1.5 mm (Crain, Peterson, & Bornstein, 1968b; see also Section III, B).

Functional connections could be demonstrated, for example, between fetal rat spinal cord and brainstem explants (Fig. 1) following formation of neuritic bridges across gaps of 1 mm during the first week *in vitro*. Simultaneous microelectrode recordings from the paired spinal cord–brainstem explants show that spontaneous discharges arising in one explant may be *regularly* followed, after a latency ranging from several milliseconds to several hundred milliseconds, by long-lasting discharges in the other explant. Selective stimulation of the dorsal root ganglion (DRG) attached to the cord explant (Fig. 1) permits clear-cut (synaptic) excitation of cord neurons without direct application of a stimulating electrode to the vicinity of the cord explant. (This procedure precludes fortuitous antidromic excitation of brainstem neurites which have bridged the gap and may then have arborized within the cord explant.) A DRG-evoked cord discharge may then be followed by a longer-lasting (> 1 second) discharge in the brainstem explant. The latency between the onset of activity in the two explants may vary widely, as occurs during spontaneous discharges, and is probably due to gradual activation of brainstem neurons through polysynaptic pathways from cord neurons, or vice versa when the brainstem explant triggers the cord. Functional connections also develop between spinal cord and cerebral explants as well as between medulla and cerebrum in culture. Bioelectric interactions between the latter tissues may be particularly complex, suggesting that patterned, rhythmic *inhibitory* as well as excitatory discharges may occur spontaneously as well as in response to local stimuli (see Section IV, and Fig. 11). The essential role of neuritic pathways in mediating the interactions between these separated CNS explants is demonstrated by the complete abolition of transmission from one explant to another after microsurgical transection of the neuritic bridge across the gap. Systematic controls have also been made in a number of cultures to eliminate the possible role of nonneural spread of current (Crain *et al.*, 1968b).

Another type of synaptogenesis which has recently been studied by these culture techniques involves the formation of neuromuscular junctions between separate explants of spinal cord and skeletal muscle. Functional motor endplates develop between fetal rodent cord neurons and adult, as well as fetal, muscle fibers (see Section IV and Fig. 10)—even with adult *human* muscle (Crain, 1970a; Crain, Alfei, & Peterson, 1970). Correlative cytologic studies during development of these neuromuscular relationships provide valuable clues to mechanisms underlying *trophic* as well as bioelectric interactions (Crain & Peterson, 1973; Pappas, Peterson, Masurovsky, & Crain, 1971; Peterson & Crain, 1970, 1972).

III. Development of Complex Organotypic Bioelectric Activities in Long-Term CNS Cultures

A. Slab Explants

1. Spinal Cord

After 2 to 4 weeks *in vitro*, a more synchronized long-lasting, diphasic, oscillatory (7–15 per second afterdischarge can be evoked in many of the rat cord explants by a single brief electric stimulus (Fig. 4, E-L *vs*. A-C). This complex response pattern is rarely detected in younger cord cultures, although it is seen in explants of neonatal cerebral cortex as early as 4 days *in vitro* (Fig. 5B). The afterdischarges appear in "all-or-none" fashion at a critical stimulus intensity (cf. Fig. 4C and D; Fig. 4F and G). They may also be evoked following facilitation of paired subthreshold stimuli at long test intervals. The oscillatory afterdischarge patterns are often relatively stereotyped, but variations in response to single stimuli of constant strength may occur (Fig. 4I–L). At times, a second oscillatory sequence of similar duration to the first appears after a silent period of .5–1 second (Fig. 4J). The repetitive discharges may continue uninterrupted for many seconds after the stimulus. They often occur synchronously over widespread regions of the explant, even after a weak stimulus localized to a few neurites close to a 10-μ stimulating electrode. Similar 5–10 per second oscillatory sequences have been evoked by single stimuli in cultures of *human* spinal cord tissues, explanted from a 6-week embryo and maintained for several months *in vitro* (Crain, 1966; Peterson *et al*., 1965).

These complex, yet stereotyped, repetitive discharges in cord explants represent organotypic functional activity of synaptic networks *in vitro* (see Section III, A,2). Nevertheless, alterations due to isolation of these small fragments from a highly integrated nervous system must always be kept in mind. Various structural and functional modifications certainly occur as the explant reorganizes *in vitro*, some of which may mimic pathological rather than normal embryological patterns *in situ* (see Section III, C). For example, the long-lasting asynchronous spike barrage responses described above (Section II, A) resemble spinal cord afterdischarges recorded *in situ* after decerebration or spinal transection (Burns, 1956, 1958; Stavraky, 1961). They also simulate the phenomena that occur during chromatolysis of cord motoneurons following ventral root section, involving an "enormous development of polysynaptic reflexes" (Downman, Eccles, & McIntyre, 1953; Eccles, 1953). This trend may be partly due to the formation *in vitro* of large numbers of collaterals on the axons of neurons which arborize and synapse profusely throughout the cord explant, especially in the neuropil layer (about 100 μ) which forms over the entire cut surface of the cord cross section (Peterson *et al*., 1965). Electron micrographs of older cord cultures reveal abundant synaptic junctions in this *de novo* neuropil (R. P. Bunge, Bunge, & Peterson, 1965). Such extensive axon-collateral sprouting during regeneration of efferent neurons after surgical isolation of CNS tissues is a characteristic phenomenon *in situ* (Hoffman, 1955; McCouch, Austin, & Liu, 1958; Purpura & Housepian, 1961; Ramón y Cajal, 1928; Weiss & Edds, 1946). Furthermore, in older cord-ganglion explants (2 weeks *in vitro*) tetanic *ventral* as well as dorsal root stimuli can trigger widespread afterdischarges in both dorsal as well as ventral cord (Table I). By 3 weeks *in vitro*, cord afterdischarges can be evoked by *single* stimuli to *either* DRG or ventral roots. Gradual disappearance of the asymmetry, seen during the first 2 weeks *in vitro*, between dorsal and ventral root modes of cord activation may be due to: (1) abundant collateral sprouting from axons of motor neurons which gradually arborize and synapse throughout the explant, especially in the *de novo* neuropil layer (see above); (2) growth of neurites from internuncial cord neurons out into the "ventral root" in these older cord culture (see also Guillery, Sobkowicz, & Scott, 1968).

2. Cerebral Cortex

The long-lasting evoked potentials in cerebral explants often show characteristic negative polarity when recorded with a microelectrode located near the original pial surface of the cortex (Figs. 5B, C; Fig. 12A; Fig. 13B–D, upper sweeps; see also Fig. 5X), and a sharp phase-reversal may occur at a critical "depth" of 200 μ to 400 μ (Crain & Bornstein, 1964). These data indicate development and maintenance in culture of at least some laminar organization of neural elements parallel to the original cortical surface. Analysis of extracellular recordings from multiple sites in the cerebral explants suggest that the superficial-negative and deep-positive slow waves represent summated postsynaptic potentials that are predominantly excitatory (depolarizing) and inhibitory (hyperpolarizing), respectively (Crain, 1964; Crain & Bornstein, 1964). This interpretation draws upon analyses of mechanisms that appear to underlie cortical evoked responses *in situ* (Eccles, 1964; Purpura, 1959). It is also in agreement with more recent intracellular recordings by Purpura, Shofer, and Scarff (1965) in neonatal cat cerebral cortex *in situ*, which demonstrate inhibitory postsynaptic potentials of "extraordinary duration," that is, 200–600 msec (see Fig. 5B, lower sweep; Crain, 1969, 1972c); (see also Purpura, 1969, 1972).

The other major type of complex bioelectric activity that appears during maturation of newborn mouse cerebral tissue *in vitro* consists of oscillatory afterdischarges similar to those described above in long-term spinal cord cultures. These afterdischarges are often well-developed by 1 to 2 weeks in culture (Fig. 5D–G) and occur more regularly than in cord explants. The cerebral repetitive afterdischarge generally consists of three to six large diphasic potentials each lasting 25–50 msec and occurring at a rate of 5–15 per second. As in the cord cultures (Fig. 4), simultaneous recordings from regions of cerebral explants located 100–400 μ apart indicate that the repetitive discharge may involve activity synchronized over large areas of the explant (Figs. $12A_5$; Fig. 13C,D). A large, early evoked potential is often followed by a long delay, prior to the appearance of a repetitive sequence of potentials of gradually increasing amplitude (Fig. 5D, G; cf. E). The response patterns are remarkably similar to those found, by Purpura and Housepian (1961), to be characteristic of slabs of neonatal cat cerebral cortex *in situ* several days after neuronal isolation (Fig. 5H). Similar oscillatory afterdischarges, with lower amplitudes, have been detected in the cerebral explants as early as 4 days *in vitro*, superimposed on prolonged (ca. 400 msec) primary evoked potentials (Fig. 5B). Although these complex repetitive discharges in cerebral slabs *in situ* and *in vitro* show marked hyperexcitability properties (Crain, 1969; Purpura, 1969), the most significant point is the mimicry displayed by the cultured tissues of intricate bioelectric patterns characteristic of organized cerebral cortex *in situ*. Analyses of similar rhythmic bioelectric activities in various regions of the CNS, *in situ*, suggest that they may be produced by complex circuits involving sequential generation of inhibitory as well as excitatory postsynaptic potentials (Andersen & Andersson, 1968; Andersen & Eccles, 1962).

B. Reaggregates of Dissociated CNS Cells

A most dramatic demonstration of intrinsic self-organizing properties of CNS neurons has recently been made utilizing small clusters of neurons after reaggregation *in vitro* of completely dissociated cells obtained from 18-day fetal mouse cerebral neocortex or 13- to 14-day spinal cord and brainstem ("presynaptic" stages: see above). After enzymatic treatment in .25% trypsin (in a Ca^{2+}- and Mg^{2+}-free physiological salt solution) and repeated pipetting, suspensions of cells in concentrations of about 10^6 cells per ml of normal culture medium were explanted onto collagen films, using .05–.1 ml per coverglass (22 mm diameter). Microscopic observation immediately following explantation confirmed that the cells had been completely dissociated prior to culture. In some cases, the cell suspension was added to coverslips on which an intact fragment of fetal spinal cord (*ca.* 1 mm^3) had been explanted 1 week earlier (Fig. 6A). Cytologic studies indicate development of characteristic neurons and glial cells (Bornstein and Model 1971), both within the clusters as well as in the neuropil and neuritic bridges connecting many of the discrete clusters (Fig. 6B). The development of abundant axodendritic and axosomatic synapses has been demonstrated by electron microscopy of these reaggregated neuronal networks, in extension of the ultrastructural studies of synaptogenesis and maturation in

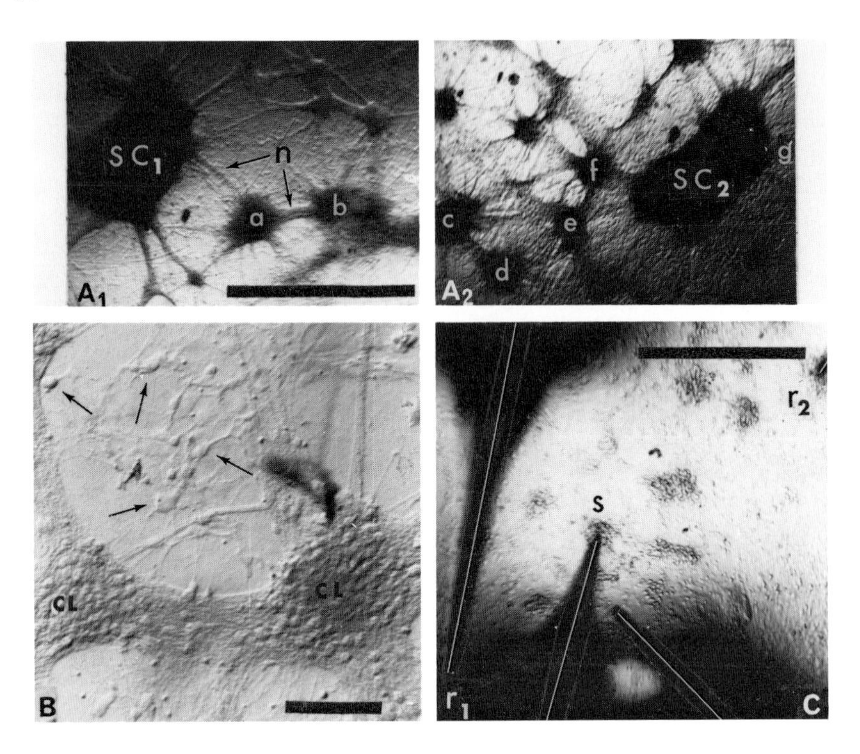

FIG. 6. Photomicrographs of cultured reaggregates of fetal mouse spinal cord, brainstem, and cerebral cortex tissues, 2 weeks after complete cellular dissociation at explantation. ($A_{1,2}$): Low power montage of a culture showing clusters of reaggregated spinal cord and brainstem cells (a–g) which developed between (and in vicinity of) two undissociated fetal mouse spinal cord cross sections (SC_1 and SC_2) explanted 1 week earlier. (Discontinuities at junction between photomicrographs A_1 and A_2 are due merely to different angles of oblique illumination used to enhance salient features of the unstained array.) Fine bundles of arborizing neurites (n) connect these clusters to one another and to the large cord explants. Microelectrode recordings from this culture showed that clusters a–g and explants $SC_{1,2}$ were all functionally connected in a complex synaptic network (Fig. 7). Scale: 1 mm. (B) Higher power view of a small region of this network including two reaggregated clusters (CL). Many neuron cell bodies can be seen both within the clusters as well as in a looser monolayer array (e.g., at arrows). Scale 100 μ (C) Photomicrograph of cultured reaggregates of fetal mouse cerebral cortex (2 weeks *in vitro*) obtained during electrophysiologic recordings (Fig. 8). In this case, the dispersed brain cells had reaggregated on a completely cell-free collagen-coated coverglass. Electric stimuli were applied via pair of stimulating electrodes, with cathode in cluster (s), and complex discharges were recorded with microelectrodes in clusters r_1 and r_2. (White line was applied over central axis of each micropipette shaft for clarity; cluster r_1 is not visible at this low magnification due to optical distortion produced by micropipettes dipping into overlying culture medium.) Scale: 1 mm. (from Crain & Bornstein, 1972 and unpublished observations).

undissociated fetal cerebral explants described above (Bornstein & Model, 1972; Model *et al.*, 1971).

After 2–4 weeks *in vitro*, complex repetitive spike discharges have been recorded, spontaneously as well as in response to electric stimuli, from dozens of discrete neuronal clusters which had become attached to the collagen-coated coverglass over an area of about 1 cm^2 (Figs. 6A; Fig. 7), and which appeared to be connected to one another by complex neuritic bridges (Crain & Bornstein, 1971, 1972). In the larger clusters containing dozens of neurons, characteristic long-lasting potentials were often observed in association with the spike barrages. The complex bioelectric potentials recorded in each cluster were clearly generated *within* the cell cluster, and they were not merely indications of impulses propagating along neurites passing through the cluster (as, for example, might occur between the two large cord explants in Fig. 6A,$SC_{1,2}$). Similar bioelectric discharges were also

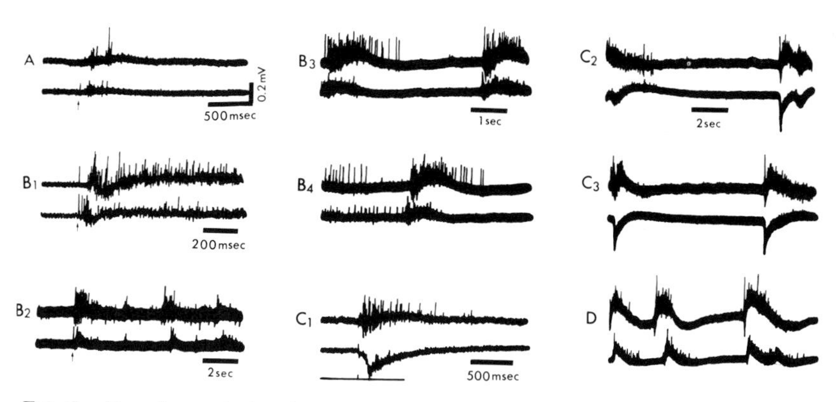

FIG. 7. Complex evoked and spontaneous bioelectric discharges in cultured reaggregates of fetal mouse brainstem and spinal cord tissues, 2 weeks after random dispersion at explantation. (A) Simultaneous microelectrode recordings of repetitive spike barrages and longlasting negative slow wave responses in two clusters of reaggregated neurons (Fig. 6A: a and g), located 3 mm apart, elicited by single stimulus applied to intervening large cord explant Fig. 6A: SG_2). (B) After introduction of strychnine (10 μg/ml), evoked discharges become greatly enchanced in amplitude, duration, and complexity (B_{12}), and similar repetitive spike and slow wave potentials now occur spontaneously and *synchronously* between these distant regions of the reaggregated neuronal network. (C_1) One recording electrode (lower sweep) relocated from cluster (g) to nearby large cord explant (SC_2); stimulus now applied to another cluster (d) midway between the two recording sites (see Fig. 6A). Note relatively long latency of positive slow wave response from large explant (lower sweep). ($C_{2,3}$) Discharges also occur spontaneously and synchronously between the cluster (a) and the cord explant (SC_2). (D) Simultaneous recordings of spontaneous discharges from two reaggregated clusters (about 3 mm apart) in another culture of dissociated brainstem and cord tissues, after introduction of strychnine. Note marked similarity of these complex repetitive spike and slow wave sequences to those recorded in the first culture (cf. $B_{3,4}$ and $C_{2,3}$: upper sweeps) (from Crain & Bornstein, 1972 and unpublished observations).

obtained from CNS reaggregates in cultures where no undissociated large explants had been included (Fig. 6C; Fig. 8).

After introduction of strychnine (1–10 μg/ml) the amplitude of these slow waves and the duration and complexity of the discharge sequences were greatly enhanced (Figs. 7B,D; Fig. 8B). All of the complex bioelectric activities were rapidly blocked, on the other hand, by raising the Mg^{2+} concentration of the medium from 1 to 5 m*M* (Fig. 8C_1), although short-latency spike potentials could still be evoked (Fig. 8C_2). The sensitivity of these reaggregated CNS neurons to pharmacologic agents is clearly similar to that observed in larger intact CNS explants (Section II), and the data indicate that functional synaptic networks have developed even after this more traumatic dissociation procedure. In some of the reaggregates, moreover, especially of cerebral cortex cells, organotypic oscillatory (ca. 10–15 per second afterdischarge patterns also occurred, spontaneously as well as in response to

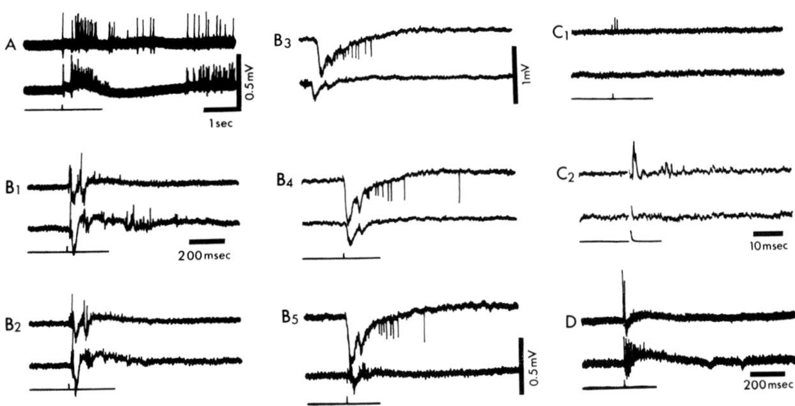

FIG. 8. Organotypic spike barrages and oscillatory afterdischarges in cultured reaggregates of fetal mouse cerebral cortex, 2 weeks after complete cellular dissociation. (A) Long-lasting intermittent bursts of repetitive spikes in two clusters of reaggregated neurons (Fig. 6C: $r_{1,2}$), located 2 mm apart, evoked by single stimulus applied to another cluster (s) midway between them. (B) After introduction of strychnine (10 μg/ml), slow wave components become greatly enhanced in amplitude and rhythmic positive potentials (ca 15 per second) appear superimposed on a long-lasting negativity ($B_{1,2}$ especially in lower sweeps). (B_3) Similar repetitive sequences also occur spontaneously and synchronously between the two clusters. Note large amplitude of these slow waves and associated repetitive spike potentials. Also note sequential increase in amplitude of spikes during later stages of the spontaneous barrage sequence (upper sweep). This is even more evident in the discharges triggered shortly afterward by single stimuli ($B_{4,5}$). Note the striking stereotyped, yet quite complex, pattern of these evoked and spontaneous discharges ($B_{3,4,5}$: upper sweeps). (C_1) After increasing Mg^{2+} concentration from 1 m*M* to 5 m*M*, all complex discharges are completely blocked, and only brief, short-latency spike potentials can be evoked (C_2). (D) Restoration of complex discharges after return to 1 mM Mg^{2+} (from Crain & Bornstein, 1972).

stimuli (cf. Figs. 8B *vs*. Figs. 4 and 5). These stereotyped, yet complex, repetitive discharge sequences have, heretofore, been observed only in well-organized undissociated CNS explants (Section IIIA,).

Furthermore, it is of great interest that the spontaneous and evoked activities in the neuronal reaggregates were often clearly synchronized, even between clusters separated by distances greater than 3 mm (Figs. 7B, D; Fig. 8B), and also between reaggregates and larger intact cord explants (Fig. 7C). The marked variation in latencies of the discharges between clusters reflect delays due to slow propagation of impulses in these fine-diameter neurites and to complex multisynaptic transmission. After introduction of strychnine, synchronization was greatly enhanced, and even some of the small clusters containing only a few neuron perikarya then showed patterned, long-lasting repetitive spike bursts occuring synchronously with more complex discharges in larger clusters.

Completely dissociated immature mammalian CNS neurons can, therefore, not only form synaptic connections after reaggregation in culture, but they can also organize from a state of random dispersion into functional synaptic networks with complex organotypic properties indicating involvement of inhibitory as well as excitatory mechanisms (see also Section VI). Since these dissociated neurons can now be studied with cytologic and bioelectric techniques during the *entire* period of regeneration and reaggregation in culture (Crain, 1973a), this method should greatly facilitate analysis of the role of each of the cells in these experimental networks in generating characteristic CNS discharge patterns. Furthermore, since histologic studies have not yet been made to determine the degree of patterned cellular organization in our neuronal reaggregates (cf. DeLong, 1970), it remains a moot question as to whether these organotypic CNS discharges can be generated by synaptic circuits with relatively unspecific neuronal connections (Crain, 1966; Crain *et al.*, 1968b; Nelson, 1967; Székely, 1966), or even by cell assemblies of randomly connected neurons with appropriate biophysical properties, as in recent computer models of CNS networks (Andersen & Andersson, 1968; Farley, 1962).

C. Limitations of CNS Cultures as Model Systems

Tissue culture techniques are still not sufficiently standardized, especially with regard to development of complex CNS netweorks with characteristic synaptic functions, and microscopic observations of the living cultures are not yet adequate to evaluate the integrity of these interneuronal relationships. Potent "biochemical lesions" may occur which involve no detectable morphologic alterations, even at the electron microscope level (see below). This is especially important to keep in mind in evaluating the functional significance of biochemical and cytological properties of cultured CNS tissues studied without correlative electrophysiologic tests on the same specimens. There are often serious variations between CNS cultures prepared under "standard" conditions even in a well-established laboratory, so that inferences about the functional integrity of *particular* explants based on bioelectric studies of this *type* of culture in another laboratory may be unwarranted extrapolations. No morphologic deficits have been detected, for example, during weeks of exposure of fetal cerebral cortex and spinal cord explants to Xylocaine at concentrations which block (reversibly) generation of all nerve impulses and characteristic synaptically mediated discharges (see Section VI).

Even under "optimal" culture conditions, of course, CNS explants will generally develop some structural and functional deficits or abnormalities relative to their *in situ* counterparts. Separation of these small fragments of CNS tissue from their normal connections with other neurons undoubtedly leads to *alterations*, at least in neuronal excitability (Crain, 1969). Isolation in culture may, moreover, selectively damage or eliminate those types of neurons in a CNS explant which are more sensitive to mechanical trauma or to chemical deficiencies in the nutrient medium. Furthermore, even if synapses do form under a particular set of conditions *in vitro*, the resulting network may be significantly unbalanced as regards normal excitatory and inhibitory components, e.g., in association with aberrant collateral sprouting (see Section III, A, I), denervation hypersensitivity, and other processes leading to development of inhibitory synaptic dominance in older CNS explants (Section V; Crain, 1969). Altered chemosensitivity of some types of neuronal membranes may also be produced by chronic exposure, during maturation, to certain metabolites which may be present at relatively high (and presently uncontrolled) concentrations in routine tissue culture media, e.g., glycine and other amino acids involved in synaptic mediation (Section V). It is of interest, in this regard, that tolerance to *d*-tubocurarine appears to develop during chronic exposure of *in vitro*-coupled cord muscle explants to this agent throughout the period when neuromuscular junctions are forming in culture (Crain & Peterson, 1971, 1973). Moreover, current use of Maximow depression-slide chambers (see Section II, A, I) involves marked alterations in the biochemical milieu during the 3- to 4-day period between feedings. Anabolites may dwindle and catabolites accumulate (including acidic pH-shifts as CO_2 levels increase). Although these environmental fluctuations have been compatible with development and maintenance of "normal" CNS morphology in culture, they may be partly responsible for some of the variability in pharmacologic sensitivity noted above. In view of all these uncontrolled parameters in the physicochemical environment of CNS cultures it is, indeed, remarkable that these isolated tissues show the degree of organotypic bioelectric properties described above, including characteristic sensitivity to at least some synapse-specific chemical tests, e.g., strychnine and Mg^{2+} (Crain, 1972a, 1972b, 1973b,c; Crain & Pollack, 1972, 1973). Systematic pharmacologic studies with chambers permitting more rigorous long-term stability and control of the culture medium, may clarify the factors responsible for the aberrant sensitivity observed following many other experimental alterations of the chemical environment (Crain, 1972c; 1973b).

In view of these present limitations in standardization of CNS explants, the burden of proof rests upon the investigator to determine the degree of organotypic function for each group of cultured CNS tissues, prepared by a particular set of culture techniques, utilizing bioelectric analyses carried out under well-defined physicochemical conditions. These direct electrophysiologic "calibrations" will provide a firm foundation for application of CNS cultures as a reproducible, experimental model system, with full cognizance of the obvious limitations of these neuronally isolated CNS tissues to studies of mechanisms underlying development of brain and behavior.

IV. Spontaneous Patterned Discharges in CNS Explants as Model of Embryonic Motility

Most of the organotypic repetitive spike barrages and complex slow waves evoked in these CNS explants by electric stimuli have also been observed to occur spontaneously, either in normal culture media or after introduction of excitatory chemical agents. Analyses of the spontaneous discharge patterns in these and other types of cultured CNS tissues indicate that "pacemaker" neurons may generate spikes sporadically, or rhythmically, and these spontaneous impulses can then trigger widespread network discharges throughout the explant, depending upon the excitability threshold of the latter system (Corner & Crain, 1969, 1972). Many of the older explants show little or no signs of spontaneous complex activity in normal culture media, although they may be rapidly activated after introduction of strychnine or other chemical agents (see Section V). It has been possible, nevertheless, to carry out systematic recordings of the temporal patterning of spontaneous complex discharges in a fairly large number of fetal rodent spinal cord and medulla explants in normal physiological salt solution (Corner & Crain, 1972). These discharges last for periods of the order of 0.1 second up to several seconds, and they may occur at regular intervals of 1–10 seconds, although activity patterns are often quite irregular (Fig. 9). Some explants also show clear periodicity in the recurrence of phases of relative activity and inactivity, with cycle times ranging up to about 10 minutes.

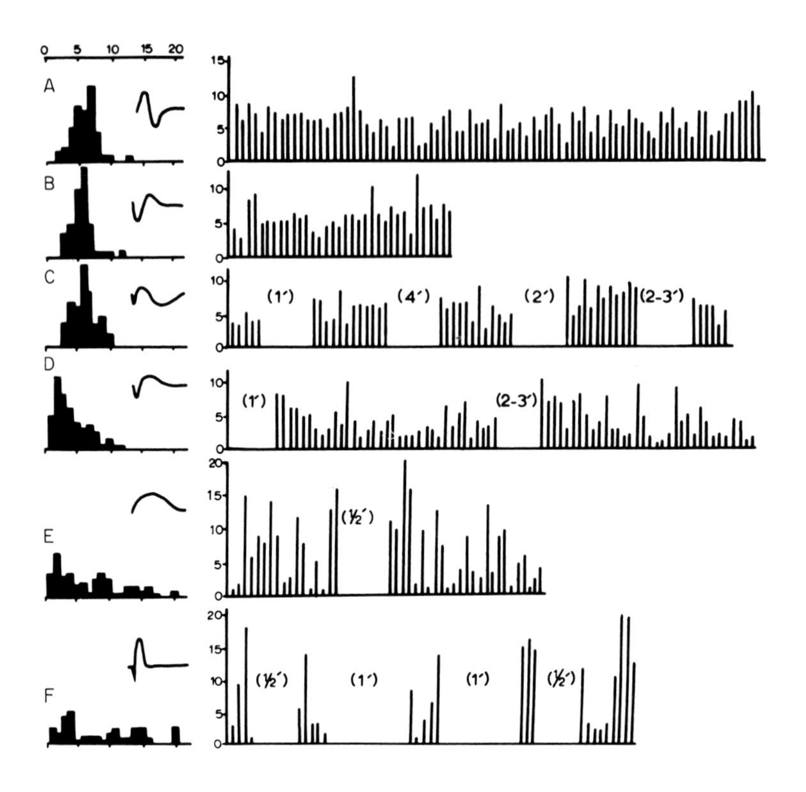

FIG. 9. Temporal patterning of several types of spontaneous complex discharges in mouse cord and medulla explants, studied for periods of $\frac{1}{4}$–3 hours. In each case, the stereotyped complex waveform is illustrated (with a 1-sec sweep-duration) in the insert between an "interdischarge interval histogram" (on left) and an "interdischarge interval tachogram" (on right). An "interdischarge interval" was defined as the time elapsed between the *end* of one complex discharge sequence and the onset of the next one. In the histograms (A-F), the "number of occurrences" is plotted against the "duration (in seconds) of interdischarge interval." In the tachograms, the "duration (in seconds) of interdischarge interval" is plotted against an abscissa consisting of a series of consecutive interdischarge intervals with arbitrary gaps indicating exceptionally long intervals ranging from .5 to 4 minutes. (A) Explant which showed continuous and relatively regular discharges (mouse cord, 19 days, i.v.). (B) *Idem* (mouse medulla, 27 days, i.v.). (C) Equally regular discharges as in (A) and (B) but with cyclic interruption of the complex activity (mouse medulla, 19 days, i.v.). (D): Culture having relatively long-lasting activity periods, in each of which the first five or so intervals last between 5 and 10 seconds, whereas for the rest of the active phase intervals shorter than 5 seconds predominate (mouse medulla, 15 days, i.v.). (E) More continuous, but extremely irregular, pattern of spontaneous potentials (mouse cord, 13 days, i.v.). (F) Irregular succession of intervals, but with frequent longer interruptions in this preparation than in record E (mouse cord, 13 days, i.v.) (from Corner & Crain, 1972).

These complex, yet stereotyped, spontaneous bioelectric discharge patterns in cultures of organized CNS tissues show remarkable mimicry of rhythmic activities which occur in the embryonic CNS *in situ*, as determined by electrophysiologic and behavioral motility studies in the intact animal. The parallels between our tissue culture model and recent microelectrode recordings of rhythmic polyneuronal burst discharges in the chick embryo spinal cord *in ovo* (Provine, 1971, 1972) are quite striking. Provine's (1971) conclusion (see also Ripley & Provine, 1972) that these "polyneuronal burst discharges are neural correlates of motility . . . (in) . . . the embryonic spinal cord" provides strong support for the relevance of the CNS tissue culture model for studies of mechanisms underlying early behavioral development (see Section V). The culture model is further strengthened by the demonstration of a similar relationship *in vitro* between spontaneous rhythmic, patterned bioelectric discharges in fetal rodent spinal cord explants and coordinated contractions of innervated skeletal muscle fibers (Fig. 10; Crain, 1970a; Crain *et al.*, 1970). Parallel cord muscle relations have also been observed in microelectrode studies of larval amphibian cultures (Corner & Crain, 1965). Further analyses of the cellular and molecular mechanisms involved in the "spontaneous" generation and spread of excitation through organotypic embryonic CNS explants may, therefore, provide valuable insights into some aspects of early behavioral development.

More complex tissue culture models are also available which may be useful for studies of the effects of higher brain centers on spinal cord activities during development (Crain *et al.*, 1968b). Rhythmic bioelectric discharges recorded in explants of fetal mouse medulla and cerebral cortex, after formation of neuritic connections *in vitro*, provide a particularly dramatic demonstration of the potentialities of this model system (Fig. 11). Spike barrages in the medulla explant can trigger characteristic oscillatory afterdischarges in the cerebral tissue, and analysis of the complex temporal patterns suggests that *inhibitory* feedback circuits may develop between and within these explants (Crain *et al.*, 1968b). Periodic generation of impulses in medulla "pacemaker" neurons appears to result not only in cerebral excitatory effects, but also in sequential generation of large inhibitory postsynaptic potentials in the cerebral explant (Fig. 11; note *positive* cerebral slow waves which often follow spike bursts in medulla). The medulla spike barrage may then be periodically self-quenched (possibly by local recurrent inhibitory networks; see Section V), thereby attenuating the inhibitory activity to the cerebral explant. In some cases, these rhythmic sequences of spike bursts alternating with silent periods in the medulla continued to occur even when cerebral activity disappeared for various intervals. At times, however, spike

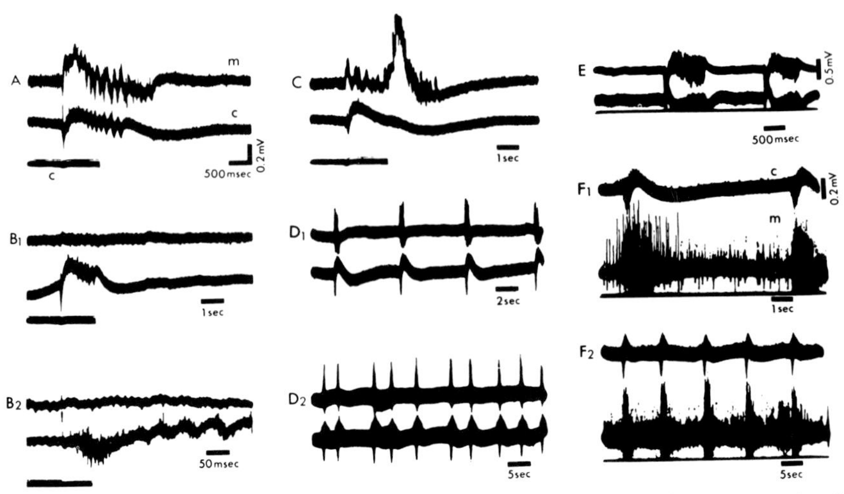

FIG. 10. Complex evoked and spontaneous discharges in coupled *fetal* rodent cord and *adult* rodent muscle explants (6- to 7-week cultures) after introduction of strychnine (10 μg/ml). (A) Simultaneous recordings of complex oscillatory (ca. 10 per second afterdischarge evoked in mouse spinal cord (second sweep: c) and in mouse muscle (first sweep: m) by single cord stimulus (third sweep: c). (B_1) After replacement of strychnine by *d*-tubocurarine (10 μg/ml), entire cord-evoked muscle response disappears while characteristic repetitive discharge still occurs in cord. At faster sweep rate (B_2), primary spike barrage in cord can be seen more clearly, followed by secondary oscillatory (15 per second) afterdischarge. (C) After return to normal medium, a complex repetitive discharge appears again in the muscle, lasting more than 4 seconds following a cord stimulus which now evokes a simpler, but still long-lasting, response in the cord. (D) Similar complex spontaneous discharges occurring rhythmically (at 3- to 5-sec intervals) and synchronously in another pair of coupled mouse cord and muscle explants under strychnine. (E) Similar spontaneous discharges in coupled explants of *mouse cord* and *rat muscle* (cf. A). (F) Similar spontaneous discharges in coupled explants of *rat* cord and *mouse* muscle. Note repetitive fibrillatory potentials continuing in muscle during intervals between synchronized cord and muscle discharges. (Muscle spikes have been retouched during first 4 seconds of second sweep in F_1; spikes during remainder of this record are barely visible, at this slow sweep rate, but their amplitude and temporal patterns are actually similar. In F_2, muscle spike bursts which occur synchronously with cord discharges have been reinforced; spikes also continue to occur, at lower frequency, during intervals between periodic discharges of cord and muscle, as in F_1) (from Crain *et al.*, 1970).

barrages from the medulla appeared to become longer lasting and less sharply interrupted by silent periods when the cerebral explant became quiescent. The latter observation raises the possibility that inhibitory feedback from the cerebral to the medulla explant may also play a role, under some conditions, in quenching medulla spike activity (Fig. 11C_1; note *negative* cerebral waves concomitant with silent periods in medulla). These remarks are, of course, highly speculative, but they provide a working hypothesis for further experiments on these complex heterogeneous neural networks, incorporating microelectrode recordings at multiple sites within each explant and correlative intracellular measurements in specific neurons (Crain *et al.*, 1968b; see also, Zipser, Crain & Bornstein, 1973).

V. Role of Inhibitory Systems in Masking Early "Behavioral Repertoire" of CNS Cultures and Embryos

The potent effect of strychnine in enhancing complex evoked and spontaneous discharges in CNS explants shortly after onset of synaptogenesis (Fig. 3C and Section II, B; Figs. 7, 8 and Section III, B) has been interpreted as evidence that inhibitory synaptic circuits may begin to function rather early in development of the central nervous system (Crain, 1969; Crain & Peterson, 1967). This view rests upon analyses of intracellular recordings in spinal cord neurons *in situ* demonstrating that low concentrations of strychnine selectively block generation of inhibitory postsynaptic potentials (Eccles, 1964). Early development of strychnine sensitivity has also been observed in many EEG studies (Bishop, 1950; Crain, 1952; Flexner, Tyler, & Gallant, 1950; see review in Himwich, 1962), and recent electrophysiological analyses suggest that *cerebral* excitatory effects of strychnine may also be mediated by selective depression of various inhibitory circuits (Bhargava & Meldrum, 1969, 1971; Pollen & Ajmone-Marsan, 1965; Pollen & Lux, 1966; Stefanis & Jasper, 1965; see review in Ajmone-Marsan, 1969), although the mechanisms of action appear to be far more complex than in the spinal cord (cf. Ajmone-Marsan, 1969; Biscoe & Curtis, 1967; Curtis, 1968; Curtis, Duggan, & Johnston, 1971).

In one of the few cases where it has been possible to obtain intracellular recordings of postsynaptic potentials in CNS neurons shortly after synaptogenesis *in situ*, i.e., in neonatal cat cerebral cortex and hippocampus (Purpura *et al.*, 1965; Purpura, Prelevic, & Santini, 1968), "extraordinary" long-duration inhibitory PSPs have been observed along with the expected excitatory PSPs. Purpura (1971) has commented, moreover, that

> the immature neocortex and hippocampus are by no means *immature* as regards the differential development of inhibitory synaptic activites. In fact, insofar as *inhibition* is concerned it must be allowed that the cerebral cortex of the neonatal kitten is virtually as "mature" as it will ever be! If, then, there is any problem that requires the immediate attention of neurobiologists interested in the development of behavior, it is the problem of defining the functional significance of the precocious and differential development of inhibition in immature cerebral cortex [pp. 31–32].

It is of interest, in this regard, that the earliest potentials recorded from fetal somesthetic cortex, in response to tactile stimulation, are predominantly surface *positive*, appearing at 43 days of gestation in the sheep (Molliver,

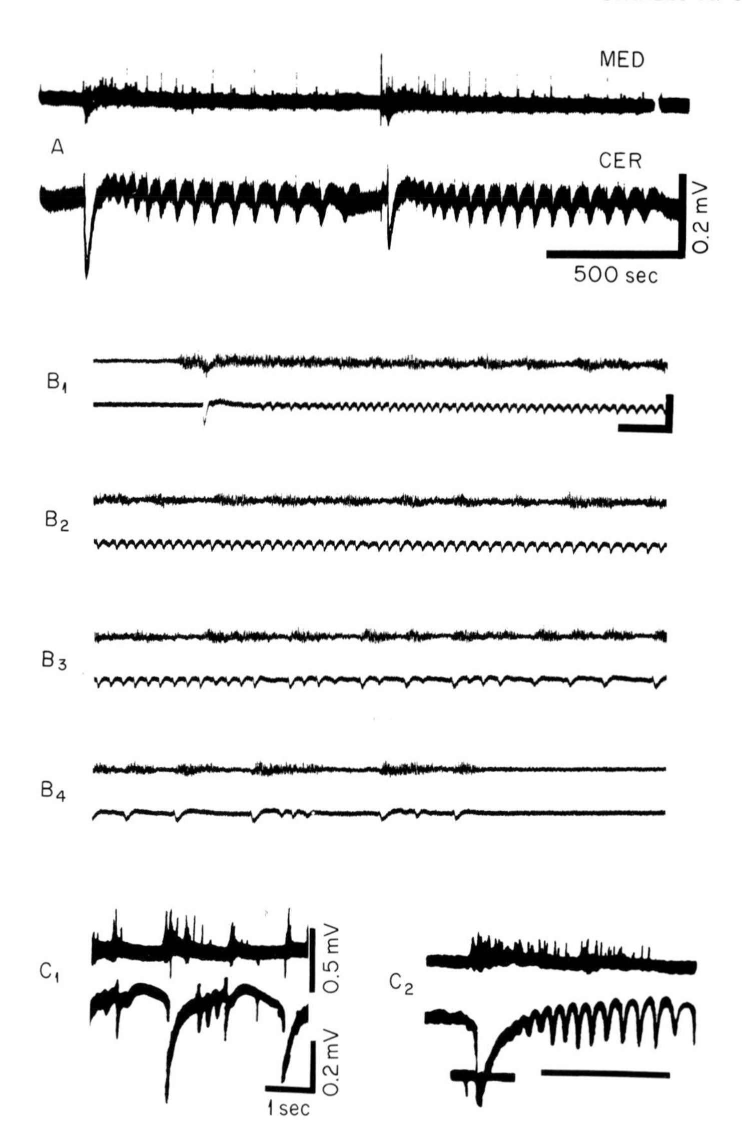

FIG. 11. Rhythmic repetitive discharges occurring synchronously between explants of fetal mouse cerebrum and medulla after formation of interneuronal connections in long-term culture (from 14-day fetus; 3 weeks *in vitro*). (A,B) Spontaneous activities of medulla and cerebral explants recorded simultaneously in closed chamber with microelectrodes positioned by sealed-in magnetically coupled micromanipulators (see Fig. 2). Note sudden onset of each medulla spike barrage (A: MED) followed closely by a complex cerebral oscillatory (ca. 15 per second) discharge sequence (A: CER). (B_{1-4}) Continuous recording of spontaneous discharges at same electrode loci as in A. Note rhythmic alterations in amplitude of medulla

1967) and at the mid-fetal stage in the dog (Molliver, in preparation). Large negative evoked potentials do not appear until several days later. Although additional electrophysiological data are required to clarify the mechanisms underlying these early surface positive potentials, a simple tentative hypothesis would be that they represent extracellular recordings of summated inhibitory (hyperpolarizing) PSPs generated by primitive synaptic networks located relatively close to the cortical surface electrode (cf. Meyerson and Persson, this volume, Molliver & Van der Loos, 1970).

Cultures of CNS tissues may provide a useful model system to study some aspects of this important problem. Extracellular microelectrode recordings at 3–4 days after explantation of mouse cerebral cortex show positive evoked potentials (Fig. 5B, C, lower sweeps) with temporal patterns remarkably similar to those of the inhibitory PSPs obtained in the neonatal cat cortex. Furthermore, introduction of low concentrations of strychnine ($10^{-6}M$) leads to appearance of prominent spontaneous and evoked slow waves in the explants, which increase in amplitude and decrease in duration during the following week *in vitro* (Crain & Bornstein, 1964), clearly resembling the changes in strychnine "sharp waves" seen during ontogenetic development of mammalian cerebral cortex *in situ* (Bishop, 1950; Crain, 1952; Himwich, 1962). Strychnine may also cause polarity inversion of *positive* evoked potentials in cerebral explants into characteristic negative slow waves of large amplitude and long duration. These phenomena can be interpreted as evidence of selective strychnine blockade of inhibitory (hyperpolarizing) PSPs, thereby unmasking excitatory (depolarizing) PSP components (Crain, 1969). On the other hand, increasing the glycine or γ-aminobutyric acid (GABA) concentration of the culture medium to $10^{-3}M$ rapidly depresses most of the complex discharges in spinal cord explants, and only simple spike bursts or short-duration responses can be evoked, even with large electric stimuli (Crain, 1972a, 1972b, 1973b, 1973c). Glycine levels in standard commercially available tissue culture media range up to $2 \times 10^{-3} M$!) These effects can be reversed after return to regular medium, and the glycine blockade (unlike a Mg^{2+} blockade—see Section II, A, 2) can be *prevented* by concomitant additions of low concentrations of

---

(FIG. 11 *continued*)
spike burst patterns and synchronization with some of the cerebral discharges, as in A. (C_1) Spontaneous discharges in another pair of medulla and cerebral explants, after coupling *in vitro*, recorded in an open moist chamber with microelectrodes positioned by conventional large micromanipulators (see Section II A, 1). Note similarity between these records and those in A and B of rhythmic spike bursts in medulla and complex oscillatory discharges occurring synchronously in cerebral explant. (C_2) Simultaneous afterdischarges evoked by single brief cerebral stimulus show same complex, yet stereotyped, patterns as recorded in sealed chamber (cf. C_2 and A) (from Crain, 1972c).

strychnine (10^{-7} to 10^{-6} *M*). Since glycine and GABA are likely to be functioning as transmitters at inhibitory synapses in the spinal cord which are selectively blocked *in situ* by strychnine and picrotoxin, respectively (Curtis *et al.*, 1971; Curtis & Felix, 1971; Curtis, Hösli, Johnston, & Johnston, 1968; Werman, Davidoff, & Aprison, 1968), this supports the view that excitatory effects of strychnine (and picrotoxin, Crain & Peterson, 1964) on cord cultures, may be due to selective interference with glycine- and GABA- sensitive inhibitory synapses in these explants. Intracellular recordings from neurons in rat spinal cord explants (2–4 weeks *in vitro*) have, in fact, demonstrated characteristic hyperpolarization potentials and membrane conductance increases following microelectrophoretic application of glycine (Hösli, Andrès, & Hösli, 1971). Similar studies of the effects of glycine, GABA, and other postulated inhibitory transmitters (and selective blocking agents) on *cerebral* explants may provide valuable data, especially in conjunction with correlative intracellular recordings, to clarify the mechanisms involved in these depressant effects, *in vitro* and *in situ*. Preliminary experiments indicate that GABA and picrotoxin are, indeed, more potent than glycine and strychnine on mouse cerebral cortex, as compared to spinal cord explants (Crain, 1972b, 1973b, 1973c).

Still more dramatic effects attributable to development of inhibitory circuits in CNS explants are observed, especially in older cultures, in cases where almost no signs of complex bioelectric acitivity can be detected in the normal culture medium. Even with large single or repetitive electric stimuli, the responses may be limited to brief spike potentials, often followed by a simple positive wave (as in Fig. 4A,D). Introduction of strychnine reveals, however, that these explants have, indeed, retained their capacity to generate elaborate, organotypic, synaptically mediated discharges (e.g., Figs. 4E-L, Figs. 10, 11), but that in normal culture media inhibitory circuits effectively quench activation of these networks, following initial generation of action potentials in some of the neurons. Direct electrophysiologic data has not yet been obtained regarding the extent to which inhibitory synapses may develop and begin to function during the *early* stages of synaptogenesis in the spinal cord of mammalian or avian embryos, *in situ*. Mature inhibitory PSPs have, indeed, been recorded during late fetal stages in the cat (Naka, 1964), and since polysynaptic circuits apparently form concomitant with the earliest detectable reflex behavior (Windle, 1934), Naka concluded that "there is no reason to suppose that the inhibitory reaction should appear later than the excitatory one . . .". Strychnine and picrotoxin have, moreover, been shown to produce convulsive limb movements in amphibian larvae (Hughes & Prestige, 1967; see also Hughes, 1968), and enhanced motility and swimming behavior has been elicited by strychnine in early fish embryos (Pollack & Crain, 1972; p. 101). On the basis of these correlative observations *in situ* and *in vitro*, the possible role of inhibitory systems during early development of behavior must be given serious consideration. This is especially important in evaluating the significance of overt motility patterns in early embryonic stages.

Interpreting the overt *motility* of the chick embryo as the major manifestation of its behavior may tend to distract one's attention away from the forest because of the rustling of the leaves on the trees. Integrated behavior of crucial survival value to the chick embryo, growing in a tightly packed shell, may involve active restraints on the mobility of a major portion of its body musculature. The early overt motility which incessantly and periodically breaks through these postulated restraints as "convulsive . . . jerky uncontrolled movements of . . . individual parts, such as head, trunk, limbs, beak, eyelids" (Hamburger, Volume I of this serial publication) may, indeed, be predominantly uncoordinated, as emphasized by Hamburger (1963, 1968, 1971; cf. Gottlieb, Introduction to Section I, this volume), but if its major functional significance is merely related to maintenance of joint movements (to preclude ankylosis, Drachman & Sokoloff, 1966), unpatterned muscle contractions may adequately fulfill this requirement. The rhythmic *temporal* patterns of these overt movements, on the other hand, certainly provide significant clues to the primitive synaptic network properties of the embryonic CNS (Corner & Crain, 1972; Hamburger, 1968, 1971; Provine, 1971, 1972; Ripley & Provine, 1972, see also Section IV and chapters by Hamburger and by Provine, first volume in this series). However, interpretation of the *spatially* uncoordinated patterns of overt muscle contractions as evidence which contradicts Coghill's (1929) generalization that "behavior . . . (in all vertebrates) . . . develops from the beginning through the progressive expansion of a perfectly integrated total pattern . . . [p. 38]" detracts from recognition of the possible existence of integrated, active CNS restraints which set limits to the mobility of the body musculature and which could be the major *behavioral* expression of these embryos during certain stages of development. These "restraints" are masked, of course, by the ubiquitous, uncoordinated overt motility of the embryo, but as Kuo (1967) has noted ". . . behavior is far more than the visible muscular movements. Besides such movements, the morphological aspect, the physiological (biophysical and biochemical) changes, the developmental history of the animals, and the ever-changing environmental context are interwoven events which are essential and integral parts of behavior [p. 25]."

Integrated CNS restraints on embryonic motility may be based on organized inhibitory synaptic circuits built into the internuncial networks of the early chick spinal cord (Crain, 1971). These diffusely distributed, endogenous negative feedback systems would serve to minimize excessive activation of the body musculature during the long period of organization and sculpturing of the CNS *in ovo* or *in utero*. In such a dynamic growth period when many neurons are selectively degenerating (Hughes, 1968), and many synaptic connections are retracting and others forming, unrestrained excitation of motor neurons could be disastrous, not only in terms of mechanical movements dangerous to the survival of the embryo in a confined, though fragile environment, but also in terms of metabolic deficits produced by such excessive muscular contractions. Although large convulsivelike movements of individual parts do, indeed, occur frequently during normal embryonic development (see above), this degree of motility may still be quite subdued relative to the capacity of the body musculature to undergo violent contractions in response to a *totally* uninhibited CNS. Organized CNS inhibitory systems may include not only those mediated by the well-established postsynaptic and presynaptic junctions (Eccles, 1964), but also any other mechanisms by which CNS neurons may *systematically* depress one another. The latter could involve, for example, diffusion of inhibitory transmitters from terminals of some types of interneurons to widely distributed chemosensitive regions on neighboring neurons (e.g., glycine- or GABA-receptor sites; see also Curtis, Hösli, & Johnston, 1967), analogous to the widespread acetylcholine-sensitivity of the skeletal muscle fiber membrane prior to formation of the neuromuscular junction (Diamond & Miledi, 1962). Perhaps embryonic CNS neurons have similarly widespread *inhibitory* transmitter sensitivities which only gradually become restricted to the sites of the inhibitory postsynaptic junctions, as occurs after denervation and reinnervation of excitatory cholinergic synapses on parasympathetic ganglion cells in the frog (Kuffler, Dennis, & Harris, 1971).

Provine's (1971) microelectrode recordings showing widespread, synchronized "burst discharges occurring throughout the rostrocaudal axis of the ventral portion of spinal cords of embryos between 6 and 20 days of age" provide, indeed, a clear-cut bioelectric correlate of the sinusoid "waves of contraction which pass through the [entire] bodies of young 4- to 6-day embryos" (Provine, first volume in this serial publication). This type of total body coordinated, patterned movements, which is the "direct precursor of swimming movements . . . in fishes and amphibians . . . breaks down soon after its inception at 4 days. Already at 5 days, only the first waves in a sequence usually go down all the way . . . [and then] the S-waves disappear altogether" (Hamburger, first volume in this serial publication). Provine's data indicate, nevertheless, maintenance of widespread burst discharges in the ventral cord throughout the *entire* period after the S-waves disappear, leaving only uncoordinated jerky movements which may involve highly variable components of the body musculature at any one moment. This "Type I" motility, as described in detail by Hamburger and Oppenheim (1967), consists of "irregular, *low amplitude* movements . . . [which] may involve all parts of the embryo simultaneously, or at the other extreme, *one part*, such as a single toe or the beak *may move, while all other parts are momentarily at rest* (italics added) [p. 175]." Why does a significant and variable fraction of the skeletal muscles remain immobile, in 5-day and older embryos, during each stereotyped burst discharge which spreads throughout the *entire* rostrocaudal axis of the spinal cord? Widespread modulation or suppression of motorneuron activity by inhibitory interneurons during these cord discharges, may, indeed, be the critical factor which accounts for this apparent discrepancy between spatial patterns of bioelectric CNS activity and overt body motility, as well as for the more general restraints on motility, e.g., relatively "low amplitudes" (see above) and long interburst intervals (Provine, 1972). (It should be kept in mind, of course, that Provine's extracellular microelectrode recordings of burst discharges probably include intermingled arrays of spike potentials generated in the *inhibitory* as well as the excitatory interneurons of these complex spinal cord networks.)

Coghill's (1940, 1943) later discussions of inhibition in relation to development of behavior indicate that his concept of "progressive expansion of . . . integrated total pattern" (see p. 97) clearly assumed a critical role for inhibitory processes.

The progressive individuation of a partial pattern within the total pattern obviously hangs on . . . organized . . . inhibition. . . . The major division of the total pattern must be under inhibition when a part acquires independence of action, and the same part can be inhibited while the major segment of the total pattern acts. So that the whole individual probably acts in every response, either in an excitatory or inhibitory way. Therefore, while overtly the individuated part acts apparently independently of the total pattern, the latter participates in its performance by inhibition [Coghill, 1943, p. 465; 1940, p. 45] (see also Paulson & Gottlieb, 1968).

Early onset of widespread, inhibitory synaptic circuits may also be the means by which stereotyped, specified neuronal cell assemblies become organized, during development, in "forward reference" (Coghill, 1929) to later functions, but without benefit of prior activity of these assemblies [in contrast to the more "plastic" cell assemblies associated with learning in Hebb's (1949) formulation; see also Section VI]. Perhaps each of these newly formed groups of nerve cells, with patterned synaptic interconnections, could be kept depressed by innervation from arborizing collaterals of a special type of inhibitory interneuron, similar to the cerebral basket cell whose "axon . . . ramifies profusely and distributes itself to 200–500 pyramidal cells, making a dense plexus enclosing the cell bodies of the pyramidal cells in a basket-like structure ending in terminal synapses [Andersen, Eccles, & Loyning, 1963, p. 542]." These inhibitory interneurons have been postulated to provide a critical component in the "inhibitory phasing" mechanism underlying synchronized rhythmic, repetitive discharges of various aggregates of adult CNS neurons (Andersen & Eccles, 1962; Andersen *et al.*, 1963), and during embryonic stages they may produce much more potent and sustained depression of the immature postsynaptic neurons in each cell assembly (see above and Section VI). These regulator inhibitory interneurons might then function as selective "switches" which would keep the complex cell assembly modules (or "mnemons," see Cherkin, 1966; Young, 1966, p. 42) "turned off" until critical endogenous or exogenous stimuli disinhibit them by direct interference with the synaptic actions of the regulator neurons at later stages of development [providing a cellular basis for "innate releasing mechanisms" (Tinbergen, 1950; see also Lehrman, 1953)].

Integrated inhibitory circuits in the CNS may develop, therefore, with widely different patterns, depending upon the specific survival requirements of each species of embryo, as emphasized in Anokhin's (1964) concept of "systemogenesis." Generalized hormonal and other determinants of the physicochemical environment of the embryonic CNS tissues provide, of course, a "range of permissive conditions" (Hamburger, 1971) under which these postulated early inhibitory systems can produce homeostatic *intra*-CNS controls which insure "from the beginning . . . [a] . . . progressive expansion of a perfectly integrated total pattern . . . [Coghill, 1929, p. 38]." This hypothesis is also consonant with Young's (1964) views regarding synaptic mechanisms underlying learning which suggest that

> in the untrained condition . . . [alternative neural] . . . pathways are held inhibited . . . by the action of small cells . . . [with] inhibitory collaterals. . . . Learning would then consist in removal of inhibition from one path. Such a mechanism recalls the suggestion that enzymes exist in an inhibited form and that demand brings them into action by disinhibition [pp. 282–284].

This similarity between selective derepression of genes and disinhibition of neuronal "mnemonic" cell assemblies may, indeed, be not only an interesting analogy but also a clue to mechanisms underlying long-term CNS activities, during ontogenetic development as well as in relation to memory and learning (see also Bonner, 1966). Validation of these postulated integrated inhibitory networks in the early embryo will require systematic microelectrode studies of the central nervous system during embryological development, *in situ*, using selective pharmacological agents, applied acutely as well as chronically, in conjunction with focal electric stimuli. Until the role of such inhibitory systems is directly analyzed, we should keep open the possibility that Coghill's generalizations regarding behavioral development may apply, not only to amphibian embryos, but also to mammalian and avian species. These comments on development of behavior in embryos may involve excessive extrapolations from the CNS tissue culture models, but it is hoped that they will provide, nevertheless, a fruitful stimulus for further experimental studies *in situ* as well as *in vitro* (see the second addendum, p. 114).

Strong support for this hypothesis has, in fact, recently been obtained in preliminary pharmacologic studies on fish embryos (common guppy, *Lebistes reticulatus*) during the development of motility and swimming behavior (Pollack & Crain, 1972). Introduction of strychnine (ca. $10^{-6}\,M$) into the fluid bathing 1- to 2-week-old embryos, after removal from the chorionic membrane, leads to increased frequency of early spontaneous (nonswimming) movements and precocious appearance of more complex movements, or both. At a developmental stage 1 to 2 days prior to the onset of normal early swimming patterns, strychnine rapidly elicits primitive swimming movements. Furthermore, at the state when primitive swimming behavior has already developed, strychnine elicits a more complex type of swimming, like that seen in older, "dormant" embryos which are able to swim immediately after release from the normally restrictive chorionic membrane. As in earlier teleost studies (e.g., Tracy, 1926), no learning period is required prior to swimming, as evidenced by the ability of embryos to swim on release from the maternal environment and restricting membranes, so long as an appropriate level of neural and muscular maturity has been attained. These observations suggest, then, that inhibitory systems may be functioning at an early stage during formation of patterned synaptic networks, at least in this type of fish embryo.

The teleost data are consonant with excitatory effects of strychnine in amphibian larvae (Hughes, 1968; see p. 96), but quite different from the preliminary pharmacologic tests on avian embryos reported by Oppenheim, Reitzel, and Provine (1972). In the latter study, no significant excitatory effects on embryonic movements or on spinal cord spike burst discharges were detected following introduction of strychnine or picrotoxin into the chick embryo until 14–15 days *in ovo*. The absence of drug effects in the younger embryos does not, of course, preclude existence of inhibitory circuits during the 4- to 14-day stages. Possibly drug diffusion barriers, lower sensitivity of immature inhibitory synapses to strychnine and picrotoxin and other pharmacologic complexities may have prevented detection of inhibitory functions. More careful observations of the initial effects of strychnine on early chick embryos have recently indicated that a transient *increase* in motility does, in fact, occur for several minutes prior to previously reported depression effects (R. Oppenheim, personal communication). Furthermore, absence of axo*somatic* synapses in the early chick embryo spinal cord (Oppenheim & Foelix, 1972) is not a reliable criterion regarding inhibitory functions (cf. Bodian, 1970), since prominent IPSPs have been recorded in neonatal cat hippocampus (Purpura *et al.*, 1968; see p. 93) at stages when only axo*dendritic* synapses could be detected by electron microscopy (Schwartz, Pappas, & Purpura, 1968). Recent studies by Curtis and

Felix (1971) indicate, moreover, that at least GABA-type inhibitory synapses may be located on *dendritic* branches of spinal cord neurons.

An analogous homeostatic inhibitory mechanism was previously proposed in connection with the regenerative response of immature (and, possibly, adult) CNS tissue to severe trauma (Crain, 1966). The large numbers of collaterals which sprout and ramify profusely from the damaged neurons (Björklund, Katzman, Stenevi, & West, 1971; Björklund & Stenevi, 1971; Purpura & Housepian, 1961; see also Section III,A, 1) may make synaptic connections primarily with neighboring *inhibitory* interneurons (Crain, 1966). This "compensatory (homeostatic) reaction . . . would neutralize the 'supersensitivity' of the partly denervated . . . efferent neurons, and thereby tend to restore the injured CNS tissue toward a more stable state compatible with continued function [Crain, 1969, p. 511]." The postulated development of inhibitory circuits early in synaptogenesis of the embryonic CNS would, of course, provide an analogous homeostatic function by minimizing unnecessary activation and motility of the organism during the normal sculpturing of the CNS.

VI. Plasticity in Stereotyped "Self-Organizing" CNS Explants

The studies of cultured CNS tissues have emphasized that development of many organotypic structures and functions appear to be so tightly coupled to genetic factors that the explants continue to organize in rather stereotyped fashion in spite of wide variations in environmental conditions, even after random dispersion of immature CNS neurons in a relatively homogeneous, unpatterned culture environment (Section IIIB). This does not at all preclude, however, development of more complex properties in these neuronal networks which are contingent upon specific environmental factors. As Dobzhansky (1968) elegantly points out,

> what is inherited is . . . a genotypic potentiality for an organism's developmental response to its environment. Given a certain genotype and a certain sequence of environmental situations, the development follows a certain path. The carriers of other genetic endowments in the same environmental sequence might well develop differently. But, also, a given genotype might well develop phenotypically along different paths in different environments. In most abbreviated terms, the observed, phenotypic variance has both a genetic and an environmental component [pp. 552–553]." (See also Birch, 1971.)

Brain tissue cultures may therefore be useful preparations to investigate the mechanisms underlying phenotypic variance of specific components of a given genotype as a function of parametric environmental alterations. It will be of interest to systematically introduce various types of extrinsic stimuli during development of these stereotyped "self-organizing" CNS explants, e.g., electric stimuli: both random as well as highly patterned (temporally as well as spatially), applied to specific afferent inputs such as neurites of sensory ganglion cells, in contrast to inputs from other CNS regions; chemical agents (diffuse or localized): hormones, enzymes, metabolic inhibitors, etc. Critical experimental alterations may reveal some aspects of the "genotypic potentiality" which are more tightly coupled to *environmental* factors, by producing selective maturation of particular neuronal circuits or cell assemblies, involving qualitative as well as quantitative changes in the network structure and functions.

Although it is probable that "the patterning of most of the long fiber systems of the CNS . . . is primarily a problem of developmental mechanics [Sperry & Hibbard, 1968, p. 42]" the "old speculation . . . continues to seem reasonable that the plastic changes imposed by function are located not in these long-axon systems but in Ramón y Cajal's type II neurons [Sperry, 1971, p. 43]" (see also Young, 1964). Many of these small interneurons with short processes are still undergoing cell division late in development and do not differentiate until a major portion of the central nervous system is already functioning, in the postnatal period (Altman, 1967; Altman & Das, 1965). Perhaps these "microneurons" are much more plastic than the long-axon "macroneurons" which differentiate at an earlier stage, when relatively little function is occurring in neighboring neurons (Altman, 1967, 1970; see also Jacobson, 1969, and this volume). Furthermore, even if the *specificity* of connections of many types of neurons is, indeed, tightly coupled to genetic factors, the *efficacy* of these synapses may be quite plastic and significantly dependent upon environmental factors. Quantitative data must be obtained to determine the critical development stage which each type of neuronal network assembly must reach through endogenous mechanisms before these systems become capable of undergoing plastic alterations in response to patterned environmental stimuli (i.e., "functional shaping," Sperry, 1965, 1971).

Attempts are now under way to detect such signs of plasticity, as a result of experimental alteration of the culture environment during development of embryonic CNS tissues, e.g., sustained changes in excitability, in bioelectric discharge patterns, in synaptic ultrastructure, etc. As a start, the possible role of spontaneous bioelectric discharges (Section IV) on early CNS development has been studied in this model system, by chronic exposure of fetal rodent spinal cord and cerebral explants to media containing Xylocaine at a concentration sufficient to block all nerve impulses during the entire period *in vitro* (Crain *et al.*, 1968a). The neurons in these drugged cultures continued, nevertheless, to develop organized synaptic networks as in normal media, and no morphologic deficits could be detected in the explants after weeks of exposure, even at the electron microscope level (Model *et al.*, 1971). Furthermore, within *minutes* after removing the blocking agent from the bathing fluid, the *first* electric stimulus applied to such a "virginal" explant often evoked an organotypic cerebral evoked potential, of large amplitude and long duration, similar to those seen in mature control explants (Figs. 12 and 13). These experiments suggest that ontogenetic development of some types of complex interneuronal CNS functions may be programmed to occur independently of prior bioelectric excitation of the cellular elements composing the system. Furthermore, after endogenous formation of such a neuronal cell assembly, in culture, it can be maintained in a quiescent state for at least several weeks and, yet, remain organized with characteristic bioelectric excitability, in mimicry of many CNS networks which appear to form in "forward reference" to their ultimate function (Coghill, 1929; see also p. 99).

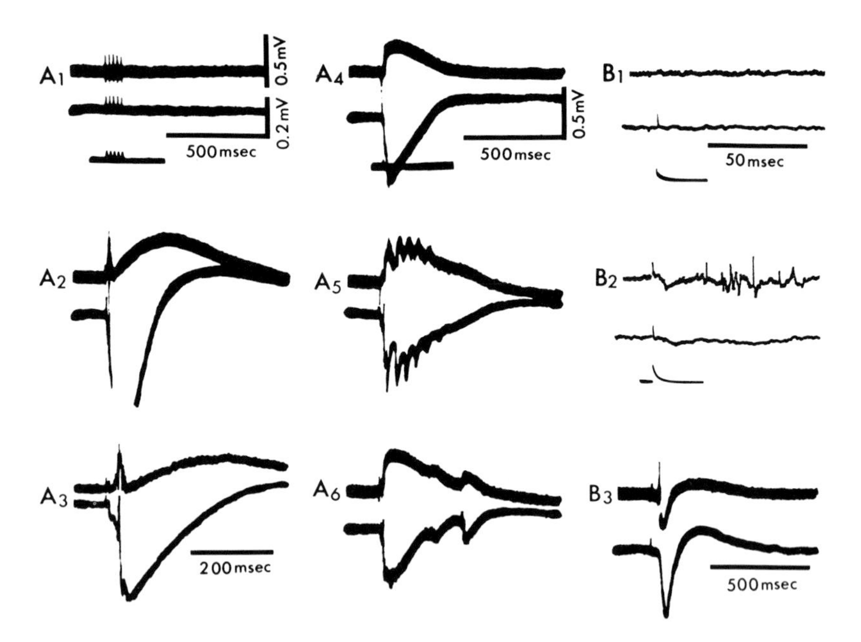

FIG. 12. Absence of bioelectric activity in 17-day fetal mouse cerebral neocortex explants during chronic (1 month) exposure to Xylocaine (50 μg/ml) and rapid recovery in normal medium. (A_1) No responses are evoked while explant is still in culture medium containing Xylocaine, even with repetitive stimuli, at high intensity. (A_2) After transfer to *simple* physiological salt solution (BSS) still containing Xylocaine at 50 μg/ml, *first* stimulus triggers characteristic cerebral evoked potential. Note long duration, large amplitude, and polarity differences (i.e., negative near original cortical surface, upper sweep; initially positive at "deeper" cortical site, lower sweep) ($A_{3,4}$) Similar responses after second and later stimuli. ($A_{5,6}$) After transfer to normal medium, responses are still more complex and longer in duration. (B_1) Absence of responses in another cerebral explant under same conditions as in A_1. (B_2) Bursts of spikes evoked by single stimulus about 2 minutes after transfer to normal medium, following acute exposure to Xylocaine at 200 μg/ml. (B_3) Characteristic "slow wave" evoked potentials appear about 1 minute later (from Crain *et al.*, 1968a).

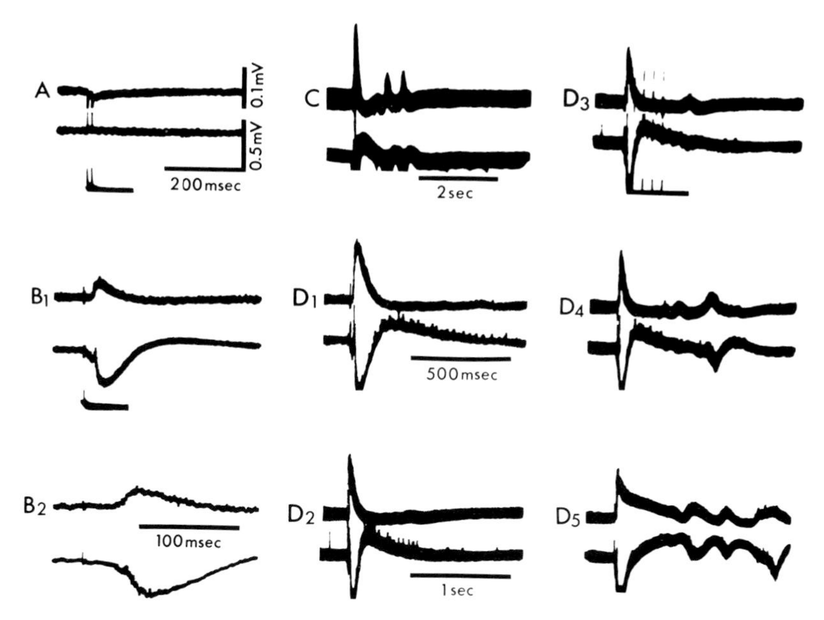

FIG. 13. Increased complexity of afterdischarges, following repetitive stimulation of cerebral explant, during recovery from chronic exposure to Xylocaine (2-day neonatal mouse; 5 days, i.v.). (A) Complete block in original culture medium containing Xylocaine (50 μg/ml). (B_1) Within a few minutes after transfer to normal medium, *first* stimulus triggers characteristic cerebral evoked potentials. Note absence of any secondary oscillatory afterdischarges; same after second stimulus (B_2). (C) After about 10 minutes of intermittent test stimuli, discharges are much more complex and longer lasting (and now appear spontaneously as well as after stimulation). ($D_{1,2}$) Recording electrodes moved to new sites in explant where no secondary oscillatory afterdischarges are evoked; note repetitive spike barrages which occur concomitant with primary slow wave response. Following brief application of repetitive (10 per second) stimuli (D_3), oscillatory afterdischarges can now be triggered by single stimuli (D_4). After further repetitive stimulation, response to single stimulus becomes still more complex (D_5). (Response durations are longer in record D_5 because excessive high-pass filtration was used in earlier records.) (from Crain *et al.*, 1968a).

Spontaneous quantal release of transmitter at presynaptic terminals may not have been blocked during chronic exposure of the CNS explants to Xylocaine or high Mg^{2+}, as in adult frog spinal cord *in situ*, where spontaneous miniature postsynaptic potentials still persist after selective block of synaptically mediated action potentials (Katz & Miledi, 1963). Spontaneous transmitter release at *inhibitory* presynaptic terminals may be particularly important in early stages of synaptogenesis, especially in the collaterals of the postulated regulator inhibitory interneurons (Section V, especially Pp. 98, 100).

The *in vitro* results are in agreement with and extend the classical *in situ* studies of Harrison (1904), Carmichael (1926), and Matthew and Detwiler

(1926) on behavioral development in amphibian embryos during chronic anesthesia (see also Gottlieb, Introduction to Section I, first volume in this serial publication). The latter experiments in the whole animal, however, did not rule out the possible role of internuncial neuronal network discharges *within* the CNS during the period of neuromuscular quiescence. The experiments by Fromme (1941), discussed by Gottlieb (Introduction to Section I first volume in this serial publication), raise the possibility that quantitative deficits in swimming behavior which appear after release from chronic anesthesia (cf. Hamburger, first volume in this serial publication) may involve sensitive synaptic circuits which are not present in our CNS explants. Alternatively, more quantitative measurements of the bioelectric properties of CNS tissues after return from chronic drug exposure to normal culture medium may yet reveal significant functional deficits parallel to those observed by Fromme *in situ*.

Although no significant changes in responses were detected in some of these virginal explants with subsequent stimuli (Fig. $12A_{3,4}$), more complex, oscillatory (5–20 per second) afterdischarges did, indeed, appear, in a few cases, during the first half hour of intermittent stimulation (Figs. 13C, D_{3-5}; see also Fig. $12A_{5,6}$; in this particular culture, however, the increased complexity of the response may have been due to more complete removal of the blocking agent prior to the latter records). Sustained increase in afterdischarges, and in spontaneous activity, has also been observed in some CNS explants, cultured in normal media, especially following brief periods of repetitive stimulation at the beginning of the electrophysiologic experiment (Crain, 1966; Crain *et al.*, 1968b). These studies, however, need to be repeated systematically, under more rigorous control of the physicochemical environment than was feasible in the earlier acute recordings in open chambers (see discussion by Crain, in Bullock, 1967), by introducing patterned stimuli during longitudinal electrophysiologic experiments on CNS explants maturing, for days or weeks, in sterile sealed micrurgical chambers (see Section II, A, 1; Fig. 2; Crain, 1970b, 1973a). The culture models may, of course, be relevant only to some of the rather primitive functional properties of the intact CNS, but in view of the remarkable organotypic bioelectric activities displayed by these isolated bits of tissue, it will certainly be worthwhile to investigate the degree to which they can develop a still more sophisticated "behavioral repertoire" relevant to studies of plasticity, learning, and memory (Horn & Hinde, 1970; John, 1967; Kandel & Spencer, 1968).

VII. Outlook

The tissue culture "window" to the brain now permits us to study many aspects of this enigmatic, intricately complicated structure in a bright new light. This combined ontogenetic and microsurgical dissection of the mammalian brain provides a dramatic geometrical simplification while retaining an extraordinary degree of organotypic function. With careful bioelectric "calibration" of cultured CNS tissues relative to their *in situ* counterparts (Section III,C), coordinated physiologic, cytologic, and biochemical studies of CNS culture models should, indeed, yield valuable insights into cellular mechanisms underlying significant aspects of neurological and behavioral development.

Acknowledgments

The author wishes to express appreciation to Dr. Murray B. Bornstein and Mrs. Edith R. Peterson (Department of Neurology, Albert Einstein College of Medicine) for their valuable cooperation in providing the cultures used for the physiologic studies described in this review. The work has been supported by grants from the National Institute of Neurological Diseases and Stroke (NB-03814, NS-06545, and NS-06735) and from the Alfred P. Sloan Foundation.

References

Ajmone-Marsan, C. Acute effects of topical epileptogenic agents. In A. A. Ward & A. Pope (Eds.), *Basic mechanisms of the epilepsies.* Boston: Little, Brown, 1969. Pp. 299–319.

Altman, J. Postnatal growth and differentiation of the mammalian brain, with implications for a morphological theory of memory. In G. C. Quarton, T. Melnechuk, & F. O. Schmitt (Eds.), *The neurosciences: A study program.* New York: Rockefeller University Press, 1967. Pp. 723–743.

Altman, J. Postnatal neurogenesis and the problem of neural plasticity. In W. A. Himwich (Ed.), *Developmental neurobiology.* Springfield, Ill.: Thomas, 1970. Pp. 197–237.

Altman, J., & Das, G. D. Post-natal origin of microneurones in the rat. *Nature* (*London*), 1965, **207**, 953–956.

Andersen, P., & Andersson, S. A. *Physiological basis of the alpha rhythm.* New York: Appleton, 1968.

Andersen, P., & Eccles, J. C. Inhibitory phasing of neuronal discharge. *Nature* (*London*), 1962, **196**, 645–647.

Andersen, P., Eccles, J. C., & Loyning, Y. Recurrent inhibition in the hippocampus with identification of the inhibitory cell and its synapses. *Nature* (*London*), 1963, **198**, 540–542.

Anokhin, P. K. Systemogenesis as a general regulator of brain development. In *The developing brain.* W. A. Himwich & H. E. Himwich (Eds.), New York: American Elsevier, 1964, Pp. 54–86.

Armstrong-James, M. A., & Williams, T. D. Post-natal development of the direct cortical response in the rat. *Journal of Physiology* (*London*), 1963, **168**, 19–20.

Baer, S. C., & Crain, S. M. Magnetically coupled micromanipulator for use within a sealed chamber. *Journal of Applied Physiology*, 1971, **31**, 926–929.

Bhargava, V. K., & Meldrum, B. S. The strychnine-like action of curare and related compounds on the somatosensory evoked response of the rat cortex. *British Journal of Pharmacology*, 1969, **37**, 112–122.

Bhargava, V. K., & Meldrum, B. S. Blockade by eserine of the cerebral cortical effects of strychnine and curare. *Nature* (*London*), *New Biology*, 1971, **230**, 152.

Birch, H. G. Levels, categories and methodological assumptions in the study of behavioral development. In E. Tobach, R. Aronson, & E. Shaw (Eds.), *Biopsychology of development.* New York: Academic Press, 1971. Pp. 503–513.

Biscoe, T. J., & Curtis, D. R. Strychnine and cortical inhibition. *Nature* (*London*), 1967, **214**, 914–915.

Bishop, E. J. The strychnine spike as a physiological indicator of cortical maturity in the postnatal rabbit. *Electroencephalography and Clinical Neurophysiology*, 1950, **2**, 309–315.

Björklund, A., Katzman, R., Stenevi, U., & West, K. A. Development and growth of axonal sprouts from noradrenaline and 5-hydroxytryptamine neurones in the rat spinal cord. *Brain Research*, 1971, **31**, 21–34.

Björklund, A., & Stenevi, U. Growth of central catecholamine neurones into smooth muscle grafts in the rat mesencephalon. *Brain Research*, 1971, **31**, 1–20.

Bodian, D. A model of synaptic and behavioral ontogeny. In F. O. Schmitt (Ed.), *The neurosciences: Second study program.* New York: Rockefeller University Press, 1970. Pp. 129–140.

Bonner, J. Molecular biological approaches to the study of memory. In J. Gaito (Ed.), *Macromolecules and behavior.* New York: Appleton, 1966. Pp. 158–164.

Bornstein, M. B. Morphological development of neonatal mouse cerebral cortex in tissue culture. In P. Kellaway & I. Petersén (Eds.), *Neurological and electroencephalographic correlative studies in infancy.* New York: Grune & Stratton, 1964. Pp. 1–11.

Bornstein, M. B., & Model, P. G. Development of neurons and synapses in cultures of dissociated spinal cord, brain stem and cerebrum of the embryo mouse. *American Society for Cell Biology, 11th Annual Meeting, New Orleans*, 1971, Abstract, p. 35.

Bornstein, M. B., & Model, P. G. Development of synapses and myelin in cultures of dissociated embryonic mouse spinal cord, medulla and cerebrum. *Brain Research*, 1972, **37**, 287–293.

Bullock, T. H. Simple systems for the study of learning mechanisms. VI. Related studies on tissue cultures. In F. O. Schmitt, T. Melnechuk, G. C. Quarton, & G. Adelman (Eds.), *Neurosciences research symposium summaries.* Vol. 11. Cambridge, Mass.: MIT Press, 1967. Pp. 253–257.

Bunge, R. P., Bunge, M. B., & Peterson, E. R. An electron-microscope study of cultured rat spinal cord. *Journal of Cell Biology*, 1965, **24**, 163–191.

Bunge, M. B., Bunge, R. P., & Peterson, E. R. The onset of synapse formation in spinal cord culture as studied by electron microscopy. *Brain Research*, 1967, **6**, 728–749.

Burns, B. D. The cause of reflex afterdischarge in the frog's spinal cord. *Canadian Journal of Biochemistry and Physiology*, 1956, **34**, 457–465.

Burns, D. B., *The mammalian cerebral cortex.* London: Arnold, 1958.

Carmichael, L. The development of behavior in vertebrates experimentally removed from the influence of external stimulation. *Psychological Review*, 1926, **33**, 51–58.

Cherkin, A Toward a quantitative view of the engram. *Proceedings of the National Academy of Sciences, U.S.*, **55**, 88–91.

Coghill, G. E. *Anatomy and the problem of behavior.* New York: Macmillan, 1929.

Coghill, G. E. Early embryonic somatic movements in birds and in mammals other than man. *Monographs of the Society for Research in Child Development*, 1940, **5**(2, Serial No. 25), 1–48.

Coghill, G. E. Flexion spasms and mass reflexes in relation to the ontogenetic development of behavior. *Journal of Comparative Neurology*, 1943, **79**, 463–486.

Corner, M. A., & Crain, S. M. Spontaneous contractions and bioelectric activity after differentiation in culture of presumptive neuromuscular tissues of the early frog. *Experientia*, 1965, **21**, 422–424.

Corner, M. A., & Crain, S. M. The development of spontaneous bioelectric activities and strychnine sensitivity during maturation in culture of embryonic chick and rodent central nervous tissues. *Archives Internationales de Pharmacodynamie et de Therapie*, 1969, **182**, 404–406.

Corner, M. A., & Crain, S. M. Patterns of spontaneous bioelectric activity during maturation in culture of fetal rodent medulla and spinal cord tissues. *Journal of Neurobiology*, 1972, **3**, 25–45.

Crain, S. M. Development of electrical activity in the cerebral cortex of the albino rat. *Proceedings of the Society for Experimental Biology and Medicine*, 1952, **81**, 49–51.

Crain, S. M. Resting and action potentials of cultured chick embryo spinal ganglion cells. *Journal of Comparative Neurology*, 1956, **104**, 285–330.

Crain, S. M. Development of bioelectric activity during growth of neonatal mouse cerebral cortex in tissue culture. In P. Kellaway & I. Petersén (Eds.), *Neurological and electroencephalographic correlative studies in infancy*. New York: Grune & Stratton, 1964. Pp. 12–26.

Crain, S. M. Muscle and nervous tissues *in vitro*: Electrophysiological properties. In E. N. Willmer (Ed.), *Cells and tissues in culture*. Vol. 2. London: Academic Press, 1965. Pp. 335–339, 344–347, 421–431.

Crain, S. M. Development of "organotypic" bioelectric activities in central nervous tissues during maturation in culture. *International Review of Neurobiology*, 1966, **9**, 1–43.

Crain, S. M. Electrical activity of brain tissue developing in culture. In H. H. Jasper, A. A. Ward, & A. Pope (Eds.), *Basic mechanisms of the epilepsies*. Boston: Little, Brown, 1969. Pp. 506–516.

Crain, S. M. Bioelectric interactions between cultured fetal rodent spinal cord and skeletal muscle after innervation *in vitro*. *Journal of Experimental Zoology*, 1970, **173**, 353–370. (a)

Crain, S. M. Long-term recordings from spinal cord explants in closed chamber with sealed-in manipulatable microelectrodes. *Journal of Cell Biology*, 1970, **47**, 43a. (b)

Crain, S. M. Tissue culture studies of developing brain function. In W. A. Himwich (Ed.), *Developmental neurobiology*. Springfield. Ill.: Thomas, 1970, Pp. 165–196. (c)

Crain, S. M. Discussion. In E. Tobach, L. R. Aronson, & E. Shaw (Eds.), *The biopsychology of development*. New York: Academic Press, 1971. Pp. 65–66.

Crain, S. M. Depression of complex bioelectric activity of mouse spinal cord explants by glycine and γ-aminobutyric acid. *In Vitro*, 1972, **7**, 249. (a)

Crain, S. M. Selective depression of organotypic bioelectric discharges of CNS explants by glycine and γ-aminobutyric acid. Soc. Neuroscience, 2nd Ann. Mtg., Houston, Texas, 1972, Abstr. p. 131 (b)

Crain, S. M. Tissue culture models of epileptiform activity. In D. P. Purpura, J. K. Penry, T. Tower, D. M. Woodbury, & R. Walter (Eds.), *Experimental models of epilepsy*. New York: Raven Press, 1972. Pp. 291–316.(c)

Crain, S. M. Microelectrode recording in brain tissue cultures. In R. F. Thompson & M. M. Patterson (Eds.), *Methods in physiological psychology*. Vol. 1. *Bioelectric recording techniques: Cellular processes and brain potentials*. New York: Academic Press, 1973, in press. (a)

Crain, S. M. Selective depression of organotypic bioelectric activities of CNS tissue cultures by pharmacologic and metabolic agents. In A. Vernadakis, & N. Weiner (Eds.), *Drugs and the developing brain*. New York: Plenum,1973 (in press). (b)

Crain, S. M. Development of complex synaptic functions in 'simple' neuronal arrays in culture. In P.N.R. Usherwood, & D. R. Newth (Eds.), *'Simple' nervous systems*. London: Arnold, 1973 (in press). (c)

Crain, S. M., Alfei, L. & Peterson, E. R. Neuromuscular transmission in cultures of adult human and rodent skeletal muscle after innervation *in vitro* by fetal rodent spinal cord. *Journal of Neurobiology*, 1970, **1**, 471–488.

Crain, S. M. & Bornstein, M. B. Bioelectric activity of neonatal mouse cerebral cortex during growth and differentiation in tissue culture. *Experimental Neurology*, 1964, **10**, 425–450.

Crain, S. M., & Bornstein, M. B. Development of organotypic bioelectric activities in cultured reaggregates of rodent brain cells after complete dissociation. *American Society for Cell Biology, 11th Annual Meeting, New Orleans,* 1971, Abstract, p. 67.

Crain, S. M., & Bornstein, M. B. Organotypic bioelectric activity in cultured reaggregates of dissociated rodent brain cells. *Science*, 1972, **176**, 182–184.

Crain, S. M., Bornstein, M. B., & Peterson, E. R. Maturation of cultured embryonic CNS tissues during chronic exposure to agents which prevent bioelectric activity. *Brain Research*, 1968, **8**, 363–372. (a)

Crain, S. M., & Peterson, E. R. Bioelectric activity in long-term cultures of spinal cord tissues. *Science*, 1963, **141**, 427–429.

Crain, S. M., & Peterson, E. R. Complex bioelectric activity in organized tissue cultures of spinal cord (human, rat and chick). *Journal of Cellular and Comparative Physiology*, 1964, **64**, 1–15.

Crain, S. M., & Peterson, E. R. Onset and development of functional interneuronal connections in explants of rat spinal cord-ganglia during maturation in culture. *Brain Research*, 1967, **6**, 750–762.

Crain, S. M., & Peterson, E. R. Development of paired explants of fetal spinal cord and adult skeletal muscle during chronic exposure to curare and hemicholinium. *In Vitro*, 1971, **6**, 373.

Crain, S. M., & Peterson, E. R. Development of neural connections in culture. In D. Drachman, & A. A. Smith (Eds.), *Symposium: The trophic function of the neuron.* New York: Annals of the New York Academy of Sciences, 1973 (in press).

Crain, S. M., Peterson, E. R., & Bornstein, M. B. Formation of functional interneuronal connections between explants of various mammalian central nervous tissues during development *in vitro*. In G. E. W. Wolstenholme & M. O'Connor (Eds.), *Ciba foundation symposium, Growth of the nervous system.* London: Churchill, 1968. Pp. 13–31. (b)

Crain, S. M., & Pollack, E. D. Restorative effects of cyclic AMP on complex bioelectric activities after acute Ca^{++} deprivation in cultured CNS tissues. *Journal of Cell Biology*, 1972, in press.

Curtis, D. R. Pharmacology and neurochemistry of mammalian central inhibitory processes. In C. Von Euler, S. Skoglund, & U. Soderberg (Eds.), *Structure and function of inhibitory neuronal mechanisms.* Oxford: Pergamon, 1968. Pp. 429–456.

Curtis, D. R., Duggan, A. W., & Johnston, G. A. R. The specificity of strychnine as a glycine antagonist in the mammalian spinal cord. *Experimental Brain Research*, 1971, **12**, 547–565.

Curtis, D. R., and Felix, D. GABA and prolonged spinal inhibition. *Nature (London) New Biology* 1971, **231**, 187–188.

Curtis, D. R., Hösli, L., & Johnston, G. A. R. Inhibition of spinal neurones by glycine. *Nature (London)*, 1967, **215**, 1502–1503.

Curtis, D. R., Hösli, L., Johnston, G. A. R., & Johnston, I. H. The hyperpolarization of spinal motoneurones by glycine and related amino acids. *Experimental Brain Research*, 1968, **5**, 235–258.

DeLong, G. R. Histogenesis of fetal mouse isocortex and hippocampus in reaggregating cell cultures. *Developmental Biology*, 1970, **22**, 563–583.

Diamond, J., & Miledi, R. A study of foetal and new-born rat muscle fibers. *Journal of Physiology (London)*, 1962, **162**, 393–408.

Dichter, M., & Fischbach, G. D. Functional synapses in cell cultures of chick spinal cord and dorsal root ganglia. *American Society for Cell Biology, 11th Annual Meeting, New Orleans*, 1971, Abstract, p. 76.

Dobzhansky, T. On genetics, sociology, and politics. *Perspectives in Biology and Medicine*, 1968, **11**, 544–554.

Downman, C. B. B., Eccles, J. C., & McIntyre, A. K. Functional changes in chromatolysed motoneurons. *Journal of Comparative Neurology*, 1953, **98**, 9–36.

Drachman, D. B., & Sokoloff, L. The role of movement in embryonic joint development. *Developmental Biology*, 1966, **14**, 401–420.

Eccles, J. C. *The neurophysiological basis of mind: The principles of neurophysiology*. London: Oxford University Press (Clarendon), 1953.

Eccles, J. C. *The physiology of synapses*. New York: Academic Press, 1964.

Farley, B. G. Some similarities between the behavior of a neural network model and electrophysiological experiments. In M. C. Yovits, G. T. Jacobi, & G. D. Goldstein (Eds.), *Self-organizing systems*. Washington, D.C.: Spartan Press, 1962. Pp. 535–550.

Fischbach, G. D. Synaptic potentials recorded in cell cultures of nerve and muscle. *Science*, 1970, **169**, 1331–1333.

Flexner, L. B., Tyler, D. B., & Gallant, L. J. Biochemical and physiological differentiation during morphogenesis. X. Onset of electrical activity in developing cerebral cortex of the fetal guinea pig. *Journal of Neurophysiology*, 1950, **13**, 427–430.

Fromme, A. An experimental study of the factors of maturation and practice in the behavioral development of the embryo of the frog, *Rana pipiens*. *Genetic Psychology Monographs*, 1941, **24**, 219–256.

Gottlieb, G. Ontogenesis of sensory function in birds and mammals. In E. Tobach, L. R. Aronson, & E. Shaw (Eds.), *Biopsychology of development*. New York: Academic Press, 1971. Pp. 66–128.

Guillery, R. W., Sobkowicz, H. M., & Scott, G. L. Light and electron microscopical observations of the ventral horn and ventral root in long term cultures of the spinal cord of the fetal mouse. *Journal of Comparative Neurology*, 1968, **134**, 433–476.

Hamburger, V. Some aspects of the embryology of behavior. *Quarterly Review of Biology*, 1963, **38**, 342–365.

Hamburger, V. Emergence of nervous coordination. IV. Origins of integrated behavior. *Developmental Biology, Supplement*, 1968, **2**, 251–271.

Hamburger, V. Development of embryonic motility. In E. Tobach, L. R. Aronson, & E. Shaw (Eds.), *The biopsychology of development*. New York: Academic Press, 1971. Pp. 45–66.

Hamburger, V., & Oppenheim, R. W. Prehatching motility and hatching behavior in the chick. *Journal of Experimental Zoology*, 1967, **166**, 171–204.

Harrison, R. G. An experimental study of the relation of the nervous system to the developing musculature in the embryo of the frog. *American Journal of Anatomy*, 1904, **3**, 197–219.

Hebb, D. O. *The organization of behavior*. New York: Wiley, 1949.

Himwich, W. A. Biochemical and neurophysiological development of the brain in the neonatal period. *International Review of Neurobiology*, 1962, **4**, 117–158.

Hösli, L., Andrès, P. F., & Hösli, E. Effects of glycine on spinal neurones grown in tissue culture. *Brain Research*, 1971, **34**, 399–402.

Hoffman, H. Axoplasm, its structure and regeneration. In W. F. Windle (Ed.), *Regeneration in the central nervous system*. Springfield, Ill. Thomas, 1955, Pp. 112–126.

Horn, G., & Hinde, R. A. *Short term changes in neural activity and behavior*. London: Cambridge University Press, 1970.

Hughes, A. F. W. *Aspects of neural ontogeny*. New York: Academic Press, 1968.

Hughes, A. F. W., & Prestige, M. C. Development of behavior in the hindlimb of *Xenopus laevis*. *Journal of Zoology*, 1967, **152**, 347–359.

Jacobson, M. Development of specific neuronal connections. *Science*, 1969, **163**, 543–547.
Jacobson, M. *Developmental neurobiology*. New York: Holt, 1970.
John, E. R. *Mechanisms of memory*. New York: Academic Press, 1967.
Kandel, E. R., & Spencer, W. A. Cellular neurophysiological approaches in the study of learning. *Physiological Reviews*, 1968, **48**, 65–134.
Katz, B., & Miledi, R. A study of spontaneous miniature potentials in spinal motoneurones. *Journal of Physiology* (*London*), 1963, **168**, 389–422.
Kuffler, S. W., Dennis, M. J., & Harris, A. J. The development of chemosensitivity in the extra-synaptic areas of the neuronal surface after denervation of parasympathetic ganglion cells in the heart of the frog. *Proceedings of the Royal Society, Series B*, 1971, **177**, 555–563.
Kuo, Z.-Y. *The dynamics of behavior development*. New York: Random House, 1967.
Lehrman, D. S. A critique of Konrad Lorenz's theory of instinctive behavior. *Quarterly Review of Biology*, 1953, **28**, 337–363.
McCouch, G. P., Austin, G. M., & Liu, C. Y. Sprouting as a cause of spasticity. *Journal of Neurophysiology*, 1958, **21**, 205–216.
Matthew, S. A., & Detwiler, S. R. The reaction of Amblystoma embryos following prolonged treatment with chloretone. *Journal of Experimental Zoology*, 1926, **45**, 279–292.
Model, P. G., Bornstein, M. B., Crain, S. M., & Pappas, G. D. An electron microscopic study of the development of synapses in cultured fetal mouse cerebrum continuously exposed to xylocaine. *Journal of Cell Biology*, 1971, **49**, 362–371.
Molliver, M. E. An ontogenetic study of evoked somesthetic cortical responses in the sheep. *Progress in Brain Research*, 1967. **26**, 78–91.
Molliver, M. E., & Van der Loos, H. The ontogenesis of cortical circuitry: The spatial distribution of synapses in somesthetic cortex of newborn dog. *Ergebnisse der Anatomie und Entwicklungsgeschichte*, 1970, **42**, 1–53.
Murray, M. R. Nervous tissues *in vitro*. In E. N. Willmer (Ed.), *Cells and tissues in culture*. London: Academic Press, 1965. Pp. 373–455.
Naka, K.-I. Electrophysiology of the fetal spinal cord. II. Interaction among peripheral inputs and recurrent inhibition. *Journal of General Physiology*, 1964, **47**, 1023–1038.
Nelson, P. G. Brain mechanisms and memory. In G. C. Quarton, T. Melnechuk, & F. O. Schmitt (Eds.), *The neurosciences: A study program*. New York: Rockefeller University Press, 1967. Pp. 772–775.
Oppenheim, R. W., & Foelix, R. F. Synaptogenesis in the chick embryo spinal cord. *Nature* (*London*) *New Biology*, 1972, **235**, 126–128.
Oppenheim, R. W., Reitzel, J., & Provine, R. The behavioral onset of inhibitory mechanisms in the chick embryo. *Society for Neuroscience, 2nd Annual Meeting, Houston*, 1972, Abstract, p. 91.
Pappas, G. D., Peterson, E. R., Masurovsky, E. B., & Crain, S. M. The fine structure of developing neuromuscular synapses *in vitro*. *Annals of the New York Academy of Sciences*, 1971, **183**, 33–45.
Paulson, G., & Gottlieb, G. Developmental reflexes: The reappearance of foetal and neonatal reflexes in aged patients. *Brain*, 1968, **91**, 37–52.
Peacock, J. H., Nelson, P. G., & Goldstone, M. Electrophysiologic study of cultured neurons dissociated from spinal cords and dorsal root ganglia of fetal mice. *Developmental Biology*, 1973, **30**, 137–152.
Peterson, E. R., & Crain, S. M. Innervation in cultures of fetal rodent skeletal muscle by organotypic explants of spinal cord from different animals. *Zeitschrift für Zellforschung und Mikroskopische Anatomie*, 1970, **106**, 1–21.
Peterson, E. R., & Crain, S. M. Regeneration and innervation in cultures of adult mammalian

skeletal muscle coupled with fetal rodent spinal cord. *Experimental Neurology*, 1972, **36**, 136–159.

Peterson, E. R., Crain, S. M., & Murray, M. R. Differentiation and prolonged maintenance of bioelectrically active spinal cord cultures (rat, chick and human). *Zeitschrift für Zellforschung und Mikroskopische Anatomie*, 1965, **66**, 130–154.

Pollack, E. D., & Crain, S. M. Development of motility in fish embryos in relation to release from early CNS inhibition. *Journal of Neurobiology*, 1972, **3**, 381–385.

Pollen, D. A., & Ajmone-Marsan, C. Cortical inhibitory postsynaptic potentials and strychninization. *Journal of Neurophysiology*, 1965, **28**, 342–358.

Pollen, D. A., & Lux, H. D. Conductance changes during inhibitory postsynaptic potentials in normal and strychninized cortical neurons. *Journal of Neurophysiology*, 1966, **29**, 369–381.

Provine, R. R. Embryonic spinal cord: synchrony and spatial distribution of polyneuronal burst discharges. *Brain Research*, 1971, **29**, 155–158.

Provine, R. R. Ontogeny of bioelectric activity in the spinal cord of the chick embryo and its behavioral implications. *Brain Research*, 1972, **41**, 365–378.

Purpura, D. P. Nature of electrocortical potentials and synaptic organization in the cerebral and cerebellar cortex. *International Review of Neurobiology*, 1959, **1**, 47–163.

Purpura, D. P., Stability and seizure susceptibility of immature brain. In H. H. Jasper, A. A. Ward, & A. Pope (Eds.), *Basic mechanisms of the epilepsies*. Boston: Little, Brown, 1969. Pp. 481–505.

Purpura, D. P., Synaptogenesis in mammalian cortex: problems and perspectives. In M. B. Sterman, D. J. McGinty, & A. M. Adinolfi (Eds.), *Brain development and behavior*. New York: Academic Press, 1971. Pp. 23–41.

Purpura, D. P. Ontogenetic models in studies of cortical seizure activities. In D. P. Purpura, J. K. Penry, D. Tower, D. M. Woodbury, & R. Walter (Eds.), *Experimental models of epilepsy*. New York: Raven, 1972. Pp. 531–556.

Purpura, D. P., Carmichael, M. W., & Housepian, E. M. Physiological and anatomical studies of development of superficial axodendritic synaptic pathways in neocortex. *Experimental Neurology*, 1960, **2**, 324–347.

Purpura, D. P., & Housepian, E. M. Morphological and physiological properties of chronically isolated immature neocortex. *Experimental Neurology*, 1961, **4**, 377–401.

Purpura, D. P., Prelevic, S., & Santini, M. Postsynaptic potentials and spike variations in the feline hippocampus during postnatal ontogenesis. *Experimental Neurology*, 1968, **22**, 408–422.

Purpura, D. P., Shofer, R. J., & Scarff, T. Properties of synaptic activities and spike potentials of neurons in immature neocortex. *Journal of Neurophysiology*, 1965, **28**, 925–942.

Ramón y Cajal, S. Degeneration and regeneration of the nervous system. Vol. 2. (Translated by R. M. May.) London: Oxford University Press, 1928.

Ripley, K. L., & Provine, R. R. Neural correlates of embryonic motility in the chick. *Brain Research*, 1972, **45**, 127–134.

Roberts, E. An hypothesis suggesting that there is a defect in the GABA system in schizophrenia. *Neurosciences Research Program Bulletin*, 1972, **10**, 468–482.

Schwartz, I. R., Pappas, G. D., & Purpura, D. P. Fine structure of neurons and synapses in the feline hippocampus during postnatal ontogenesis. *Experimental Neurology*, 1968, **22**, 394–407.

Skoglund, S. Growth and differentiation with special emphasis on the central nervous system. *Annual Review of Physiology*, 1969, **31**, 19–42.

Sperry, R. W. Embryogenesis of behavioral nerve nets. In R. L. De Haan & H. Ursprung (Eds.), *Organogenesis*. New York: Holt, 1965. Pp. 161–186.

Sperry, R. W. How a developing brain gets itself properly wired for adaptive function. In E. Tobach, L. R. Aronson, & E. Shaw (Eds.), *Biopsychology of development*. New York: Academic Press, 1971. Pp. 27–44.

Sperry, R. W., & Hibbard, E. Regulative factors in the orderly growth of retinotectal connexions. In G. E. W. Wolstenholme & M. O'Connor (Eds.), *Ciba foundation Symposium, Growth of the nervous system*. London: Churchill, 1968. Pp. 41–52.

Stavraky, G. W. *Supersensitivity following lesions of the nervous system*. Toronto: University of Toronto Press, 1961.

Stefanis, C., & Jasper, H. Strychnine reversal of inhibitory potentials in pyramidal tract neurons. *International Journal of Neuropharmacology*, 1965, **4**, 125–138.

Székely, G. Embryonic determination of neural connections. *Advances in Morphogenesis*, 1966, **5**, 181–129.

Tinbergen, N. The hierarchical organization of nervous mechanisms underlying instinctive behavior. *Symposium of the Society for Experimental Biology*, 1950, **4**, 305–312.

Tracy, H. C. Development of motility and behavior reactions in the toadfish. *Journal of Comparative Neurology*, 1926, **40**, 253–369.

Weiss, P., & Edds, M. V. Spontaneous recovery of muscle following partial denervation. *American Journal of Physiology*, 1946, **145**, 587–607.

Werman, R., Davidoff, R. A., & Aprison, M. H. Inhibitory action of glycine on spinal neurons in the cat. *Journal of Neurophysiology*, 1968, **31**, 81–95.

Windle, W. F. Correlation between the development of local reflexes and reflex arcs in the spinal cord of cat embryos. *Journal of Comparative Neurology*, 1934, **59**, 487–505.

Young, J. Z. *A model of the brain*. London: Oxford University Press (Clarendon), 1964.

Young, J. Z. *The memory system of the brain*. Berkeley: University of California Press, 1966.

Zipser, B., Crain, S. M., & Bornstein, M. B. Intracellular recordings of complex synaptically mediated discharges in explants of fetal hippocampal cortex during maturation in culture. *Federation Proceedings, Federation of American Societies for Experimental Biology*, 1973, **32**, 420.

Addenda

Intracellular recordings from explants of fetal mouse hippocampal cortex have recently demonstrated characteristic sequences of excitatory and inhibitory postsynaptic potentials during generation of organotypic patterned oscillatory discharges in long-term cultures (Zipser, Crain and Bornstein, 1973; *cf.* p. 75).

A disinhibition hypothesis similar to the material on p. 100 oriented primarily on the adult CNS was recently proposed by Roberts (1972) and provides further support for the views expressed in this manuscript (pp. 97–102). It was prepared for the Symposium on Prenatal Ontogeny of Behavior and the Nervous System in December 1971. On the basis of extensive neurochemical and pharmacologic studies of inhibitory systems in adult CNS, Roberts (1972) suggests that "in behavioral sequences, innate or learned, genetically preprogrammed circuits are released to function at varying rates and in various combinations by inhibition of neurons that are tonically holding command neurons in check. The activity of such circuits would be regulated by neurons exerting tonic inhibitory effects on the command neurons. . . . The successful operation of [such] a nervous system . . . requires a coordination of neural activity that can determine from birth, *or even before*, the ability of an individual to prevent the too-frequent firing of preprogrammed circuits of behavioral options spontaneously or maladaptively. . . . (italics added) [pp. 468–475]."

PROBLEMS OF NEURONAL SPECIFICITY IN THE DEVELOPMENT OF SOME BEHAVIORAL PATTERNS IN AMPHIBIA

GEORGE SZÉKELY

Department of Anatomy
University Medical School
Pécs, Hungary

I. Introduction

A current effort in neurological research is to try to find the structural background of neural activities. Due to our ignorance concerning the delicate architecture of the central nervous system, one is often compelled to look at the nerve center under investigation as a black box with a wiring diagram known only fragmentarily. It is rather hazardous to complete the wiring diagram on the basis of the input–output relationship of the black box. Nevertheless, such efforts may result in nicely constructed conceptual nervous systems and attractive interpretations of the animal's behavior. Once the concept is stated, a number of experiments can be devised, which, up to a certain point, may support the idea unambiguously. The numerous biological "facts" obtained from experiments, then, are liable to turn the concept itself into a "fact," and it is not always easy to infer from the haze of data whether or not the kind of nervous system envisaged does exist.

Nevertheless, in the course of experiments the central nervous system may be interrogated in a number of different ways, and the answer it gives depends very much on how the question is posed. To the question of whether specific interconnections governed by mutual chemoaffinity of like neurons may account for an observed neural activity, the answer will, very probably, be yes. If, on the other hand, the question is put more searchingly and one asks whether specific interconnections sufficiently account for the animal's behavior under investigation, the answer may, quite conceivably, suggest neural mechanisms other than the biochemical specificity of neurons. In this presentation I shall try to direct the inquiry toward three phenomena that are known in the literature as (1) the corneal specificity, (2) the cutaneous local sign specificity, and (3) the myotypic specificity, or "homologous muscle response" phenomenon.

II. Corneal Specificity

In a famous experiment Weiss (1942) grafted an eye into the place of the otic capsule in newt larvae. After metamorphosis a regular lid closure (corneal) reflex could be elicited in the ipsilateral eye of the host by tactile stimulation of the grafted cornea. The interpretation of the phenomenon was that the corneal tissue differs, probably in its biochemical nature, from the surrounding skin tissue. These differential properties were imparted to the sensory neurons which, in turn, changed their central connections to establish synapses with central nerve cells of matching properties. Thus, an appropriate reflex chain developed to evoke the corneal reflex from the wrong place. The result was corroborated in other experiments (Kollros, 1943; Székely, 1959), in which the eye was grafted into the caudal head region (Fig. la), and it has been regarded as a model experiment in verifying the "organ-specific modulation" of sensory neurons by the periphery. It is clear that the concept presupposes a series of specific synaptic linkages involving a chain of highly specified sensory neurons, interneurons, and motor neurons.

The corneal reflex consists of eye withdrawal and passive closure of the eye lids in amphibia. In development the first appearance of the reflex coincides in time with the maturation of the effector side: the abducens nucleus and the retractor muscles of the eye ball (Kollros, 1943; Weiss, 1942). This occurs a few days before metamorphosis, and the reflex can be evoked at relatively high threshold from the cornea at that time. Later the threshold decreases and the reflexogenic area expands, covering a region from the snout to the ear capsule at metamorphic climax. In adult urodeles the area shrinks slightly, and the ear zone is normally insensitive in evoking the corneal reflex. This area corresponds roughly to the sensory field of the ophthalmic division of the trigeminal nerve. In underfed urodele larvae, however, the reflex appears in smaller animals, though later in time than during normal development, and the reflexogenic area expands as far caudal as the base of the gills, involving a skin area supplied by the sensory fibers of the vagus nerve. The expanded reflexogenic area persists in the adult. In addition to some vaguely defined head jerks and general escaping movements, the only reflex which can be invariably elicited from the head region is the closure of the eye lids in urodeles. In anura a wiping reflex of the forelimb can also be evoked from the same reflexogenic area.

The center for the corneal reflex is not precisely known. Kornacker (1963) investigated the synaptic activity in the medulla of the frog following local stimulation of the head. He came to the conclusion that the afferent limb of the corneal reflex consists of small diameter sensory fibers, which terminate laterally to the larger diameter fibers in the region of the descending trigeminal nucleus, directly on the remote dendrites of the abducens motor neurons. The supposition that the corneal reflex is mediated through a monosynaptic pathway is not very likely for the following reasons. First, in the frog's spinal cord cutaneous sensory fibers appear to establish only polysynaptic connections with motor neurons (Simpson, 1969). Second, monosynaptic activation of spinal motor neurons occurs through the fast conducting (large diameter) sensory fibers in the frog (Czéh & Székely, 1971a), suggesting the involvoment of muscle afferents. Third, Kornacker's calculations for a monosynaptic pathway is based on the extracellularly recorded motor response to snout nerve stimulation, which activates primarily the large diameter sensory fibers. The conduction velocity of larger fibers comfortably allows for a polysynaptic pathway, and his data give no information concerning motor activation when small diameter fibers only are stimulated. Fourth, the presence of a wiping reflex, which can be elicited from the same reflexogenic area, is also suggestive of a more complicated reflex center. The afferent limb for the wiping reflex runs in the descending trigeminal tract and releases the reflex from the second spinal cord segment. The wiping reflex normally appears at higher threshold, but in mesencephalic animals it can be evoked with the same stimulus strength as the corneal reflex. The two reflexes can be separated by graded barbitural anesthesia to which the corneal reflex is less sensitive (Kornacker, 1963). For these reasons it is safer to conclude that the center for the corneal reflex corresponds in extension to the descending trigeminal nucleus, probably with a strong involvement of the reticular formation neurons within this region. This localization would agree with that experienced in human pathology.

This center is certainly more complex than could be described unambiguously with the blueprint of a two- or three-neuron reflex arc. Furthermore, whether the response is a lid closure alone or is associated with the wiping reflex, head jerks, and perhaps general escaping reactions depends on the stimulus strength. This phenomenon is called reflex irradiation in the Sherringtonian reflexology, and it is one of the characteristic properties of the so-called withdrawal reflexes of the spinal cord. In fact, the corneal reflex may be looked upon as a typical withdrawal reflex which appears first in response to nociceptive stimuli, since the cornea is the most sensitive part of the head. Another feature of withdrawal reflexes is that the excitatory state of the reflex center influences both the threshold of the response and the size of the area from which it can be evoked. If the skin were wounded at the edge of the reflexogenic area, the threshold should be lowered, and the area evoking the reflex in Ambystoma should expand. As a matter of fact, in his original paper Weiss (1942) has offered this alternative interpretation, but it was ruled out since the corneal reflex could be elicited from the grafted cornea several months after operation. The increase in quantity of afferent inflow resulting from the stimulation of a certain locus may be regarded as equivalent in its effect with that of increasing the central excitatory state. This can easily be achieved by transplanting an extra eye within, or outside of, the reflexogenic area. On the basis of Detwiller's (1936) experiments, it can reasonably be assumed that the growing eye graft in the head of the larva attracts sensory fibers from the surroundings. The fiber terminals are more exposed in the corneal epithelium than in the surrounding skin, and the increased amount of afferent impulses to the stimulation of the grafted cornea results in a lower threshold and an expanded reflexogenic area. This train of speculation, taken together with the assumption that a relatively larger number of sensory fibers supplied the smaller head of these animals, could account for the expanded reflexogenic area of underfed Ambystoma larvae in Kollros' (1943) experiment. In this case, as well as the case of an extra eye grafted in the caudal head region, the sensory fibers emerge from the vagus nerve; nevertheless, their central processes terminate in the descending trigeminal nucleus, in other words, in the same reflex center as those of the ophthalmic nerve.

The first answer the nervous system gives is that the corneal reflex is very probably a threshold phenomenon, and it may not be a perequisite to graft an organ of specific character in order to evoke the reflex from an abnormal place. This answer is based on an number of assumptions, but the following experiment will provide some support. If a limb is grafted into the caudal part of the head in newt larvae, and a regeneration blastema is produced by amputating the foot of the grafted limb at about metamorphosis, a corneal reflex can be elicited from the blastema with approximately the same stimulus strength as that from a grafted cornea (Fig. 1b). As regeneration proceeds, the threshold increases, and with complete regeneration of the foot the area is no longer effective in evoking the reflex. Reamputation of the foot enables a blink reflex to be elicited again from the new blastema. As the animal grows

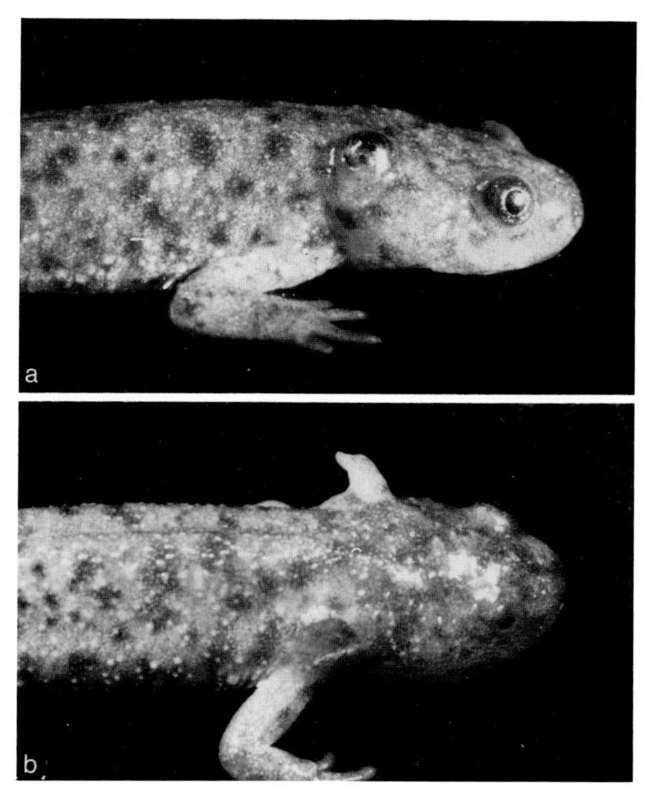

FIG. 1. *Pleurodeles waltlii*. In (a) a supernumerary eye, and in (b) a limb is grafted into the caudal region of the head. The limb bears a regeneration blastema. Both grafts are innervated by the sensory fibers of the vagal nerve, and mechanical stimulation of both the grafted cornea and the regeneration blastema results in a corneal reflex of the ipsilateral normal eye.

older, the resulting new blastema remains ineffective, and this time (2–3 months after metamorphosis) coincides with the incapability of the blastema to rebuild a new foot (Székely, 1959). It is obvious that the blastema and the cornea do not share the same biochemical specificity; nevertheless the type of their innervation seems to be identical. It is known that the corneal epithelium is innervated by an abundance of free nerve terminals which emerge from a rich nervous plexus underneath the epithelial layer, and Hay (1960) was able to show similar nerve terminations in the regeneration blastema. In a series of experiments, Singer (1952) has shown that nerve fibers invade the epidermis of a blastema in considerably greater numbers than are observed in normal skin, and a critical density of innervation is required to complete the regeneration of a limb in urodeles. The coincidence of the incapability of the blastema to regenerate the foot with the lack of reappearance of the blink reflex strongly suggests that a critical ammount of sensory impulses must be sent into the center to evoke a blink from an abnormal place, be this a grafted eye or a blastema, or remote skin of an unusually small head of an underfed animal.

A variety of interpretations may be given to these observations. To regard the corneal reflex merely as a threshold phenomenon would oversimplify the problem. The limb skin adjacent to the blastema, and the regenerated foot, both with the same "critical amount" of innervation, are ineffective in evoking the corneal reflex. Another alternative which may be considered is that nerve impulses generated by terminals of a low grade of differentiation have a tendency of spreading in the center, and if they are released in a sufficient quantity, they may manage to reach the abducens nucleus even from the vagal sensory area. A more pretentious interpretation, however, not mutually exclusive with the former from a quantitative point of view, would be that similar cues may be coded into sensory messages generated by similar types of nerve terminals, and that the center posseses the ability to dispatch the similar messages to the same motor neurons. The next section will dwell on this latter neural mechanism in somewhat more detail. Either way, the only safe conclusion we may draw is that these experiments, in their present state, do not yield any reliable information concerning synaptic events in the central nervous system.

III. Cutaneous Local Sign Specificity

The frog wipes its back with the hindlimb and its belly with the forelimb to remove an unpleasant stimulus from the skin. This is called the wiping reflex and is controlled by the spinal cord. A spinal or a mesencephalic frog discloses the reflex more readily than an intact frog. The animal, therefore, does not learn how to locate the site of a stimulus, but this capability is apparently built in to the structure of the spinal cord, presumably in the form of specific reflex arcs. To explain the development of these and similar specific reflex arcs, Sperry (1951) has put forward the idea of cutaneous local sign specificity. The fundamental implication of the idea is that the integument undergoes a refined differentiation in the course of development, with a resulting distinction of any one point of the skin from the others on the basis of a biochemical or physicochemical specificity. This differential specificity is supposed to be fieldlike in nature and at least biaxial in dimension. In these fields the specificity is envisaged as a quantitative gradient along each axis, but these quantitative gradients differ qualilatively from each other along their separate axes. Thus, the coordinates of an anteroposterior and a dorsoventral field define any given point of the skin in the trunk region. These specific local skin properties are then stamped upon the sensory nerves innervating different skin areas, and the sensory fibers become specified by the periphery. In the center a similar process of specification takes place, and the neurons become specified according to their positions within the neural axis. The subsequent establishment of central synaptic patterns is determined by the mutual chemoaffinity between specified sensory fibers and matching neurons. We may note that the local sign specificity is actually a more sophisticated version of the theory of "organ-specific modulation" of neurons mentioned in the previous section.

To test Sperry's idea on the wiping reflex, Miner (1956) cut out a transverse strip of skin reaching from the midline down to the belly in tadpoles (*Rana pipiens*), and reimplanted it with a 180° rotation. The white belly skin developed on the back and the darkly pigmented dorsal skin on the belly. After metamorphosis the frogs produced misdirected reflexes: they wiped on the belly upon stimulation of the dorsally placed belly skin, and the wiping was aimed at the back when the dorsal skin was stimulated on the belly. Recently, Jacobson and Baker (1969) repeated these experiments and recorded the same erroneous reflexes. They could also show a normal pattern in the peripheral innervation of the rotated skin. These results appear to support unequivocally the idea of local sign specificity.

Jacobson and Baker (1969; Baker & Jacobson, 1970) have extended Miner's experiments in many other respects. Investigating its development, the first normal wiping reflex appears at stage XX of Taylor and Kollros (1946), that is, about the beginning of metamorphosis. It consists of forelimb wiping aimed at stimulation sites on the head. Within about 4–5 days, the full complement of wiping reflexes develops. An important finding made by these authors is that the skin has to be rotated prior to stage XV (that is, about 12 days before stage XX) in order to obtain misdirected reflexes from the graft. In about one half of the animals the first responses are normal. The misdirected reflexes appear a few days later, first in small spots of the rotated skin. These initially small reflexogenic areas for erroneous responses gradually expand and cover most of the graft's surface. Usually, normal reflexes can be evoked from the edges of the graft, and the marginal strip giving normal reflexes is wider in animals with smaller skin grafts. Small patches of interchanged back and belly skin invariably give normal reflexes. Similarly, animals with a strip of back skin rotated 180° in the anteroposterior axis wipe correctly on the site of stimulation. Two more observations seem to be pertinent along with the above data. Jacobson and Baker (1969) rerotated the skin graft which gave previously misdirected reflexes in nine young frogs. Four of them showed normal reflexes only, and five retained the former erroneous reflex pattern from the rerotated graft. In a separate series of experiments, Baker (1970) performed the same back-to-belly skin rotation experiment on two other anuran species (*R. catesbiana* and *R. clamitans*), and in both cases the animals disclosed normal reflexes from the rotated skin area.

If we try to interpret all these data in Sperry's terminology, a number of conflicts emerge. Some of these may be pointed out. (*a*) It was unequivocally stated that the skin rotation must be done prior to stage XV in order to observe maladaptive responses, yet half of the juvenile frogs with rerotated skin exhibited normal reflexes. This implies that the tadpole's skin loses the capacity to modulate sensory nerves in the last third of the larval period, but the frog's skin resumes this capacity to a certain extent, after metamorphosis. If this were so, then one half of the tadpoles operated upon later than stage XV ought to have shown misdirected reflexes, but they did not. (*b*) Baker's finding that in two other frog species reversed reflexes did not accompany the skin reversal is relevant to this problem. He proposed three alternatives to account for the results. First, cutaneous specification might have occurred in these species earlier in development than in *R. pipiens*. From a general embryological point of view this is not very likely, since both *R. clamitans* and *R. catesbiana* have a longer larval period, and one would expect prolonged differentiation processes. Second, the maladaptive behavior might have appeared later in a postmetamorphic age. He tested his animals for 3 months after metamorphosis and found exclusively normal reflexes. Third, the misdirected reflexes may be a species-specific occurrence confined to *R. pipiens*. This would imply that the spinal cord of the other two species must elaborate the wiping reflexes all by itself. The fact that the marginal strip of a skin graft usually gave normal reflexes led Miner (1956) to the conclusion that nerves which innervated the normal skin and also invaded the graft were responsible for this effect. A cut made around the grafted skin greatly abolished the normal responses. Jacobson and Baker's (1969) experiment, on the other hand, clearly indicates that nerves from the normal skin did not invade the graft, and the receptive fields of individual skin nerves met and abutted at the graft edges in the case of back-to-belly inverted skin (cf. Fig. 4 of Jacobson & Baker, 1969). There seems to be a contradiction between the two findings, and the neuronal specificity theory does not offer any help in resolving the discrepancy. Furthermore, the observation that the marginal strip for normal reflexes is wider in animals with smaller skin grafts cannot be accounted for on the basis of neuronal specificity. A possible supposition, that some agent(s) of the skin responsible for synaptic rearrangements in the center can diffuse easier into a small graft than into a large one, would predict that initially narrow marginal strips would widen with time. However, just the reverse happens in Jacobson and Baker's experiment. The marginal strips for normal reflexes and the inefficacy of small interchanged back and belly patches are suggestive of a quantitative factor in the sense that a critical size of the rotated skin surface, or in other words, a critical number of sensory fibers, is required to convey the peripheral message to the center in order to evoke misdirected responses. Here we suggest an interpretation of nervous function similar to that made in the previous section. (*c*) The normal reflexes invariably shown by animals with a strip of back skin rotated 180° in the anteroposterior direction would imply, in Sperry's terminology, that the anteroposterior axis does not really exist in the specific field gradients of the integument. Cues for the anteroposterior position of any skin area may be attributed to the anatomy of sensory nerves in the sense that they carry peripheral information into their corresponding spinal segments. Here we would have a system in which the "longitude" (the anteroposterior axis) of a point is defined by a conventional neural mechanism, and the "latitude" (the dorsoventral axis) by the specificity of the skin. One can go a step further and ask whether a neural mechanism other than neuronal specificity could not account for the latitude location as well. We shall see later that this can be done.

These data confronted in the above manner confuse rather than disentangle the problems of misdirected wiping reflexes. In his masterfully written book, Gaze (1970) discusses the shortcomings of the neuronal specificity theory and offers an alternative interpretation involving peripheral as well as central specification of connections of cutaneous sensory nerves. Starting from the histogenetic degeneration that occurs in the spinal ganglia of Xenopus larvae through stages 53–59 (Prestige, 1965), a time span which roughly corresponds to stages VII–XVII in *R. pipiens*, he proposes a selective connection of the sensory fibers with the periphery. Cells are produced in a large excess in the spinal ganglia, and those which fail to connect with the skin or terminate in the wrong place, degenerate. If the skin is replanted with reversed dorsoventral axis, most of the nerve fibers regenerate obviously into the wrong place, and they perish. New fibers grow out, of the large excess of reserve cells and those arriving at the correct place survive. It may be noted that this interpretation presupposes that both the central and peripheral processes of sensory neurons are predestined for their terminal sites. The idea is rather attractive, for the period of cell turnover coincides in time with the period of successful skin rotation. Yet the following experiment refutes the general validity of this interpretation and adds to the confusion.

The experiments were performed on tadpoles of the European species *R. esculenta*. They react much in the same way to skin rotation as do those of *R. pipiens*: they develop misdirected wiping reflexes. In the adult frog the cutaneous nerves emerge from the trunk spinal nerves at four levels in the dorsoventral direction, and they innervate four more or less distinct stripes of the skin (Fig. 2.). From the area innervated by nerves 1 and 2, wiping reflexes aimed at the back can be evoked. Stimulation of the area of

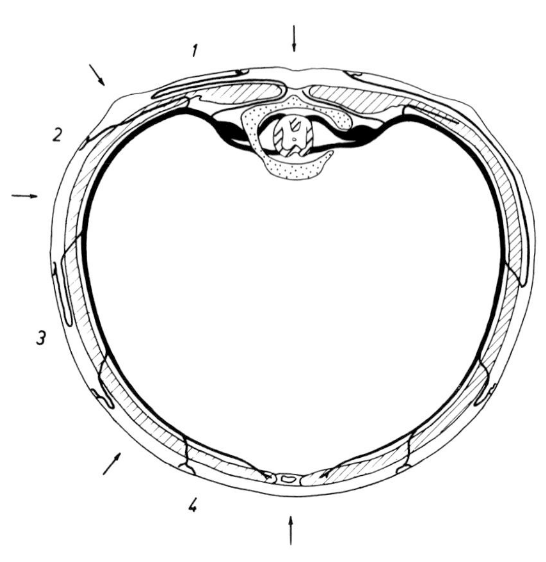

FIG. 2. Schematic representation of the cutaneous nerves in the trunk region of the frog. The left side shows the normal arrangement. Arrows indicate the border of skin areas innervated by nerves 1, 2, 3, and 4, respectively. Note that area 3 is supplied by two nerves, the lower one of which is the *deep* nerve 3. On the right side the nerve crossunion 3—1 is shown; the distal end of nerve 3 is sutured to nerve 1. For technical reasons, nerve 2 was cut out during the operation.

nerve 3 gives rise to wiping on the side, and if the area of nerve 4 is stimulated, the animal rubs the belly either with fore- or hindlimb, depending on whether the stimulus is applied to the belly cranially or caudally (Fig. 3.).

Nerves 1 and 3 are sufficiently long to permit crossunions of two different kinds in adult frogs. In the first experimental group the distal ends of each nerve 3 of spinal segments V, VI, and VII were separated from the skin and sutured to each nerve 1, which had been cut at the site of emergence from the dorsal musculature (3–1 crossunion). For technical reasons nerve 2 was cut also. Since the fascia closed quickly over the proximal stumps of the cut nerves, regeneration of nerves 1 and 2 did not occur. However, the regenerating fibers of nerve 3 were guided by the distal stumps of nerve 1 to the back skin (right side of Fig. 2). The animals were tested 3–5 months after operation. Most of the skin area innervated now by nerve 3 gave correct wiping reflexes, as if nerve 3 had become "respecified" by the dorsal skin in adult frogs. In many animals the spinal nerve of segment VI, and sometimes that of segment V, gave origin to a second (deep) cutaneous nerve 3 which, being attached to the skin more ventrally, escaped detection at the time of operation. From the receptive area of deep nerve 3, both correctly aimed and misdirected reflexes could be evoked. The latter consisted of wiping on the belly either with the hindlimb, or more frequently with

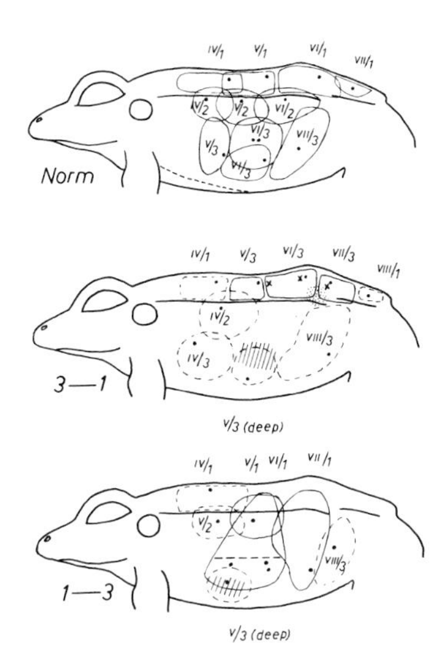

FIG. 3. Receptive fields of sensory nerves in normal and in operated animals. Roman numerals refer to the segmental origin, and Arabic numerals to the dorsoventral sequence of the nerves. Dots indicate the points at which the nerves enter the skin. On the top, a normal animal is shown. Note the receptive field of the deep nerve VI/3. The broken lines demarcate the belly skin area from which forelimb reflexes can be evoked. In the middle a representative case of the 3—1 nerve crossunion is shown. The operation was made at the V, VI, and VII segmental level. Receptive fields of nerves V/3, VI/3 and VII/3, respectively, are delinated by solid lines on the back skin. Dashed lines demarcate the receptive fields of the adjacent intact nerves. The cross-marks and the dotted area on the back skin indicate places from which misdirected reflexes (wiping on the side) could be evoked. From the hatched area within the receptive field of deep nerve V/3, belly wipings with the forelimb could be elicited. Otherwise, the reflexes were found to be normal. No nerves to the empty area in the middle were found, although this area gave normal reflexes to strong electrical stimuli. On the bottom, a 1—3 nerve crossunion is represented. Nerve V/1 grew into the place of the nerve VI/2 which was cut out at operation, and nerve VI/1 invaded the distal stumps of nerves V/3 and VI/3. Note the large receptive fields of nerves VI/1 and VII/1. From the area above the dashed line in the field of nerve VI/1, back wipings were evoked. Under this line, and anywhere else, the reflexes were correctly aimed, with the exception of the hatched area from which forelimb reflexes could occasionally be elicited. The median strip of the back skin (empty) was innervated by contralateral nerves 1, and contralateral reflexes aimed at the corresponding contralateral points could be evoked from this area.

the forelimb. It could frequently be observed that following a single stimulus the frog wiped first on the place of stimulation with the hindlimb, then vigorously rubbed the belly with the forelimb. Detaching nerve 4 from the skin did not abolish the misdirected reflexes. If the tests were performed carefully on mesencephalic animals, tiny spots or small areas could be found on the back skin innervated by nerve 3, from which the animal produced a reflex aimed at the side, that is, the reflex corresponded to the original function of the innervating nerve. Usually, the larger the receptive field of the intact deep nerve 3, the larger were the areas for misdirected reflexes, and occasionally one or two belly wipings could also be evoked from such spots of the back skin.

The results of the second group, in which the distal ends of nerve 1 were sutured to nerve 3 (1–3 crossunion), were not as conclusive. As the investigation of the receptive fields indicated, the regenerating fibers invaded the areas of innervation of nerves 3, 2, and 1. From the darkly pigmented skin the animals invariably wiped on the back, from the transitory zone between the darkly pigmented and the white belly skin, the reflex was aimed at the site of the stimulus. If the deep nerve 3 was present, belly wipings could also be evoked from its receptive field, though not as frequently as in the former group. Misregeneration and collateral sproutings were checked by careful dissection and by establishment of the receptive fields of both the crossunited and the neighboring intact nerves.

It seems almost hopeless to try to interpret these observations on the basis of the neuronal specificity theory. We shall try, rather, to look into the spinal cord and present an alternative explanation for "recognition" of local sign in the skin, based on the geometry of the dorsal horn and on impulse pattern transmission. The receiving zone for primary afferent fibers in the spinal cord is the dorsal part of the dorsal horn, more precisely laminae I, II, and III of Rexed (1952), which incorporate the area commonly called the substantia gelatinosa (SG). Unfortunately, almost nothing is known of this part of the frog's spinal cord. However a considerable body of work was done recently on the cat's spinal cord (Ralston, 1968; Scheibel & Scheibel, 1968; Szentágothai, 1964), which reveals the complexity of this neural structure. We may use these data to get an impression of the intricacy of sensory information processing right in the first relay station. In doing so, we have to keep in mind that a frog is obviously not a cat; nevertheless fundamental differences in the structure of the spinal cord would not be expected between these two remote species.

As shown in the left side of Fig. 4, laminae II and III consist of small neurons with rich dendritic arborizations which are quite narrow in the mediolateral direction, but expand considerably in the sagittal plane. Their axons enter the Lissauer tract, and run a distance of one to four segments giving off several collaterals to the same laminae. The neurons are arranged in columns and are so closely packed that Scheibel and Scheibel's (1968) estimation of all number runs up to 250–300 cells/$10^6 \mu^3$. The output elements of this self-contained system are provided by the neurons of laminae IV. They are moderately large cells whose dendrites penetrate the entire depth of the SG radially and cover a conic area with the apex pointing at the cell body. This system receives a double input from the dorsal root. *Coarse cutaneous sensory fibers* which enter the dorsal fasciculus send collaterals to the base of layer III. The preterminal parts of their collaterals break up into rich, flame-shaped arbors which penetrate the SG in radially oriented columns, and extend for several hundred micra in the longitudinal direction with a restricted lateral expansion. With the dendritic arborization of cells in laminae II and III they form continuous sheets of neuropil in the sagittal plane, but the adjacent sheets are separated from each other in the transversal plane (right side of Fig. 4).

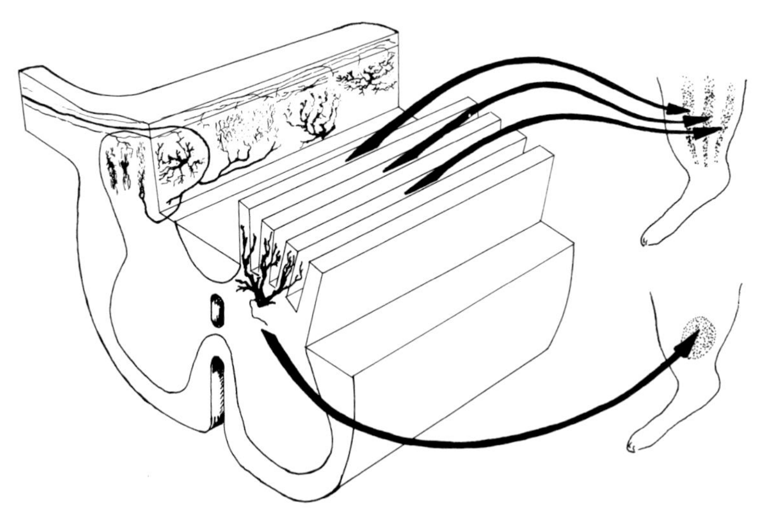

FIG. 4. Diagrammatic representation of the structure of the substantia gelatinosa, the gelatinosal neuropil sheets, and the postulated cutaneous sensory field of a lamina IV neuron. On the left side, a dorsal root is shown through which a thick and two thin sensory fibers enter the cord. The thick fiber terminates in a "flame-shaped" end formation, which is shown in cross section in the transverse plane, and in longitudinal section in the longitudinal plane of the block diagram. The thin fibers travel in the Lissauer tract and give off collaterals to lamina II. In the transversal plane two, and in the longitudinal plane, three neurons represent the neuronal population of laminae II and III. Their axons enter the Lissauer tract (shown with the last neuron), and the collaterals recur to the same laminae. The dendritic arborizations of these neurons and the terminals of the sensory fibers constitute the neuropil sheets. The neuron at the deepest level of the longitudinal plane represents the longitudinal dendritic arborization of a lamina IV neuron. On the right side the dorsal part of the white matter is removed, and the four longitudinal crests symbolize four neuropil sheets. In the transverse plane the dendrites of a lamina IV neuron penetrate three neuropil sheets. On the extreme right three arrows point to three dotted stripes on a cat's leg, and these stripes are presumed to have a primary central representation as linear continua along the corresponding neuropil sheets. The lamina IV neuron with its conically shaped dendritic domain samples the sensory input from these three neuropil sheets. Hence the neuron represents a small closed field in the periphery (right lower corner). Redrawn from Figs. 14 and 15 of Scheibel and Scheibel (1968).

The *fine cutaneous sensory fibers* enter the Lissauer tract, where they divide into ascending and descending branches spanning over a distance of five to six segments. Preterminal fibers penetrate the SG from the main branches and terminate in lamina II with dense endarborizations which cap the dorsal margins of the longitudinal neuropil sheets. In electron micrographs numerous complex synaptic formations and axoaxonic engagements, the assumed structural substrate for presynaptic inhibition, can be seen, especially in the dorsal part of the neuropil sheets (Ralston, 1968; Réthelyi & Szentágothai, 1969). There are several other interesting structural features of the SG, for which the reader is referred to the original articles. A resourceful functional conjecture proposed by Scheibel and Scheibel (1968) on this structure may be mentioned here. If each neuropil sheet represents a linear sensory continuum of some portion of the skin surface, then the lamina IV neurons penetrating a number of adjacent neuropil sheets collect information from a small closed area of the skin (Fig. 4).

Returning to the frog and looking for similarities in the structure of the two (cat and frog) spinal cords, one is troubled by the scarcity of data on the latter animal. The presence of the structure homologous to the mammalian SG is well established in the frog (Joseph & Whitlock, 1968; Kennard, 1959; Ramón y Cajal, 1909; Silver, 1942). Electron microscope studies in progress in this department are suggestive of similar complex synaptic organizations in this part of the frog's spinal cord, as described for the cat. The projection of small diameter fibers to a well-localized area capping the dorsal horn has already been described by Ramón y Cajal (1909). In our prelimminary investigation tracing degeneration after dorsal root section with the Fink-Heimer method, we found the distribution of degenerated terminals in the SG to be very similar to that described by Szentágothai (1964) in the cat, which suggests a similar terminal arborization of the cutaneous afferents. The bifurcating dorsal root fibers encompass as many as eight to nine segments in *R. pipiens* (Liu & Chambers, 1957), and five to six segments in *R. catesbiana* and *Bufo marinus* (Joseph & Whitlock, 1968). A marked difference between the two spinal cords is that primary afferent fibers do not reach the ventral horn in the frog (Joseph & Whitlock, 1968 and our material), and the motor neuron dendrites, on the other hand, extend up to the dorsal surface of the cord (Sala y Pons, 1892) and presumably receive monosynaptic activation only from muscle afferents (Czéh & Székely, 1971a; Simpson, 1969). It seems reasonable to assume, as a working hypothesis, that the frog's spinal cord is basically similar to the cat's cord.

Let us try to account first for the normal development of the central connections of cutaneous fibers. The trunk skin is innervated by the sensory fibers of spinal nerves III to VII. According to their anatomical positions, the majority of the cutaneous afferents terminate in the gelatinosal neuropil sheets of the corresponding segments, but in gradually decreasing number they reach the region of the hindlimb and forelimb segments as well. Information fed into the longitudinal continuum of the neuropil sheets is processed and sampled by neurons of the subjacent layers in the manner suggested by Scheibel and Scheibel's diagram (Fig. 4). The lamina IV neurons transmit the information to lamine V and VI (Wall, 1966), and the strict geometry of these latter neurons emphasized by Scheibel and Scheibel (1968) is suggestive of further processing before information passes these laminae. Depending finally on the segmental location where all these neural events take place, the appropriate motor pattern will be molded by similar information processing of interneurons and motor neurons in the ventral horn to indicate the craniocaudal position of the cutaneous stimulus. This mechanism would replace Sperry's anteroposterior gradient field of chemospecificity.

A similar argument can be made with respect to the local sign along the dorsoventral axis. It is known that the dorsoventral sequence of a dermatome projects in a lateromedial order on the SG (Szentágothai & Kiss, 1949). An observation made on lizard embryos (Szentágothai & Székely, 1956) suggests that mechanical factors play an essential role in the development of this dermatomal projection. At early stages of development the bipolar sensory neuroblasts are more or less segregated into two groups according to the orientation of their longitudinal axes. Those which send the peripheral process into the dorsal ramus of the spinal nerve (and thus innervate the back skin) assume a horizontal orientation, and those which innervate the belly skin via the ventral ramus are oriented with their long axes close to the vertical plane. As a consequence of this orientation, the dorsal root fibers decussate at the entrance to the spinal cord, and fibers innervating the back skin hit the ventral part, while fibers from the belly skin terminate in the dorsal part of the SG, which occupies a vertical position at this stage of development (Fig. 5). Later as the dorsal and lateral funiculi develop, the SG turns in the horizontal plane with the original ventral edge pointing laterally; hence the lateromedial representation of the dorsoventral axis of a dermatome in the SG. The decussation of the primary afferent fibers has been observed since in chicken and frog embryos as well.

Assuming a similar projection of cutaneous fields on the SG in the frog, the dorsoventral localization of stimulus points can be envisaged in the manner suggested by Fig. 6. In the scheme an extensive overlap is supposed to exist in the projection of neighboring cutaneous nerves. This is not justified in view of Scheibel and Scheibel's (1968) finding in the lumbosacral enlargement of the cord, where the transverse discreteness of the neuropil sheets is the most pronounced. However, these sheets merge into a more

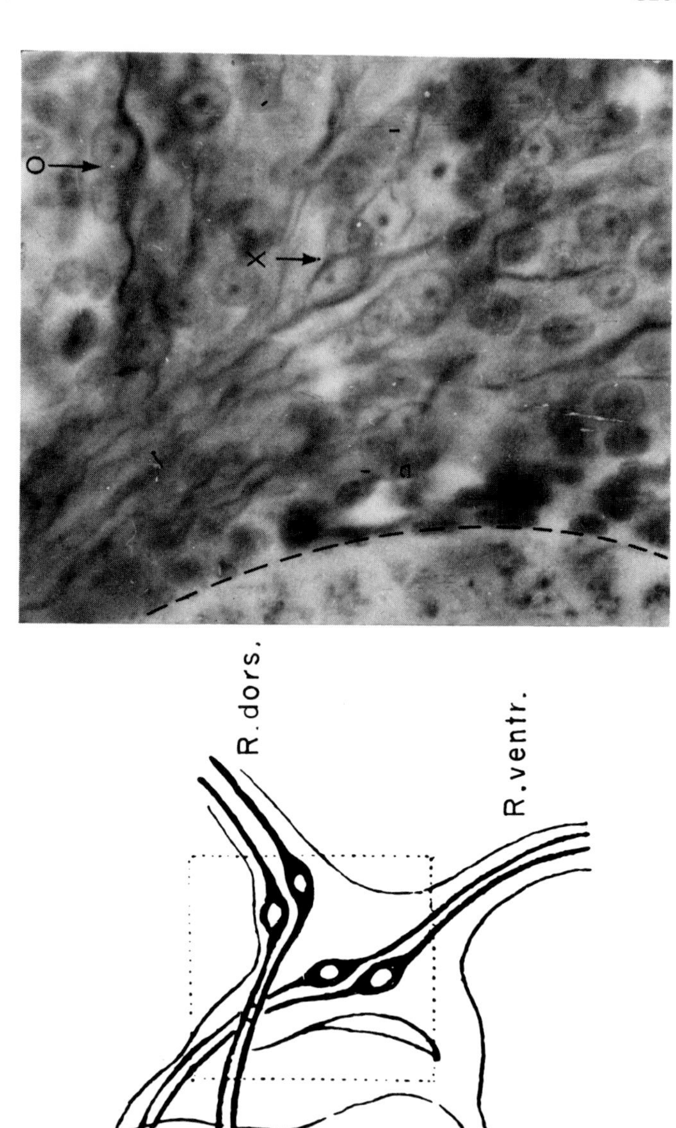

FIG. 5. Diagrammatic and photographic representation of decussating dorsal root fibers in the lizard embryo. In the photograph sensory neurons of the ramus dorsalis (○ →) and ramus ventralis (x →) are shown with arrows. A broken line indicates the border of the spinal cord.

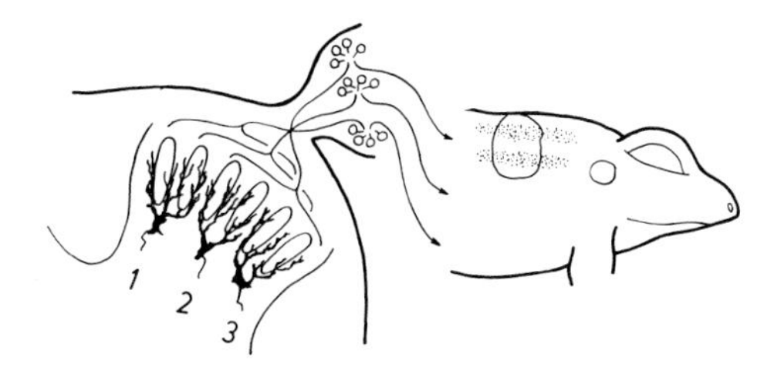

FIG. 6. Explanatory diagram for the "recognition" of cutaneous signs in the dorsoventral direction in the frog. The left side of the diagram represents the dorsal horn of the spinal cord. Lamina IV neurons are represented by 1, 2, and 3, which send their dendrites to the neuropil sheets. These latter are represented by oval areas. It is assumed that the three cutaneous nerves (dorsal, middle, and ventral) project on the lateral, middle, medial neuropil sheets, respectively. The brackets indicate the possible extent of excitation when a signal arrives through the corresponding nerve. Small circles in the spinal ganglion represent sensory neurons, and the intent of the illustration method is to indicate that each nerve contains a number of fibers. The two dotted stripes on the back of the frog are presumed to have a primary central representation as linear continua along the two lateral neuropil sheets, and neuron 3 collects information in the manner suggested in Fig. 4 from the closed field outlined by solid lines.

diffuse neuropil domain at the thoracic level, and the diagram need not necessarily mean the actual arborization of individual sensory fibers. Rather we intend to indicate the probable extent of the spread of the excitatory state in the center on stimulation of a nerve; this may be mediated also by the returning axon collaterals of neurons of the SG. If a stimulus is injected through, for instance, a back nerve, the highest level of excitation will develop in the most lateral neuropil sheet, and neuron 3 of lamina IV will forward the information (which evokes a back wiping). This mechanism presupposes that at least the majority of the fibers of the back nerve should terminate in the most lateral neuropil sheet. The primary axon orientation of sensory ganglion neuroblast, that is, the actual termination pattern of fibers, is inadequate to assure the exact localization of stimulus points in the dorsoventral direction. In order to bring about a good localization, the proposal of a second factor, which will be called a physiological factor, is necessary. We propose that different impulse patterns arise from different skin areas, and that the neurons of the SG are sensitive in different degrees to the different impulse patterns. In the present example the back nerve carries an impulse pattern which is characteristic of the back skin, and to which neurons in the lateral sheets are most sensitive. The physiological factor controls in this way the spread of excitation in the SG and corrects for faulty anatomical connections. In other words, this proposal suggests that the cutaneous local sign in the dorsoventral direction is coded by both anatomical and physiological characteristics of receptors and sensory fibers and is decoded by means of both anatomical and physiological characteristics of central neurons.

With this proposition we have arrived at a rather problematic realm of neurophysiology, and the opponents to the idea would certainly make up a much longer list than the supporters. The "impulse pattern theory" in its up-to-date form, as contrasted to the theory which assigns specific receptors to specific cutaneous sensory modalities, was first proposed by Sinclair (1955) and Weddel (1955), and an attractive comprehensive review on the problem was given by Melzack and Wall (1962). In short, the theory maintains that a single impulse provides no information for the center. The mass of impulses arriving in a center is patterned in both space and time, and the central neurons, or neuron sets, due to their characteristic anatomical and physiological properties, are differentially sensitive to different impulse patterns. The temporal pattern, which can be studied with mathematical techniques (Moore, Perkel, & Segundo, 1966), is stamped upon a series of impulses by the multifarious transduction properties of skin receptors, by their different rates of adaptation, and by the different conduction velocities of their nerve fibers. The distribution of the endarborizations of central processes, together with the receiving dendritic arbor of central neurons, provides the spatial pattern. A variety of neural codes based on different features of a series of impulses is extensively discussed by Mountcastle (1967). The significance of the anatomical and physiological properties of neurons in the analysis (decoding) of input patterns, and the physiological consequences of various degrees of convergence and divergence is lucidly discussed by Bullock (1965) and Melzack and Wall (1965). Recently, an important role has been attributed to gating mechanisms effected by presynaptic inhibtion (Wall, 1966) and to filtering mechanisms at the axonal branching points (Chung, Raymond, & Lettvin, 1970) in shaping the course of different impulse patterns. It is not feasible to survey all the relevant aspects of the input pattern mechanism, and the reader is referred to the literature (see also Gerard & Duyff, 1964) for further details; nevertheless, the assumption is that the course of a series of impulses is determined by dynamic physiological factors within the framwork of a multichoice anatomical pathway in the center.

Let us now investigate what happens if a dorsoventral strip of skin is rotated by 180°, and let us also try to account for the results first in terms of neuronal specificity. The theory maintains the rearrangement of synapses. According to Fig. 6, this would imply that the central processes of the back nerve switch over and terminate now in the medial neuropil sheets. The conflicts listed under (*a*), (*b*), and (*c*) arise under this assumption. The nerve crossunion experiments add one more to these conflicts. If for instance, nerve 3 is sutured to nerve 1 to innervate the dorsal skin area, then as the result indicates, most of the nerve 3 fibers should have been respecified. This implies again that the central fibers of nerve 3 abandon their sites of termination and displace the fibers of nerve 1 to occupy their synapsing sites in the lateral neuropil sheets. A number of termination sites (those of nerve 3) would remain unoccupied in the middle neuropil sheets, and one would expect that the central fibers of nerve 4 would expand their area of termination and occupy the empty synapsing sites, as Sperry's gradient theory would imply. Quite a similar event actually occurs in the case of retinotectal projection of double-nasal and double-temporal eyes in the Xenopus toad (Gaze, Jacobson, & Székely, 1965). If this had happened, then one should have been able to evoke wiping of the side to the stimulation of the belly, unless one assumes a series of transneuronal respecification, which is rather unlikely. We may remember that exactly the reverse happened: the frog wiped the belly when the side (deep nerve 3) was stimulated. It is obvious that the assumption of synaptic rearrangement takes us nowhere.

Returning to our proposition that the dorsoventral localization of a stimulus point depends on anatomical and physiological factors, the rotation of the skin primarily means the change of input patterns. That is, if the dorsum is covered with ventral skin, the back nerve conveys a series of impulse patterns characteristic of the belly nerve. By the action of different gating and filtering mechanisms, the excitation is directed toward the medial sheets, suppressed in the lateral sheets, and the frog wipes the belly. The same events take place with the belly nerve, which innervates the back skin. The most lateral and medial sheets, which represent a mid-dorsal and mid-ventral strip of the skin, receive fibers only from the back nerve and belly nerve, respectively. In these sheets the anatomical factor obviously predominates, and the actual connections determine the direction of impulse transmission. Hence a fringe remains at the midline, both dorsally and ventrally, from where normal reflexes can be evoked after skin rotation. It is also clear that in smaller skin grafts the fringes for normal reflexes are larger, and a critical size of rotated skin area is required for misdirected reflexes, as shown recently by Baker and Jacobson (1970). A similar argument can be made to interpret the results of the nerve crossunion experiments. If nerve 3 is switched over in the periphery to innervate back skin, its fibers convey an impulse pattern characteristic of back skin. The excitation will be suppressed in the middle neuropil sheets and shifted toward the lateral sheets. However, in a few places in the middle sheets the anatomical factor prevails, and the animal produces side wipings to the stimulation of a few points on the dorsal skin. It is clear that these points are larger when a large deep nerve 3 occurs, because in this case nerve 3 contains fewer fibers and has a smaller central representation area, where the level of excitation is suppressed by the impulse pattern arising from the back skin. In one or two sheets the central representation areas of nerve 3 and deep nerve 3 (which conveys the appropriate impulse pattern) overlap, and the excitation of this area by the fibers of the crossunited nerve 3 may occasionally be effective in evoking a wipe of the side. A similar argument can account for the belly wipes evoked from the skin area of the intact deep nerve 3. The level of excitation is low in the middle neuropil sheets, and impulses carried by the deep nerve 3 more effectively excite the medial sheets, where the central areas of deep nerve 3 and nerve 4 overlap.

While the impulse pattern theory seems to resolve most of the conflicts mentioned above, it cannot answer the question: why is the skin rotation ineffective in bringing about rotated reflexes if the operation is done at late larval stages? Perhaps some factors in the periphery may be responsible for the discrepancy, and their exploration would help to disentangle the problems of wiping reflexes. It must be stressed that we have no data to support the supposition that the different skin areas generate different impulse patterns in the frog. Unfortunately, nothing is known about the frog's skin receptors. A few preliminary investigations made in this department revealed different numbers and caliber spectra, in the 1-to-10-μ diameter range, in cutaneous nerves. Nerve fibers of different size may innervate different skin receptors, and the density of innervation is definitely different by a factor of 3 to 5 in different skin areas. These scarce data are obviously insufficient, and the interpretation based on impulse pattern theory is as conjectural as that based on neural specificity theory, and neither of them can claim more support than that other. However, the former idea has the advantage over the neuronal specificity theory in that it can be tested directly on frogs.

IV. Myotypic Specificity

In an impressive series of experiments performed on axolotls, Weiss (1937a, 1937b, 1937c, 1937d) has found that extra limbs grafted into the brachial region and innervated by branches of the brachial plexus moved in a coordinated manner and synchronously with the normal limb. It was also shown that whichever segment of the cord, or whichever branch of the brachial plexus, gave rise to the innervation, the supernumerary limb moved in the same way. The only compelling prerequisite was that the brachial plexus contribute with a branch, however small, to the innervation. Various axial orientations of the grafted limb in an otherwise normal, or deafferented, animal did not influence the coordinated and synchronous movements. With the aid of tissue culture experiments (Weiss, 1934, 1945) the role of various "tropisms," and hence the establishment of selective neuromuscular connections, was excluded, and it was assumed that the regenerating nerve fibers invaded the extra limb in a haphazard manner. The results were interpreted in terms of what is known as *myotypic modulation*, or homologous muscle responses. By this is meant that individual limb muscles possess specific biochemical properties which distinguish them from each other and which are imparted to the innervating motor neurons through the axon. This makes the neuronal surface more receptive to a certain kind of synaptic ending than to another. The motor neurons become attached to the central motor apparatus in such a way that they will fire at the time appropriate for the function of the innervated muscle. That is why, according to the hypothesis, homologous muscles of the normal and grafted limb contract simultaneously, and the two limbs move synchronously. Evidence in favor of the idea continued to accumulate, and from normal functional restitution following nerve crossunions in fish to synchronous movements of duplicated digits in man, all were ascribed to myotypic modulation of motor neurons (for references, see Weiss, 1955). Recently in a series of experiments performed on kittens, Eccles, Eccles, and Magni (1960) tried to find electrophysiological correlates of myotypic modulation at the neuronal level. Using the size and frequency of monosynaptic excitatory potentials to indicate that an identified motor neuron was stimulated by afferent fibers of the same or a synergistic muscle, they were able to show a redistribution of monosynaptic connections according to the scheme of myotypic modulation following crossunion of the tibial and peroneal nerves. In a later experiment, however, the unsatisfactory results of the statistical analysis of the data led the authors to regard their findings as not sufficiently conclusive to support Weiss' idea (Eccles, Eccles, Shealy, & Willis, 1962).

Despite contradictions inherent in the theory it has stood firmly for decades. The first doubt emerged from experiments performed on fish (Sperry & Deupree, 1956). When pectoral fin muscles were connected experimentally with the nerves to the pelvic fin muscles, the functional restitution was rather poor. The authors came to the conclusion that failure in functional recovery could be due either to failure of the regenerating pelvic nerves to establish functionally effective connections with pectoral muscles, or to incapacity of pelvic motor neurons to undergo modulation. A similar observation was made in urodele larvae, in that movements of limbs innervated by heterotopic spinal cord segments were characteristic of the innervating segments rather than the anatomical construction of the limb (Székely, 1963). This phenomenon was more prominent in the chick with a grafted leg at the place of the wing, or with the lumbosacral cord segments substituted for the brachial segments. It was shown that despite the normal histology of neuromuscular connections, limbs with heterotopic innervation could perform coordinated movements, but to a very limited extent, although irregular twitches of muscle fibres could be observed all over the limb (Straznicky, 1963, and unpublished observations). These data indicate that hind limb muscles are unable to modulate motor neurons, and suggest that the pattern for forelimb and hindlimb movement is rigidly laid down in the structure of the respective spinal cord sections in urodeles and chick. In subsequent experiments performed on the external ocular muscles (Sperry & Arora, 1965) and fin muscles (Mark, 1965) of the chichlid fish, it has also been found that the muscles were unable to alter the function of motor neurons. The authors have explicity concluded that functional recovery was due to the appropriate anatomical reconstitution of neuromuscular connections following the experimental derrangement of the nerves. Selectivity in the development of neuromuscular connections during ontogenesis has been inferred also from spinal cord transplantation experiments performed on Pleurodeles larvae (Straznicky & Székely, 1967). In his recent paper, Mark (1969) has pointed out the multiterminal innervation of muscle fibers in amphibians and fishes to account for selective reinnervation, which occurs in these lower vertebrates but does not occur in mammals. Recalling the fact that myotypic modulation is restricted to motor neurons in the limb-moving segments of the spinal cord, and the data of Nicholas and Barron (1935) and Székely and Czéh (1967) that most of the limb muscles are represented in every limb-moving segment, an alternative interpretation for the synchronous movement of the two limbs seems to be obvious: any branch of the brachial plexus carries nerve fibers for almost every limb muscle, and selective nerve ingrowth insures the formation of the right neuromuscular connections. However, this interpretation is based on indirect evidence and is still unable to account for the finding that a distal limb nerve is capable of reinnervating the whole limb (Weiss, 1937b).

The results of the three experiments described below indicate that the synchronous movement of the normal and grafted limbs is a trivial phenomenon which does not warrant any conclusion concerning neural events that may happen either in the periphery or in the center. The experiments involve muscle action potential recordings from right limb muscles in freely moving newts. The technique has been described in detail elsewhere (Székely, Czéh, & Vörös, 1969). In the first (1) experiment, the recordings were made from intact animals, and it indicates a very complicated interaction that occurs between functionally opposing muscles (Székely *et al.*, 1969). In the second (2) experiment, the ventral roots of the brachial plexus were cut in different combinations, and the myograms of such partially innervated limbs indicate that a rhythmic output pattern is conveyed by each root of the brachial plexus (Székely & Czéh, 1971b). In the third (3) experiment, the recordings were made simultaneously from normal and grafted limbs (Czéh & Székely, 1971b), and, as will be shown below, the assumption of homologous response phenomenon could not be corroborated.

1. Figure 7 shows the myogram recorded from an intact animal. The muscles were chosen so that they represented four pair of antagonists in the conventional sense. Two of them, *Acromialis-Latissimus* and *Dorsalis scapulae-Pectoralis*, belong to the shoulder girdle; *Brachialis-Extensor ulnae* are arm muscles, and *Flexor digitorum-Extensor digitorum* are forearm muscles. Upward-pointing arrows indicate when the limb leaves the ground. At the downward-pointing arrows, the limb is on the ground again; thus the narrow space between upward- and downward-pointing arrows indicate the phase of protraction, and the wide space between them represents the phase of retraction. A pertinent feature of the myogram is the delicate interaction of synergistic as well as antagonistic muscles in the act of walking. With the exception of *Dorsalis scapulae*, the muscles are active, though with presumably different strength, during both protraction and retraction, and there is extensive overlap in their activities. This activity pattern of the muscles

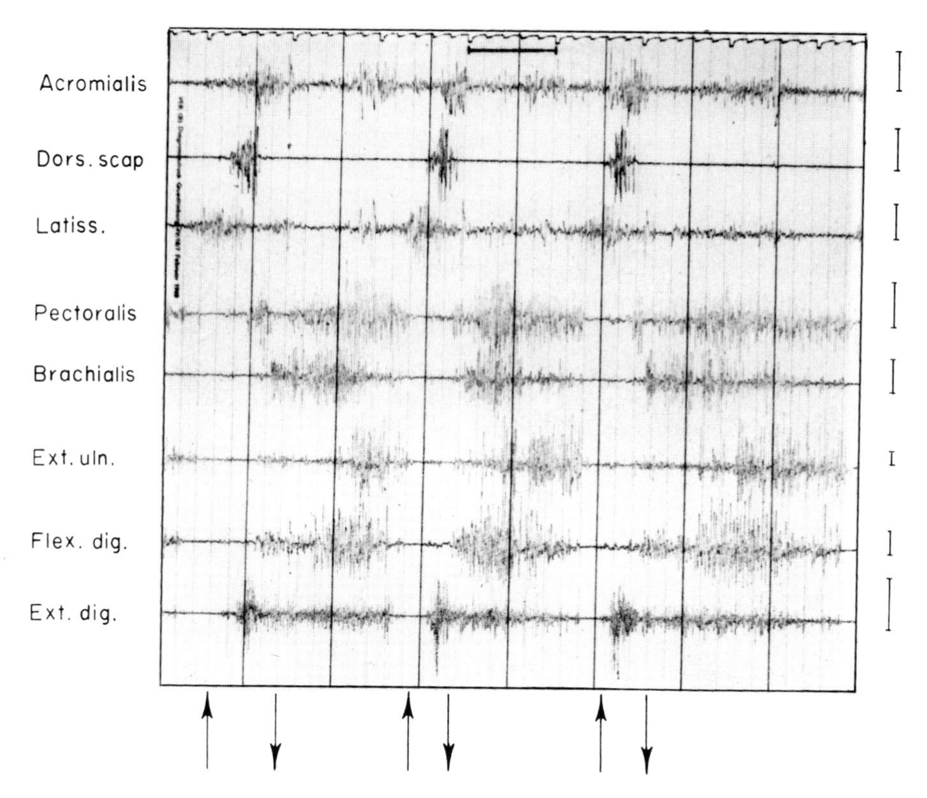

FIG. 7. Normal myogram recorded from eight forelimb muscles in freely moving *Ambystoma mexicanum*. Upward-pointing arrows indicate when the limb is off of the ground and downward-pointing arrows when the limb is on the ground. Time calibration on top is 1 second, voltage calibration on extreme right corresponds to 100 μV.

seems to be programmed somehow in the structure of the limb segments of the spinal cord, since it is maintained after deafferentation of one or both forelimbs (Székely *et al.*, 1969), and also in the case when this part of the spinal cord is isolated and transplanted with a limb into a common tunnel made in the dorsal fin of axolotl larvae (Székely & Czéh, 1971a). The myograms clearly demonstrate extensive co-contractions which were neither recognized nor taken into consideration in the construction of the "theoretical myochronograms" derived from moving pictures to show the sequence of muscular contractions (Székely & Czéh, 1967; Weiss, 1941). These myograms, therefore, contain a strong warning against drawing conclusions concerning the timing of individual muscle activities in a complex movement like stepping. The large overlap in muscle activities raises the question: which of the muscles may be regarded as "homologous" pairs, as opposed to those with differently timed activities, in the normal and the extra limb? As a matter of fact, the activity of any muscle may coincide with that of any other of the arm and forearm muscles during the "homologous response."

2. The forelimb moving section of the spinal cord consists of segments III, IV, and V, and the ventral root emerges with two rootlets from the third and fourth segments in Ambystoma. This anatomical arrangement makes it possible to transect the ventral roots in six different combinations (Fig. 8), and to investigate the muscle activity pattern in partially innervated limbs. The results are discussed in detail elsewhere (Székely & Czéh, 1971b); only a few pertinent points will be mentioned here. As can be seen in the diagram (Fig. 8), segment III controls predominantly protraction activity, in segment V retraction activity prevails, and in segment IV the two activities are almost balanced. Furthermore, a weak retraction activity can also be found in segment III, and segment V controls also protraction activity of two muscles. (We succeeded in recording from two hand muscles in two animals, which revealed both protraction and retraction activities in the limb innervated only by segment V.) With the exception of *Acromialis*, *Dorsalis scapulae*, and *Brachialis*, which are not represented in segment V, the rest of the muscles are represented in every one of the three limb moving segments. The movement of limbs innervated by either part of segment IV was close to normal, whereas in limbs with innervation from segment III or V only protraction or retraction, respectively, could be observed. Therefore, the movement observed behaviorally does not reflect accurately the activity pattern recorded: incomplete patterns may bring about movements that appear to be normal, and weak muscle activities may not result in visible movement. From these observations the following inferences can be made. (*a*) Each limb-moving spinal cord segment generates a rhythmic output pattern which contains commands for both protraction and retraction activi-

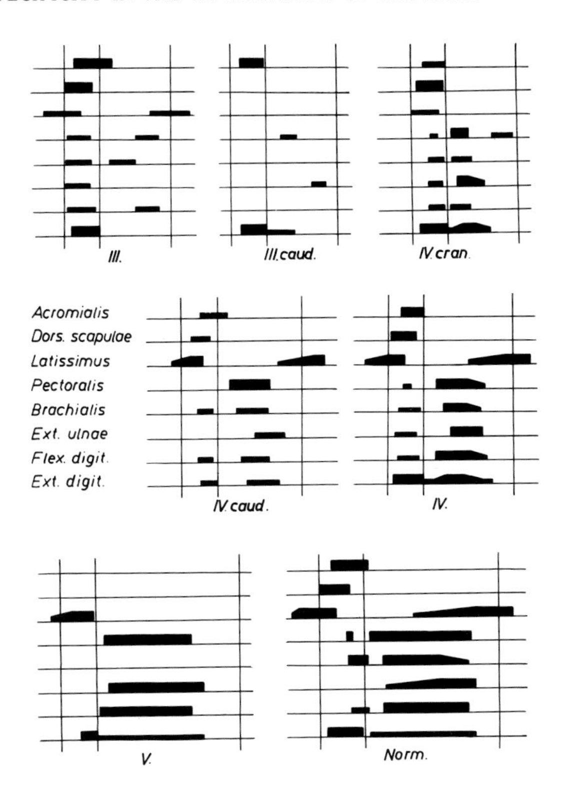

FIG. 8. Diagrammatic representation of myograms recorded from partially innervated limbs in *Ambystoma mexicanum*. Vertical lines demarcate the phase of protraction (narrow space) and retraction (wide space). Subscripts show the origin of innervation to the limb. III. = third segment of the spinal cord; III. caud. = caudal part of the third segment; IV. cran. = cranial part of the fourth segment; IV. caud. = caudal part of the fourth segment; IV. = entire fourth segment; V. = fifth segment; Norm. = intact animal. Black stripes indicate muscle activities. The width of the stripes indicates the height of the amplitude in an arbitrary scale. The names of muscles in the middle refer to the corresponding lines for each myogram.

ties. Furthermore, any major branch of the brachial plexus, or virtually any muscle nerve for that matter, carries these two commands in a rhythmic manner. (*b*) If the nerve fibers establish selective connections with the appropriate muscle, then an extra limb innervated by one of the three segments should yield the function and the muscle activity pattern characteristic of the innervating segment. (*c*) Since any segmental nerve conveys a rhythmic output pattern, and minor irregularities in activity of individual muscles presumably do not interfere with limb movement, an extra limb innervated by a single segment may show coordinated movements in synchrony with the normal limb even if the normal anatomy of neuromuscular connections is not completely reestablished.

3. These inferences were tested in the third experiment which was performed on Ambystoma. About 6 weeks after the animals hatched, extra limbs were grafted into a position such that they became innervated either by the third, by the fourth, or by the fifth spinal nerve, respectively. The movement of the limbs was regularly observed, and muscle activities were recorded in adults from the following four pairs of homologous muscles: Normal (*N*) *Brachialis* transplanted (*T*) *Brachialis*, *N Extensor ulnae T Extensor ulnae*, *N Flexor digitorum T Flexor digitorum*, and *N Extensor digitorum T Extensor digitorum*. Only one animal recovered in which the extra limb was innervated by the third nerve alone. The limb showed strong protraction and noticeable retraction activity. Protraction activities prevail in the myogram (Fig. 9), and in this respect it is comparable with the normal activity of segment III (cf. Fig. 8). A strong retraction activity can also be seen in *N Brachialis* and *T Extensor digitorum*, and somewhat more weakly in *T Extensor ulnae*, and these activities would not be expected on the basis of the second experiment. The two muscles which show the best homologous responses are *N Brachialis* and *T Extensor digitorum*.

In the second group the grafted limb was innervated by the fourth nerve in only two of the nine animals, in three animals the fifth nerve contributed with a small branch to the graft's innervation, and in the remaining animals both limbs received mixed innervation from two or three segments. Despite the various sources of nerve supply, both the limb movement observed and the activity pattern recorded are close to normal. The most beautiful homologous responses were shown by an animal in which the graft received innervation only from segment IV (Fig. 10); nevertheless, there are irregularities in the arm muscles, especially in the activity of *T Brachialis*. In all myograms a number of irregular patterns appeared in which heterologous muscles contract simultaneously, or there was a phase shift in the activities of homologous muscles.

In the third group the graft was supplied by the fifth nerve alone in five animals; in two other cases the fourth nerve contributed a very small branch to the innervation. The shoulder and the elbow remained motionless in these cases, and only two animals performed elbow movements coinciding with protraction. Figure 11 shows the muscle activity of an animal in which the graft received innervation only from segment V, and the elbow was motionless. The activity patterns of the forearm muscles of the grafted and normal limb are regular in that the normal muscles show a normal activity minus the activity of segment V. The arm muscles show irregular patterns, especially *T Extensor ulnae*, which is active during the entire walking step, and resembles in this respect the activity of *Latissimus*. The prevalent extensor

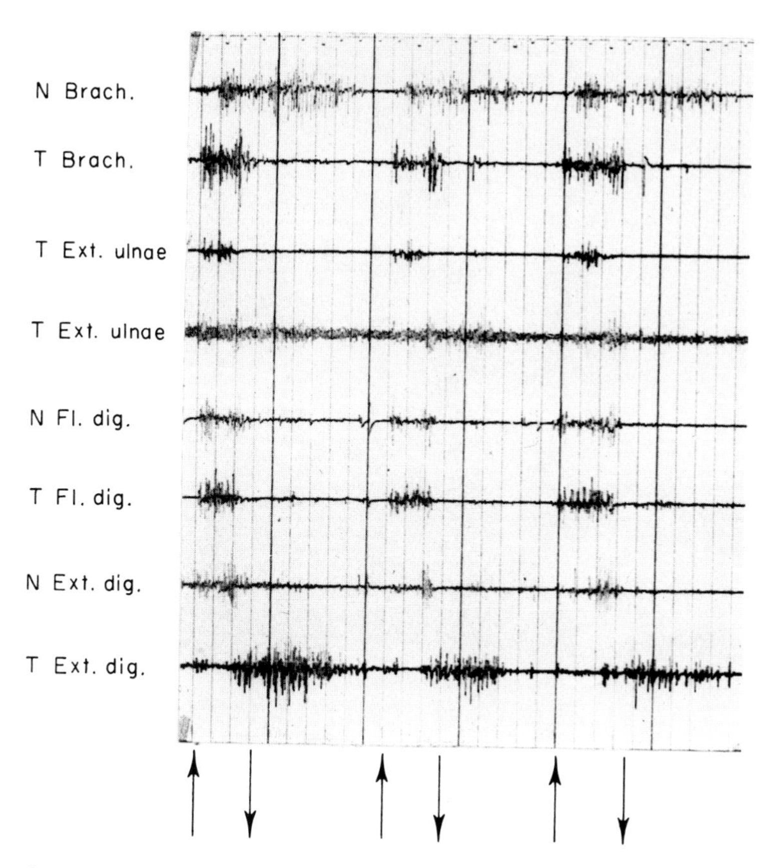

FIG. 9. Myogram recorded from four pairs of homologous muscles of the normal (N) and transplanted (T) limbs in *Ambystoma mexicanum*. The transplanted limb was innervated by the third spinal nerve. Arrows indicate protraction and retraction. See text for details.

activity may account for the immobility of the elbow. In another animal the limb performed the best synchronous movement in this group, but the muscle activity pattern, with the exception of *N Brachialis*, is highly irregular (Fig. 12). The pattern of *T Brachialis* and *N Extensor ulnae* is characteristic of that of a normal *Extensor digitorum*, and the two muscles contract synchronously. The conspicuous protraction activity of *T Brachialis* explains the elbow movement during protraction.

Other aspects of the results are described elsewhere (Czéh & Székely, 1971b). The point most relevant to the present discussion is that in the muscle activity pattern of the grafted limbs, the activity of the innervating segment was not reflected exactly as would have been expected from inference (*b*).

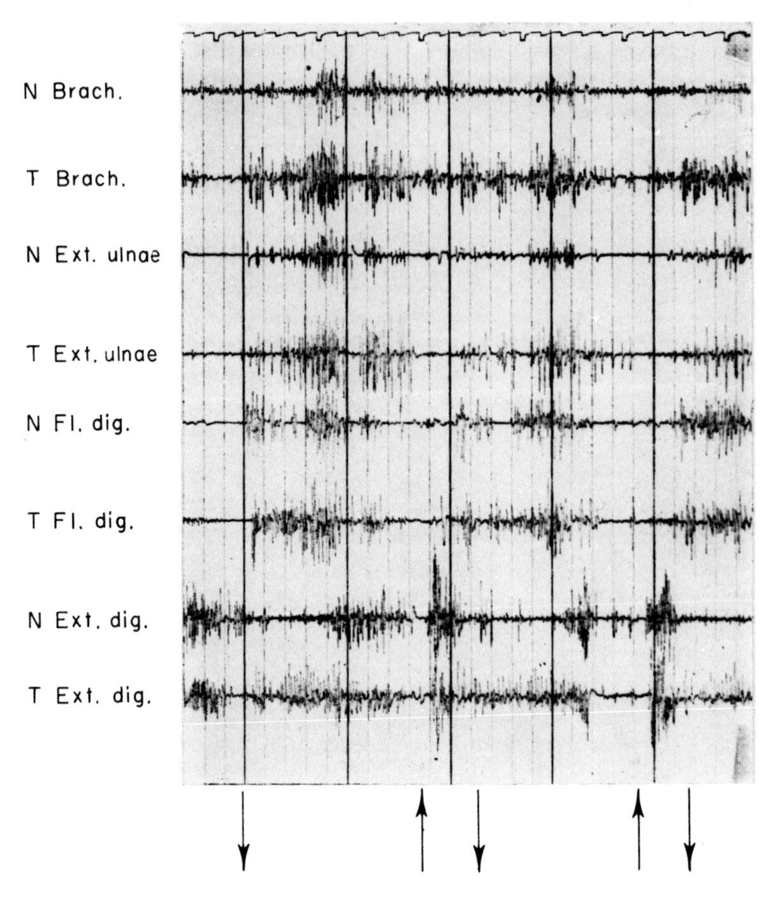

FIG. 10. The transplanted limb was innervated by the fourth spinal nerve. With the exception of *T Brachialis*, the myogram is close to normal.

A second important result is that nonhomologous muscles were found to contract synchronously about as often as did homologous muscles. This disproves inference (*b*), indicates that the premise of selective nerve regeneration is wrong, and suggests that the muscle reinnervation occurs on a statistical basis. This suggestion speaks in favor of inference (*c*), that a complete anatomical restoration of neuromuscular connections is not a prerequisite condition of coordinated movements of the grafted limb.

Because one feels intuitively that a coordinated limb movement requires an appropriate distribution of muscle strength during ambulation, the third inference, that despite random ingrowth of nerve fibers the grafted limb moves in a coordinated manner and in synchrony with the normal limb,

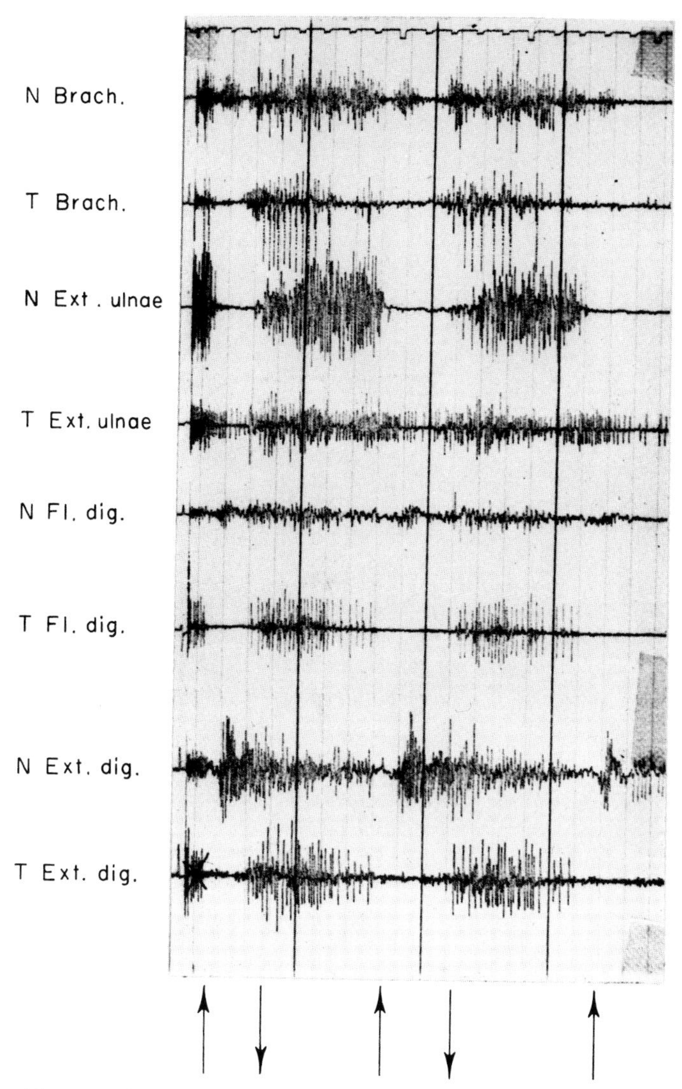

FIG. 11. The transplanted limb was innervated by the fifth spinal nerve, and it was motionless at the elbow. Note the uninterrupted activity of *T Extensor ulnae*. The sum of activities of *N Flexor digitorum* and *T Flexor digitorum* and that of *N Extensor digitorum* and *T Extensor digitorum* gives a normal activity pattern (cf. Fig. 7).

needs a little more comment. It was interesting to observe that when the animal moved quietly in water, the grafted limb seldom produced any movement. On the other hand, if a restrained animal performed vigorous escape movements with the four normal limbs, the graft remained motionless in

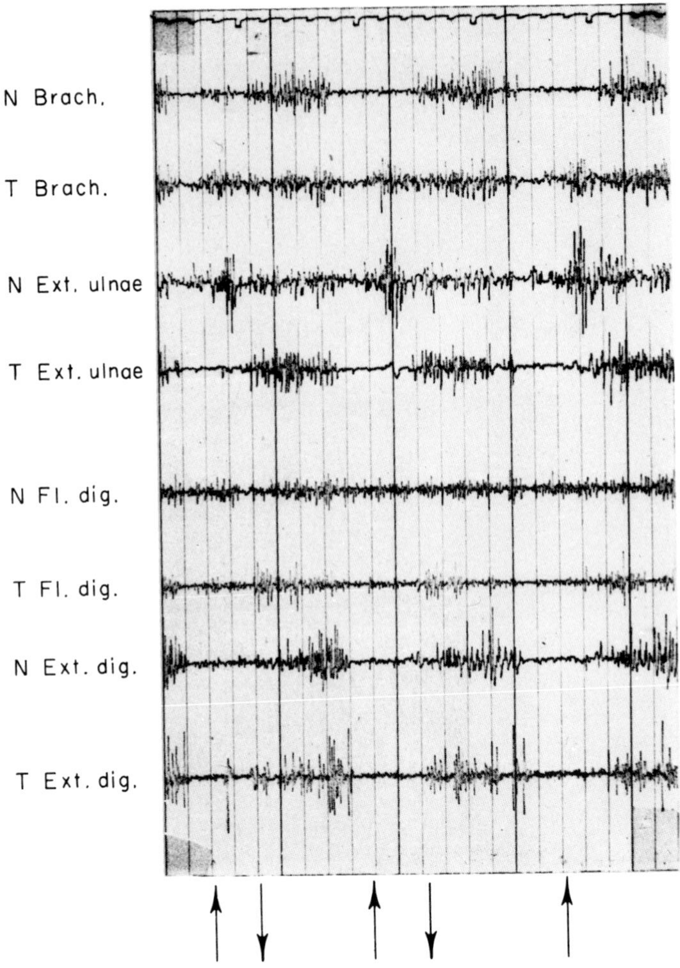

FIG. 12. In addition to a branch from the fifth spinal nerve, the transplanted limb probably received innervation from uncontrollable sources as well. The elbow also participated in the movement. Note the *Extensor digitorum*-like activity of *T Brachialis* and *N Extensor ulnae* (cf. Fig. 7).

clonic rigidity perpendicular to the body. It seems that the appropriate distribution of muscle strengths was confined within narrow limits, such that the limb could take part only in smooth ambulation of the animal over even ground. Even in this case the grafted limb was very feeble and would certainly have been incapable of propelling the body, and the light weight of the fine recording wires was frequently sufficient to stop its movements. It was a steplike movement rather than a real stepping. One cannot escape the impression that once a limb gets moving in response to rhythmic impulses, which it receives from any branch of the brachial plexus, then as a result of its anatomical construction the only complex movement the limb is capable of performing is the walking step. And this can be simulated with consecutive electric stimulation of nerves 3, 4, and 5.

V. Summary and Conclusions

In the present review we have surveyed the results and interpretations of three basic experiments on which the theory of neuronal specificity has largely been based. As has been shown, the corneal specific modulation is very probably a threshold phenomenon. Even if the explanation is not quite so simple, certainly neural mechanisms other than the neuronal specificity must lie in the background. The interpretation of the cutaneous local sign specificity in terms of neuronal specificity has brought up so many conflicts that we have been compelled to seek for an alternative interpretation. We dwelt long on this subject because the interpretation suggested here is no less conjectural than is the theory of neuronal specificity. The third case, that is, the myotypic specification, could be explained on the basis of the peculiar functional capacity of the limb-moving spinal cord segments to generate rhythmic output to which the limb responds with a steplike movement. That is why the phenomenon itself cannot be demonstrated with the ocular muscles, because the activities of the two centers, limb moving and occulomotor, are basically different. There are a great many other experiments to which I did not refer, all of which appear to support the neuronal specificity theory (Jacobson, 1971; Sperry, 1965; Weiss, 1955). The most notable of these is the amazingly fine grain of retinotopic organization in the projection of optic fibers onto the optic tectum, which is restored during regeneration and after eye rotation in accordance with the scheme of the theory. However, if one starts to pose questions in a more inquiring way, one soon finds out that the optic fiber regeneration (Gaze & Jacobson, 1963), the projection of double-nasal and temporal "compound" eyes (Gaze *et al.*, 1965), and the intricate structural complexity of the visual centers (Székely, 1971) raise serious difficulties for the theory. The introduction of gradient fields in an effort to moderate the rigidity of a chemically overspecified system is of little help in rescuing the general validity of the theory. The theory of gradient fields cannot be applied as a theory to interpret the experimental result in this case, but merely to describe the phenomenon in a more sophisticated fashion, primarily because the notion maintains the fundamental but never enunciated assumption of the neuronal specificity theory, viz., that neurons are simple relay elements, which they definitely are not.

In fact, it was not new experimental data, but rather new ideas which cast doubt on the concept that the organization of the nervous system is controlled by the specific chemoaffinity properties of billions of neurons. At the advent of the theory, when the nervous system was viewed largely as a blueprint drawing, the assumption of specific neuronal interconnections formed on a basis of chemoaffinity was indeed a rather attractive, and almost compelling, hypothesis. Rejection of this hypothesis, however, does not imply that we must swing to the opposite extreme and postulate a random model of interneuronal connections. This would ignore a large body of anatomical, physiological, and behavioral evidence. Many fascinating articles in these two volumes (Hamburger; Oppenheim; Provine—in Volume 1 indicate that embryos of different species start moving with a characteristic motor pattern. Many of these behavioral patterns (e.g. hatching) are very complicated, and the embryos acquire their characteristic motility before having been exposed to environmental influence. The determination of the movement pattern of limbs before the functional stage may also be mentioned in this connection (Straznicky, 1963; Székely, 1963). The species-specific and stable character of the early motilities are suggestive of a specific structural organization in the nervous system.

If we abandon the specific chemoaffinity theory, the question of how the characteristic structural organization of the nervous system develops remains open. In an earlier paper (Székely, 1966) a proposal was made concerning the organization of intercellular connections in neuron assemblies on the basis of morphological characteristics (such as cell density, geometry of dendrite arbors, distances, form of contact, convergence, etc.) of the components. A form-function relationship was suggested in the sense that the well-defined shape and form of neurons may lead to a structural organization which endows a given neural center with a characteristic function. The frog's retina was mentioned as an example. Lettvin, Maturana, Pitts, and McCulloch (1961) made an interesting study to correlate the operational groups at the output of the retina with the various anatomical groups of ganglion cells. Another example may be the fascinating histological works of Scheibel and Scheibel (1968) on the spinal cord. As mentioned above, due to their characteristic dendritic arborization, the dorsal horn neurons are capable of sampling information in a rather specific way from the neuropil sheets of the substantia gelatinosa, and it is not necessary (moreover one wonders whether it would be realistic) to assume specific interconnections among these neurons. The strict geometry of neurons and axonal end arborizations determines the interneuronal connections, not explicitly, but rather in a statistical sense.

The very attractive pictures produced by the Scheibels tempts one to make generalizations and to suppose that the organization of the ventral part of the spinal cord may be controlled by a similar mechanism. The strict geometry of motor neurons and of the innumerable interneurons may control the structural organization of the assembly, in which one or a few functions characteristic of the structure are prewired through interconnections established on a statistical basis. To make a fashionable comparison, the system works as a computer with a number of inbuilt subroutines which are called up by the program. In the structure of the spinal cord, a number of "subroutines" may be similarly built in, and information of the environment arriving in the form of different patterns of input and processed by the sensory side of the cord evokes a set of subroutines and puts them together into a characteristic motor pattern, which can be either a wiping reflex or ambulation. It is well known from studies of neurohistogenesis that the cell patterns of nervous centers is determined in early embryonic life. This may be the very point where genetics plays its role to determine the structural characteristics of different centers. At this point one stops and asks how far these generalizations may be extended to account for the structure and function of higher nervous centers as well, and how far genetic factors may be responsible for the development of behavior. If the close structure–function relationship can be accepted, then, paraphrasing Gottlieb's introductory remarks (in Volume 1), the development of the basic patterns of behavior is strictly predetermined, but they evolve in an epigenetic way. The statistical aspect of the structural organization, on the other hand, leaves ample space for a probabilistic development of more complex and integrated behavioral patterns, also in an epigenetic fashion, under environmental influences.

It is impossible to give the outline of an idea about the structural organization of the nervous system in the space of a single paragraph, and we are already far beyond our data with these brief conjectures and generalizations. The problem is not only that we know so little about the morphology and physiology of individual neurons, let alone neuronal assemblies, but the main difficulty is that we do not know anything about the language of the nerve cells. In other words, we do not know what kinds of impulse series provide information for the nervous system, and which are the criteria by which the nerve cell, and not the experimentor, distinguishes one impulse pattern from another. It seems, however, that by collecting more and more quantitative data, with both morphological and physiological techniques, from the sorts of recombination experiments from which the concept of neuronal specificity emerged, we may finally learn how the nerve cells talk to each other. And if we ever succeed in making progress in this or in any other direction, merit is due to the proponents of the specificity theory, who, with their ingeniously devised experiments, focused our attention on the crucial points of neurogenesis.

Acknowledgment

The author wishes to express his gratitude to Madge E. Scheibel and A. B. Scheibel for consent to redraw two of their excellent pictures. Thanks are due to the Company of Biologists Limited, Cambridge, England, and to the Publishing House of the Hungarian Academy of Sciences for permission to use Figure 1 and for Figs. 5, 7, 9, 10, 11, and 12, respectively.

References

Baker, R. E. Behavioral reflexes in *Rana catesbiana* and *Rana clamitans* with large skin grafts. *Journal of Comparative Neurology*, 1970, **173**, 129–136.

Baker, R. E., & Jacobson, M. Development of reflexes from skin grafts in *Rana pipiens*: Influence of size and position of grafts. *Developmental Biology*, 1970, **22**, 476–494.

Bullock, T. Mechanisms of integration. In T. H. Bullock & G. A. Horridge (Eds.), *Structure and function in the nervous system of invertebrates*. San Francisco: Freeman, 1965.

Chung, S.-H., Raymond, S. A., & Lettvin, J. Y. Multiple meaning in single visual units. *Brain Behavior and Evolution*, 1970, **3**, 72–101.

Czéh, G., & Székely, G. Monosynaptic spike discharges initiated by dorsal root activation of spinal motoneurons in the frog. *Acta Physiologica*, 1971, **39** 401–406. (a)

Czéh, G., & Székely. G. Muscle activities recorded simultaneously from normal and supernumerary forelimbs in Ambystoma, *Acta Physiologica*, 1971, 287–301. (b)

Detwiler, S. R. *Neuroembryology: An experimental study*. New York: Macmillan, 1936.

Eccles, J. C., Eccles, R. M., & Magni, F. Monosynaptic excitatory action on motoneurones regenerated to antagonistic muscles. *Journal of Physiology* (*London*), 1960, **154**, 69–88.

Eccles, J. C., Eccles, R. M., Shealy, C. N., & Willis, W. D. Experiments utilizing monosynaptic excitatory action on motoneurones for testing hypotheses relating to specificity of neural connections. *Journal of Neurophysiology*, 1962, **25**, 559–580.

Gaze, R. M. (Ed.) *The formation of nerve connections*. London: Academic Press, 1970.

Gaze, R. M., & Jacobson, M. A study of the retinotectal projection during regeneration of the optic nerve in the frog. *Proceedings of the Royal Society, Series B*, 1963, **157**, 420–448.

Gaze, R. M., Jacobson, M., & Székely, G. On the formation of connexions by compound eyes in Xenopus. *Journal of Physiology* (*London*), 1965, **176**, 409–417.

Gerard, R. W., & Duyff, J. W. (Eds.) Information processing in the nervous system. Proceedings of the International Union of Physiological Sciences.Vol. 3. XXII.International Congress, Leiden, 1962. Amsterdam: Excerpta Medica Foundation, 1964.

Hay, E. D. The fine structure of nerves in the epidermis of regenerating salamander limbs. *Experimental Cell Research*, 1960, **19**, 299–317.

Jacobson, M. *Developmental neurobiology*. New York: Holt, 1971.

Jacobson, M., & Baker, R. E. Development of neuronal connections with skin grafts in frogs: behavioral and electrophysiological studies. *Journal of Comparative Neurology*, 1969, **137**, 121–142.

Joseph, B. S., & Whitlock, D. G. Central projection of selected spinal dorsal roots in Anuran amphibians. *Anatomical Record*, 1968, **160**, 279–288.

Kennard, D. W. The anatomical organization of neurons in the lumbar region of the spinal cord of the frog (*Rana temporaria*). *Journal of Comparative Neurology*, 1959, 447–468.

Kollros, J. J. Experimental studies on the development of the corneal reflex in amphibia. III. The influence of the periphery upon the center. *Journal of Experimental Zoology*, 1943, **92**, 121–142.

Kornacker, K. Some properties of the afferent pathway in the frog corneal reflex. *Experimental Neurology*, 1963, **7**, 224–239.

Lettvin, J. Y., Maturana, H. R., Pitts, W. H., & McCulloch, W. S. Two remarks on the visual system of the frog. In W. A. Rosenblith (Ed.), *Sensory communication.* New York: Wiley, 1961.

Liu, C. N., & Chambers, W. W. Experimental study of anatomical organization of frog's spinal cord. *Anatomical Record,* 1957, **127**, 326.

Mark, R. F. Fin movement after regeneration of neuromuscular connections: an investigation of neuromuscular specificity. *Experimental Neurology,* 1965, **12**, 292–302.

Mark, R. F., Matching muscles and motoneurones. A review of some experiments on motor nerve regeneration, *Brain Research,* 1969, **14**, 245–254.

Melzack, R., & Wall, P. D. On the nature of cutaneous sensory mechanisms. *Brain,* 1962, **85**, 331–256.

Melzack, R., & Wall, P. D. 1965. Pain mechanisms: A new theory. *Science* 1965, **150**, 971–979.

Miner, N. Integumental specification of sensory fibres in the development of cutaneous local sign. *Journal of Comparative Neurology,* 1956, **105**, 161–170.

Moore, G. P., Perkel, D. H., & Segundo, J. P. Statistical analysis and functional interpretation of neuronal spike data. *Annual Review of Physiology,* 1966, **28**, 493–522.

Mountcastle, V. B. The problem of sensing and the neural coding of sensory events. In G. C. Quarton, T. Melnechuk, & F. O. Schmitt (Eds.), *The neurosciences: A study program.* New York: Rockefeller University Press, 1967.

Nicolas, J. S., & Barron, D. H. Limb movements studied by electrical stimulation of nerve roots and trunks in Amblystoma. *Journal of Comparative Neurology,* 1935, **61**, 413–431.

Prestige, M. C. Cell turnover in the spinal ganglia of Xenopus laevis tadpoles. *Journal of Embryology and Experimental Morphology,* 1965, **13**, 63–72.

Ralston, H. J. The fine structure of neurons in the dorsal horn of the cat spinal cord. *Journal of Comparative Neurology,* 1968, **132**, 275–302.

Ramón y. Cajal, S. *Histologie du système nerveux de l'homme et de vertébrés.* Vols. I & II. Paris: Maloine, 1909.

Réthelyi, M., & Szentágothai, J. The large synaptic complexes of the substantia gelatinosa. *Experimental Brain Research,* 1969, **7**, 258–274.

Rexed, B. The cytoarchitectonic organization of the spinal cord in the cat. *Journal of Comparative Neurology,* 1952, **96**, 415–496.

Sala y Pons, C. Estructura de la médula espinal de los Batracios, 1892. Cited by S. Ramón y Cajal, *Histologie du système nerveux de l'homme et de vertébrés.* Paris: Maloine, 1909.

Scheibel, M. E., & Scheibel, A. B. Terminal axonal patterns in cat spinal cord. II. The dorsal horn. *Brain Research,* 1968, **9**, 32–58.

Silver, M. L. The motoneurons of the spinal cord of the frog. *Journal of Comparative Neurology,* 1942, **77**, 1–40.

Simpson, J. F. On how a frog is not a cat. Unpublished doctoral dissertation, Massachusetts Institute of Technology, 1969.

Sinclair, D. C. Cutaneous sensation and the doctrine of specific energy. *Brain,* 1955, **78**, 584–614.

Singer, M. The influence of the nerve in regeneration of the amphibian extremity. *Quarterly Review of Biology,* 1952, **27**, 169–200.

Sperry, R. W. Regulative factors in the orderly growth of neural circuits. *Growth Symposia,* 1951, **10**, 63–87.

Sperry, R. W. Embryogenesis of behavioral nerve nets. In R. L. De Haan & H. Ursprung (Eds.), *Organogenesis,* New York: Holt, 1965.

Sperry, R. W., & Arora, H. L. Selection in regeneration of the oculomotor nerve in the chichlid fish Astronotus ocellatus. *Journal of Embryology and Experimental Morphology,* 1965, **14**, 307–317.

Sperry, R. W. & Deupree, N. Functional recovery following alterations in nerve muscle connections of fishes. *Journal of Comparative Neurology,* 1956, **106**, 143–158.

Straznicky, K. Function of heterotopic spinal cord segments investigated in the chick. *Acta*

Biologica, 1963, **14**, 145–155.
Straznicky, K., & Székely, G. Functional adaptation of thoracic spinal cord segments in the newt. *Acta Biologica*, 1967, **18**, 449–456.
Székely, G. The apparent "corneal specificity" of sensory neurons. *Journal of Embryology and Experimental Morphology*, 1959, **7**, 375–379.
Székely, G. Functional specificity of spinal cord segments in the control of limb movements. *Journal of Embryology and Experimental Morphology*, 1963, **11**, 431–444.
Székely, G. Embryonic determination of neural connections. *Advances in Morphogenesis*, 1966, **5**, 181–219.
Székely, G. The mesencephalic and diencephalic optic centres in the frog. *Vision Research*, 1971 *Supplement*, **3**, 269–279.
Székely, G., & Czéh, G. Localization of motoneurones in the limb moving spinal cord segments of Ambystoma. *Acta Physiologica*, 1967, **32**, 3–18.
Székely, G., & Czéh, G. Activity of spinal cord fragments and limbs deplanted in the dorsal fin of urodele larvae. *Acta Physiologica*, 1971, 303–312. (a)
Székely, G., & Czéh, G. Muscle activities of partially innervated limbs during locomotion in Ambystoma. *Acta Physiologica*, 1971, 269–286. (b)
Székely, G., Czéh, G. & Vörös, G. The activity pattern of limb muscles in freely moving normal and deafferented newts. *Experimental Brain Research*, 1969, **9**, 55–62.
Szentágothai, J. Neuronal and synaptic arrangements in the substantia gelatinosa Rolandi. *Journal of Comparative Neurology*, 1964, **122**, 219–239.
Szentágothai, J., & Kiss, T. Projection of dermatomes in the substantia gelatinosa. *AMA Archives of Neurology*, 1949, **62**, 734–744.
Szentágothai, J., & Székely, G. Zum Problem der Kreuzung der Nervenbahnen. *Acta Biologica*, 1956, **6**, 215–229.
Taylor, A. C., & Kollros, J. J. Stages in the normal development of *Rana pipiens* larvae. *Anatomical Record*, 1946, **94**, 7–23.
Wall, P. D. The laminar organization of the dorsal horn and effects of descending impulses. *Journal of Physiology (London)*, 1966, **188**, 403–423.
Weddel, G. Somesthesis and the chemical senses. *Annual Review of Psychology*, 1955, **6**, 119–136.
Weiss, P. In vitro experiments on the factors determining the course of one outgrowing nerve fiber. *Journal of Experimental Zoology*, 1934, **68**, 393–448.
Weiss, P. Further experimental investigations on the phenomenon of homologous response in transplanted amphibian limbs. I. Functional observations. *Journal of Comparative Neurology*, 1937, **66**, 181–209. (a)
Weiss, P. II. Nerve regeneration and the innervation of transplanted limbs. *Journal of Comparative Neurology*, 1937, **66**, 481–535. (b)
Weiss, P. III. Homologous response in the absence of sensory innervation. *Journal of Comparative Neurology*, 1937, **66**, 537–548. (c)
Weiss, P. IV. Reverse locomotion after the interchange of right and left limbs. *Journal of Comparative Neurology*, 1937, **67**, 269–315. (d)
Weiss, P. Self-differentiation of the basic patterns of coordination. *Comparative Psychological Monographs*, 1941, **17**, 1–96.
Weiss, P. Lid-closure reflex from eyes transplanted to atypical locations in Triturus torosus: Evidence of a peripheral origin of sensory specificity. *Journal of Comparative Neurology*, 1942, **77**, 131–169.
Weiss, P. Experiments on cell and axon orientation *in vitro*: the role of colloidal exudates in tissue organization. *Journal of Experimental Zoology*, 1945, **100**, 353–386.
Weiss, P. Nervous system (Neurogenesis). In B. H. Willier, P. A. Weiss, & V. Hamburger (Eds.), *Analysis of development*. Philadelphia: Saunders, 1955.

A PLENTITUDE OF NEURONS

MARCUS JACOBSON

Department of Biophysics
The Johns Hopkins University
Baltimore, Maryland

I. Introduction

We have two distinct, but related problems concerning any theory of the development of the nervous system. First, how is the structure and function of the nervous system determined and controlled genetically, either directly or indirectly during development? Second, to what extent and by what means is the nervous system modified by the experience of the individual?

It is undeniable that there is an extensive body of data concerning the invariant structure and functions of neurons that can be readily understood from the standpoint of genetic control of neuronal development: a simple deterministic relationship between genes and the neural substrates of behavior. The nature of these neurons and their development could be fully understood only if one were in possession of sufficient facts. It is equally undeniable that there is a great body of data showing the variability of neuronal structure, function, and behavior which indicates what best may be described as a probabilistic rather than a deterministic mode of neuronal ontogeny. Regardless of the facts at our command, we could never be certain of the behavior of these neurons, and our knowledge would forever remain a statistical prediction.

It is my opinion, therefore, that the next development in neurobiology will be a theory of neuronal development that combines the deterministic and probabilistic aspects. The purpose of the following speculative theory is to give foundation to this synthesis and to show that this leads to a shift in emphasis and a change in our ideas of the role of individual experience in the development of the brain.

In my conjectures about development of the brain, I am aware that it is most unlikely that what I have to offer is entirely original. There may be specialists who could trace antecedents of any of the thoughts I have to offer. We should bear in mind Dr. Johnson's remark to the effect that of these things we can no longer say anything new that is true, or anything true that is new. But we can undoubtedly arrange old thoughts in new relationships to each other, and we are obliged, each time we reconsider them, to see them in the light of our own times. That is my main reason for writing this article.

I have not illustrated my thesis with numerous concrete examples, for that would reduce its force and distinctness as a theory. The essential thesis is that neurons develop in two complementary modes which together permit all possible neuronal functions to be represented: functions that are innately predetermined as well as those that develop as a result of individual experience. In the first mode of development, neurons can express their functions only in a predetermined way as highly predictable patterns of behavior which are characteristic of each species. In the second mode of development, neurons form populations with such diverse potentials that all possible contingencies of function can be realized, including forms of behavior that are unpredictable or aleatory. In the latter mode of neuronal ontogeny, we postulate that there are neurons, especially in the human brain, in which the range of conceivably diversity of structures and functions is exhaustively exemplified. From this *plenum formarum* some neuronal functions and not others will be actualized. This is what Arthur O. Lovejoy has called "the principal of plenitude", namely that whatever can exist must somewhere actually exist, so that there is a maximization of diversity to the limit of logical possibility.

One way in which potential neuronal functions may be actualized is by selecting those which match certain functional criteria, for example, by selecting those neurons which respond preferentially to specific patterns of sensory stimulation. According to this view, the functional potential of these neurons is predetermined in the embryo, but the selective actualization of the functions of certain neurons occurs as a result of individual experience. Although the actualization of neuronal functions may be very great, it is nevertheless limited in man, and even more limited in the lower animals. No single brain evinces a complete realization of all the possibilities of neuronal structure and function. That is, existence is limited to things that actually can coexist because they are compatible or mutually interdependent, and are not contradictory or mutually exclusive. Thus, for the brain of each species, the possible things that are selected from the plenum of possibilities comprise the brain which has actually evolved in that species. As we shall show, brain evolution has occurred as a result of mutations that affected the brain either directly or indirectly, and conferred adaptive advantages on the species. Such neural variants might have arisen in different ways, according to whether they involved the neurons that develop under tight genetic control (Class I neurons) or whether they involved neurons whose development is mainly controlled by exogenous influences such as hormones or sensory stimulation (Class II neurons). Discrete morphological changes in the brain resulting from mutations that directly alter Class I neurons result in what may be called the fine tuning of brain evolution, whereas mutation affecting Class II neurons, whether by changing their sensitivity to exogenous conditions, or by changing the biochemical conditions under which the neurons develop, result in multiform changes in brain functions and behavior.

II. Two Modes of Neuronal Ontogeny

I have made a distinction between Class I neurons whose structure and functions are severely constrained genetically and thus invariant, and Class II neurons with greater variability (Jacobson, 1969, 1970a, 1970b). These have been termed macroneurons and microneurons by Altman (1967). Others have also recognized the value of making a distinction between these two classes of neurons in the cerebral cortex, namely pyramidal cells which have relatively invariant structural and functional characteristics and whose axons project elsewhere (Class I), and Golgi Type II cells which exhibit great variability and connect locally (Globus & Scheibel, 1967b; Scheibel & Scheibel, 1970). The distinction follows and extends the classification into two types of neurons made nearly a century ago by Golgi (1886). Class I neurons are identified as the large neurons with long axons that form the primary afferent and efferent pathways of the nervous system. They constitute what may be termed the hard wiring of the brain. In contradistinction, Class II neurons are thought to develop under lax genetic constraints, and thus to exhibit greater variability and have indeterminate or probabilistic patterns of connectivity. They are interneurons which perform integrative functions between the primary afferent and efferent systems. In each part of the nervous system Class I neurons are generated and differentiate before Class II neurons (Altman, 1967; Angevine, 1970; Jacobson, 1970b). This rule about the time of origin of neurons provides a simple method of neuronal identification and a means of distinction between the two classes by labeling them with tritiated thymidine at different stages of development (Sidman, 1970).

This conception has the advantage that it provides an explanation for the great diversification of Class II neurons without the need for invoking any detailed genetic specifications of the hundreds or even thousands of recognizable neuronal phenotypes. It is postulated that these Class II neurons develop freely, with little genetic control of the details of their morphology and connectivity. Genetic control is assumed to extend merely to those cellular components that are essential for the life of the cell. The morphological details, especially the pattern of axonal and dendritic branching and the location of synapses on the surface of the neuron, are all determined by the contingencies of development, that is by probabilistic epigenetic factors. One consequence of this, which will be amplified later, is that slight modifications resulting from gene mutations will be insignificant against the background of variability that arises from other causes in Class II neurons. Only changes in the external conditions to which Class II neurons are sensitive or changes in the sensitivity of these neurons are likely to produce changes of behavior which may affect the evolution of the species.

Contingencies such as the availability of space and the levels of nutrients, hormones, and other conditions of the cellular environment play important roles in modifying the differentiation of Class II neurons. If, in addition, the production of such neurons occurs in excess, the availability of space and nutrients will limit the number of cells that can be generated or can survive to maturity. Such a developing system will show adaptive changes similar to those that have been observed in populations of cells or organisms that are engaged in a Darwinian struggle for survival under conditions of restricted space, nutrients, and other environmental factors. The development of Class II neurons in my theory would bear a striking resemblence to the process of survival of the fittest individuals in a population showing small but significant individual differences. The surviving neurons will become more and more closely matched with the functional requirements of the organism but will have a progressively reduced reserve of potential functions. In the case of neuronal ontogeny, the small but significant differences between neurons arise inevitably, because the contingencies of development are unique for each neuron and result in their diversification during development. From this diversity, certain neurons are selected for survival on the basis of their response to extrinsic factors such as sensory stimulation or hormonal stimulation. The function of these stimuli is permissive, in the sense that they merely constitute a functional validation of preexisting neuronal structures.

III. Constructive and Destructive Forms of Neuronal Plasticity

We shall note that neuronal plasticity may be constructive or destructive. The constructive process may either take the form of functional potentiation of preexisting structures or of the development of new neuronal structures. The destructive form of neuronal plasticity may be a functional restriction, or a structural atrophy, or even death of the neuron. Restriction may proceed partially or to completion in different neurons. The restriction of functional potential is inherent in Class I neurons, which have invariant and unmodifiable functions from the beginning of their existence. Class II neurons have multiple functional potentials which become progressively restricted during their lives. Once the restriction of functional potential has been completed, the neuron is regarded as unipotential and functionally unmodifiable. The progression from the multipotential to the unipotential condition is irreversible, but occurs at different rates and at different times in various parts of the nervous system. Therefore, the modifiability of neurons can only diminish and not increase. The theory of neuronal plentitude holds that the functional potential of individual neurons as well as of assemblies of neurons is maximal in the earlier stages of development and progressively diminishes with experience and learning.

Changes in the nervous system that occur during sensory stimulation and experience are usually regarded as constructive modifications. Altman (1967) has proposed that experience in the newborn mammal stimulates proliferation of "microneurons." His studies, although landmarks on the way to an understanding of the role of experience on neurogenesis, have certain limitations which prevent unreserved acceptance of their conclusions. It does not seem that postnatal sensory stimulation can play a large role in altering *neuronal* proliferation in mammals (although it may have an effect on gliogenesis and synaptogenesis), because neurogenesis has ceased completely in the neocortex before birth (Berry & Rogers, 1966), and with the exception of neurons formed in the olfactory bulbs, hippocampal formation, cerebellar cortex, and brainstem nuclei, the majority of neurons of all types appear to originate prenatally. Rather, the significance of the time of neuronal ontogenesis that is emphasised here is that the neurons that are first in the field are less variable and less modifiable than those that are last in the field (but not necessarily formed postnatally), and that the latter are more susceptible to destructive as well as to constructive changes resulting from experience. Moreover, these effects may be produced directly by nervous activity or indirectly via the endocrine system. As there appears to be no way in which neuronal activities may affect the proliferation of neuroepithelial germinal cells directly, any effect of experience on neural cell proliferation has to be mediated by hormones, which have been shown to have destructive as well as constructive effects on the brain. Thus, Hunt and Jacobson (1971) have shown that prolactin or somatotropin increase brain cell number by reducing cell death as well as by increasing cell proliferation. By contrast, corticosterone administered to newborn mice reduces brain cell number, probably by both reducing proliferation and by increasing death of brain cells (Howard, 1968).

The new physiological activities that result from experience are thought to be due to growth of axons or dendrites, neogenesis of synaptic connections, or functional enhancement at synapses (Cragg, 1968). Such constructive changes do not preclude the possibility that an excessive number of connections develop initially and that sensory stimulation selectively maintains some connections, while the others are eliminated or repressed, as Mark (1970) has postulated. The evidence is inadequate to show either that experience controls the initial development of neuronal connections or that it facilitates and maintains previously formed connections. These two hypothetical mechanisms are not mutually exclusive; both are viable possibilities to be demonstrated or refuted experimentally. The concept that emerges in this article is that the effects of experience, whether mediated directly by neurons or indirectly by hormones, are likely to be destructive as well as constructive. Synaptic growth and transmission may be decreased as well as increased, and neural metabolism may be enhanced or repressed as a result of sensory-motor activity. The net effect of experience may thus be a selective elimination of synapses and of neurons in the richly interconnected population of neurons that normally develop in the brain of the naïve creature.

The effects of experience are usually greatest in the young animal at "critical periods" during which specific kinds of stimulation are necessary for development to continue normally. Quite specific defects in behavior occur if the animal has not been properly stimulated during the critical period, but even a brief period of stimulation may be sufficient. At present, our difficulty in understanding this phenomenon is largely due to inadequate knowledge of what occurs in the nervous system during such "critical periods." We know that the functional specificity of the sensory systems must have developed, and that the central nervous system must have developed to an advanced stage before stimulation can have any effects, but we do not know what is added or subtracted as a result of the type of stimulation that is obligatory during the "critical period." Two examples may be sufficient to indicate how the specific stimuli that are required during "critical periods" may have a permissive rather than a constructive function.

As is well known, male sexual behavior in mammals is determined to a large extent by testosterone acting on the brain during a short critical period which lasts for 10 days after birth in the rat. Castrated rats develop male sexual behavior some weeks after receiving an injection of testosterone on the day after birth, but female behavior ensues if the androgen is not administered during the first 10 days after birth (Gorski, 1966; Harris & Levine, 1965). The expression of male sexual behavior is due to the action of testosterone on neurons that have not been fully identified but which must be present in both sexes, and merely remain functionally unexpressed in females.

It seems to have escaped notice that Class II neurons bear the brunt of the influences of hormones, metabolic or nutritional disturbances, and sensory stimulation. These exogenous influences come into play late in development after the histogenesis and differentiation of Class I neurons has largely been completed but during the period of genesis and differentiation of Class II neurons in many regions of the brain. Changes in extracellular conditions during the period of development of Class II neurons may alter their proliferation, could determine the number that survive or die, and perhaps in fluence the functions of the surviving neurons.

IV. Neuronal Evolution in Relation to Ontogeny

Because the two classes of neurons are subject to different kinds of controls during development, it follows that genetic mutations may have different effects on Class I and Class II neurons. As Rensch (1960) puts it,

> Quite often, phylogenetic transformation seems to be brought about by the addition of new phases to the ontogenetic development; this has been referred to as anabolies by Sewertzoff (1931) and as hypermorphosis by DeBeer (1940). The frequency of this phenomenon seems to be due to the fact that alterations of early and intermediate stages of ontogeny will more readily be wiped out by selection; more developmental reactions are disturbed by such alterations than by mutants adding new phases to the final stage of the morphogenesis [Rensch, 1960, p. 253].

There are numerous ways in which mutations may alter the brain and behavior. Mutations may affect the nervous system directly or may have an indirect effect on the peripheral sensory or motor organs, endocrine system, or on general physiological functions primarily involving the kidneys, liver, or any other organ. Mutations affecting nonneural systems, if they have any neurological effects, are much more likely to alter the development of Class II neurons than to affect Class I neurons. By virtue of their normally great variability and redundancy, Class II neurons are buffered against the effects of changes in their morphology resulting directly from genetic mutations. However, mutations may have large effects on the structure and functions of Class II neurons if they alter neuronal sensitivity to hormones, metabolic agents, or to sensory stimulation, or if the mutations change the factors to which the neurons are sensitive. Mutations of Class II neurons may be accepted if they produce no significant changes in functions. These neutral mutations may have resulted in the great diversity and variability of Class II neurons. However, mutations that are neutral under one set of conditions may become of evolutionary significance if the environmental conditions change. Thus the great reserve of potentially advantageous mutations that are embodied in Class II neurons gives them tremendous significance in conferring rapid adaptive capacity in the face of changes in the environment. As Stebbins (1966) has demonstrated, this type of evolutionary change in the adaptive value of a mutation as a result of a change in the environment is almost independent of mutation rate or population size.

Because Class I neurons are committed to perform specific and invariant functions, and because of their strategic locations at the input and output and as essential links between parts of the nervous system, mutations that affect even a small number of these neurons will result in significant changes in behavior. However, these changes are much more likely to be deleterious than beneficial. This is one reason for the remarkably conservative evolution of Class I neurons. A striking example of a mutation that affects only a small group of Class I neurons and which has a deleterious effect on binocular vision has been found in Siamese cats (Guillery, 1969; Guillery & Kaas, 1971). Guillery has also found that albino rats and ferrets, as well as Siamese cats, have a genetically determined anomaly of chiasmal crossing of optic nerve fibers. In the mutants, some optic nerve fibers that arise from ganglion cells in the temporal half of the retina cross over at the chiasma to the opposite side of the brain, whereas they normally grow into the same side.

In this example, the mutation has selectively altered the growth trajectory of axons of a small group of retinal ganglion cells. Mutations may alter behavior significantly if they involve even a small number of large neurons with long axons, such as retinal ganglion cells, motoneurons, or Purkinje cells. On the other hand, mutations that act indirectly on Class II neurons, via the endocrine system, for example, will affect relatively large numbers of neurons. Even when the effect is selective, as in the action of testosterone on the brain, large numbers of neurons are affected in several brain regions, in the hypothalamus and cerebrum. The effects of mutations of Class II neurons are likely to be protean and yet compatible with normal brain function. By contrast, mutational effects on Class I neurons are almost invariably harmful. Any agents that modify Class I neurons will have disadvantageous effects unless they produce very small modifications. Large modifications of Class II neurons are relatively more easily tolerated.

An example of the tolerance of the nervous system to large changes in Class II neurons is provided by some recent experiments that R. K. Hunt and I have performed on frogs. We found that injections of prolactin or somatotropin into frog tadpoles resulted in up to 70% increase in the total number of brain cells (Hunt & Jacobson, 1971). Some regions, such as the optic tectum, showed even greater increases in the number of cells, and yet we could see no obvious changes in neural functions or behavior. Preliminary studies have shown that the number of retinal ganglion cells is not increased, and that other types of Class I neurons, such as spinal and cranial motoneurons, are also unaffected by prolactin or somatotropin administered to tadpoles. We may draw similar inferences from the results of administration of somatotropin to the mouse fetus, reported by Zamenhof and his associates (Zamenhof, Mosley, & Schuller, 1966). The fact that behavior of the mice was not obviously altered, although the number of brain cells had been significantly increased, suggests that Class I neurons had not been affected by the hormone.

The foregoing considerations lead us to recognize that the two classes of neurons play different roles in the evolution of behavior. These differences in the evolutionary roles of neurons are correlated with differences in their modes of development. Class I neurons are the first to develop and form what may be thought of as a skeleton to which Class II neurons are later attached. Thus, slight modification of Class I neurons have cumulative effects which may become deleterious at later stages of development. The majority of mutations affecting Class I neurons are expected to be disadvantageous, and in fact are so. Class II neurons, by contrast, develop only after the main plan of the nervous system has been sketched in by Class I neurons. Small modifications of Class II neurons are unlikely to result in significant changes in brain function. However, during the period of development of Class II neurons the organism is undergoing large changes both internally and in relation to the external environment, and the Class II neurons are sensitive to many of these changes. Mutations affecting nonneuronal systems may thus alter the conditions under which Class II neurons develop, and in fact, the development of Class II neurons is greatly influenced by exogenous conditions which include sensory stimulation.

V. The Functions of Experience

The following example illustrates the role of sensory stimulation in the development of neurons in the mammalian visual cortex. Recent work has shown that the developing cortical neurons are extremely sensitive to visual deprivation. Binocularly driven cells in the visual cortex of the kitten are present at birth, but disappear unless the animal has a period of normal vision, with both eyes working together, during the fourth to sixth week after birth (Hubel & Wiesel, 1965). During this critical period the cortical cells are very sensitive to the effects of visual deprivation, and even a few hours of monocular occlusion results in a reduction in the number of binocularly activated cortical cells (Hubel & Wiesel, 1970). Although the visual cortical neurons are binocularly connected and retinotopically arranged at birth, they appear to lack the specificity of adult neurons with regard to the orientation, direction of movement, and binocular disparity of visual stimuli. Barlow and Pettigrew (1971) have recently shown that these functional specificities of visual cortical neurons are absent in the newborn cat, and only begin to appear at the fourth week after birth if the animal has had normal visual experience, but fail to develop in visually deprived kittens. As is now well known from the work of Hirsch and Spinelli (1970, 1971) and Blakemore and Cooper (1970), the visual cortical neurons of the kitten develop orientation specificities that match the orientations of bar-shaped visual stimuli to which the kitten has been exposed, and the cortical cells fail to respond to stimulus orientations which they have not experienced during the critical period.

These reports do not show whether development of the functional characteristics of visual cortical neurons is due to constructive or destructive processes, or to a combination of these. The process may be constructive in the sense that visual experience stimulates the formation of new connections between the visual cortical cells. However, it is also possible that the development of specific visual cortical functions is a destructive process, and that the immature visual cortical neurons have multiplex connectivity which becomes pruned or tuned by selective elimination of excessive connections. There are thus two ways in which we might conceive of functional neuronal adaptation. Sensory stimulation may stimulate the initial formation of neuronal connections, or experience might diminish the preexisting plenitude of neuronal branches and connections. In both cases the changes are adaptive; that is, they fit the creature more adequately to survive in its natural habitat or even in conditions which are completely abnormal, such as those imposed by sensory deprivation or enrichment in the laboratory.

In the inexperienced animal, the neurons of the visual cortex must be capable of being changed, either by gaining new functions, or by selective reduction of their preexisting functions, into the functional types that are found in the adult. The fact that there is a small number of such functional types and that neurons with the same functions are not randomly distributed but are arranged in vertical columns in the cerebral cortex shows that the immature, inexperienced neurons are not equipotential but must have innate predispostions to assume specific functions. If so, it is merely a small step to postulate that visual cortical neurons in the newborn animal are already precommitted to specific functional roles in sufficient diversity to include all types found in the adult. The full development and even survival of each neuron is contingent on sensory stimulation which matches the trigger features and other functional characteristics of each neuron. These functional characteristics are predetermined in the fetus but are selectively actualized by sensory stimulation. Under normal conditions of visual experience, most neurons in the visual cortex receive sufficient stimulation to ensure their final development according to their predetermined function. Restriction of visual experience results in the full development of only those neurons whose functional characteristics match the restricted visual stimuli, while the remainder will either remain undeveloped or will atrophy and die. If visual experience results in a reduction of the initially redundant connections, inexperienced animals will have more synapses, and probably more neurons, than experienced animals of similar genetic background.

VI. Neuronal Modification by Selective Depletion

The prediction is that experience will result in a reduction in the number of synapses and probably in an increase in their size and enhancement of their functions. These changes will be difficult to show by recording with microelectrodes in the brain because of the small and biased sample of neurons that can be studied by that method. Anatomical methods that permit unbiased sampling of neurons and synapses are preferable to those that are highly selective. Thus, the observation that visual deprivation results in a reduction of the spines on the apical dendrites of pyramidal cells in the visual cortex (Globus & Scheibel, 1967a; Valverde, 1967) is of limited value because it is restricted to a single type of neuron in a population consisting of many types, and because it fails to distinguish between a redistribution of synapses and an absolute reduction in the number of synapses. Experience may have opposite effects on different neurons in the same part of the brain. Thus, Cragg (1967) found that when rats that had been reared in the dark were exposed to light, the synapses in the superficial layers of the visual cortex became larger and less numerous, while those in the deep cortical layers became smaller and more numerous. Fewer and larger asymmetrical axodendritic synapses were also found in layer III of the occipital cortex of rats reared under conditions of sensory-motor enrichment than in littermates reared in a less stimulating environment (Möllgaard, Diamond, Bennett, Rosenzweig, & Lindner, 1971). These results support the hypothesis that sensory stimulation reduces the plenitude of synapses in some parts of the brain.

The theory of neuronal plenitude suggests that functional adaptation takes the form of a selective maintenance or functional validation of neuronal connections and a functional deterioration or even structural atrophy of the unused connections. That is not to say that constructive changes may not occur *pari passu* with the selective depletion of preexisting neuronal structures. The maturation of the nervous system involves an increase in the total number of synapses in all regions that have been studied. This synaptogenesis is almost certainly determined innately as part of the normal developmental program, and there is no admissible evidence showing that synapses from *de novo* as a result of sensory stimulation or electrical activity in the nervous system.

The initial formation of synapses must involve two types of interactions: cooperative and competitive. Cooperative interactions include the cytochemical affinities between pre- and postsynaptic membranes that result in selective formation of synapses (Sperry, 1963), as well as the trophic effects that are illustrated by the interactions between nerve and muscle (Guth, 1968) and nerve and sensory cells (Jacobson, 1971). These connections develop on the basis of a temporospatial pattern of genetic control. Competitive interactions involve a "struggle" between the excess number of presynaptic elements for connection with a limited number of postsynaptic sites. This process of competitive struggle for survival may include not only the survival of the fittest neurons, but also of the fittest axonal and dendritic branches and their synaptic connections. The effect of these interactions is to reduce the initial redundancy, to selectively promote the development of neuronal structures that can coexist because they are mutually compatible or mutually interdependent, and not contradictory or mutually exclusive. The reduction of structures, including synapses which this theory predicts, results in an increased matching of the functions of the nervous system with the conditions of the world in which the creature lives. As Herbert Spencer put it, it is a process which brings the inner and outer relations of the organism into closer correspondence.

VII. Nativism and Empiricism in the Light of the Theory of Neuronal Plenitude

This theory also has reference to the dispute between the nativists and empiricists about what is given to the nervous system by nature and what is acquired by nurture. The obligatory interaction between the organism and its environment, and therefore, the interdependence of nature and nurture, is a well-known theme. I shall mention only how it relates to the theory that I am advancing here.

In this theory the nativist philosophy applies to Class I neurons which develop deterministically according to a preestablished ontogenetic pattern. The empiricist philosophy applies to Class II neurons whose development is contingent upon a multiplicity of factors which can only be expressed in terms of probabilities. The range of functions and structures of the first class of neurons is limited by genetic controls, and these in turn are the products of evolutionary selection. Diversification of the second class of neurons is restricted only by the contingencies of space, nutrition, and mutual interactions within the developing brain. The functional expression, and even the actual survival of this second class of neurons, is determined by the experience and sensory stimulation of each individual. Their development is an adaptive process whereby only those functions become expressed that are called up in the organism by the contingencies of its daily life and are necessary for its normal activities and survival. According to this theory, the capacity for neuronal function is inherent, but neurons can express themselves functionally only in conformity with the needs of the individual creature which are determined by its environment. On this theory, neuronal capacities are imminent and they are expressed or are actualized in response to functional demands, that is, by selective functional validation of preexisting neuronal structures. Given a sufficiently large number and diversity of neurons, there is a high probability that they will be capable of subserving every contingency of functional activity that is required for the normal life and survival of the organism.

I do not pretend to have proved the above theory; all I claim is that, like any useful theory, it is not incompatible with the known facts, and it clarifies some problems that hitherto could not be explained by other theories. Not least important is that this theory makes certain predictions about the number and diversity of neurons in the developing brain that should permit its refutation, for I believe that the possibility of refutation is an essential element of any theory that is to be worthy of serious consideration. As Nietzsche put it: "It is certainly not the least charm of a theory that it is refutable; it is precisely thereby that it attracts the more subtle minds."

VIII. Summary

The nervous system of vertebrates consists of a very large number of nerve cells of great morphological and functional diversity. Many more nerve cells are produced during normal development than survive to function in the mature animal. There is a competition between neurons which results in the elimination of some neurons in part or whole. It is argued that the survival of developing nerve cells is contingent upon their functional fitness. The final state of the developing nervous system is a dynamic equilibrium which results from cooperative and competetive interactions between its components. The cooperative interactions occur between neurons that have genetically predetermined affinites. These may take the form of a structural and functional congruence of neurons that develop synaptic connections. The competitive interactions between neurons of diverse functional capabilities result in the survival of those with functional and structural congruence and the elimination of neurons that are mutually incompatible.

The first neurons to be generated and to differentiate in any part of the nervous system have invariant structure and functions which are genetically predetermined. These Class I neurons form a framework into which the Class II neurons, which are formed later, are inserted. Class II neurons develop under the influence of exogenous stimuli mediated by the sense organs and nerves and by hormones. The quality, quantity, and timing of stimulation are critical determinants of the development, and even survival, of Class II neurons.

There is a principle of developmental genetics to the effect that gene mutations modifying early stages of development are likely to have greater effects, usually deleterious, than mutations altering later stages of development. When this principle is applied to neuronal ontogeny it is shown that large, rapid changes in Class II neurons may be tolerated and may be of benefit to the individual, but modifications of Class I neurons are brought about slowly by the accumulation of small advantageous changes during evolution. Moreover, because the details of morphology are of much less functional significance in Class II than in Class I neurons, many more neutral mutations, which do not significantly alter function, will become fixed in the former than in the latter. The accumulation of such neutral mutations in Class II neurons endows them with potentially adaptive capacities. Mutations that are neutral or functionally insignificant under one set of environmental conditions may be functionally advantageous when the conditions change and may enable the organism to adapt rapidly to changed conditions.

References

Altman, J. Postnatal growth and differentiation of the mammalian brain, with implications for a morphological theory of memory. In G. Quarton, T. Melnechuk, & F. O. Schmitt (Eds.), *The neurosciences: A study program.* New York: Rockefeller University Press, 1967.

Angevine, J. B.; Jr. Critical cellular events in the shaping of neural centers. In F. O. Schmitt (Ed.), *The neurosciences: Second study program.* New York: Rockefeller University Press, 1970. Pp. 62–72.

Barlow, H. B., & Pettigrew, J. D. Lack of specificity of neurones in the visual cortex of young kittens. *Journal of Physiology* (*London*), 1971, **218**, 98P–100P.

Berry, M., & Rogers, A. W. Histogenesis of mammalian neocortex. In R. Hassler & H. Stephan (Eds.), *Evolution of the Forebrain.* New York: Plenum, 1966. Pp. 197–205.

Blakemore, C., & Cooper, G. Development of the brain depends on the visual environment. *Nature* (*London*), 1970, **228**, 477–478.

Cragg, B. G. Changes in visual cortex on first exposure of rats to light: Effect on synaptic dimensions. *Nature* (*London*), 1967, **215**, 251–253.

Cragg, B. G. Are there structural alterations in synapses related to functioning? *Proceedings of the Royal Society, Series B*, 1968, **171**, 319–323.
DeBeer, G. R. *Embryos and ancestors*. London: Oxford University Press, 1940.
Globus, A., & Scheibel, A. B. The effect of visual deprivation on cortical neurons: a Golgi study. *Experimental Neurology*, 1967, **19**, 331–345. (a)
Globus, A., & Scheibel, A. B. Pattern and field in cortical structure: the rabbit. *Journal of Comparative Neurology*, 1967, **131**, 155–172. (b)
Golgi, C. *Sulla fina anatomia degli organi centrali del sistema nervoso*. Milano: *U. Hoepli, 1886.*
Gorski, R. A. Localization and sexual differentiation of the nervous structures which regulate ovulation. *Journal of Reproduction and Fertility, Supplement*, 1966, **1**, 67–88.
Guillery, R. W. An abnormal retinogeniculate projection in Siamese cats. *Brain Research*, 1969, **14**, 739–741.
Guillery, R. W. & Kaas, J. H. A study of normal and congenitally abnormal retinogeniculate projection in cats. *Journal of Comparative Neurology*, 1971, **143**, 73–100.
Guth, L. "Trophic" influences of nerve on muscle. *Physiological Reviews*, 1968, **48**, 645–687.
Harris, G. W., & Levine, S. Sexual differentiation of the brain and its experimental control. *Journal of Physiology* (*London*), 1965, **181**, 379–400
Hirsch, H. V. B., & Spinelli, D. N. Visual experience modifies distribution of horizontally and vertically oriented receptive fields in cats. *Science*, 1970, **168**, 869–871.
Hirsch, H. V. B., & Spinelli, D. N. Modification of the distribution of receptive field organization in cats by selective visual exposure during development. *Experimental Brain Research*, 1971, **13**, 509–527.
Howard, E. Reduction in size and total DNA of cerebrum and cerebellum in adult mice after corticosterone treatment in infancy. *Experimental Neurology*, 1968, **22**, 191–208.
Hubel, D. H., & Wiesel, T. N. Binocular interaction in striate cortex of kittens reared with artificial squint. *Journal of Neurophysiology*, 1965, **28**, 1041–1059.
Hubel, D. H., & Wiesel, T. N. The period of susceptibility to the physiological effects of unilateral eye closure in kittens. *Journal of Physiology* (*London*), 1970, **206**, 419–436.
Hunt, R. K., & Jacobson, M. Neurogenesis in frogs after early larval treatment with somatotropin or prolactin. *Developmental Biology*, 1971, **26**, 100–124.
Jacobson, M. Development of specific neuronal connections. *Science*, 1969, **163**, 543–547.
Jacobson, M. Development, specification and diversification of neuronal connections. In F. O. Schmitt (Ed.), *The neurosciences: Second study program*. New York: Rockefeller University Press, 1970. Pp. 116–129. (a)
Jacobson, M. *Developmental neurobiology*. New York: Holt, 1970. (b)
Jacobson, M. Formation of neuronal connections in sensory systems. In W. R. Lowenstein (Ed.), *Handbook of sensory physiology*. Vol. I. Berlin & New York: Springer-Verlag, 1971.
Mark, R. F. Chemospecific synaptic repression as a possible memory store. *Nature* (*London*), 1970, **225**, 178–179.
Möllgaard, K., Diamond, M. D., Bennett, E. L., Rosenzweig, M. R., & Lindner, B. Quantitative synaptic changes with differential experience in rat brain. *International Journal of Neuroscience*, 1971, **2**, 113–128.
Rensch, B. *Evolution above the species level*. New York: Columbia University Press, 1960.
Scheibel, M. E., & Scheibel, A. B. Elementary processes in selected thalamic and cortical subsystems: The structural subsystems. In F. O. Schmitt (Ed.), *The neurosciences: Second study program*. New York: Rockefeller University Press, 1970. Pp. 443–457.
Sewertzoff, A. N. *Morphologische Gesetzmässigkeiten der Evolution*. Jena: Fischer, 1931.
Sidman, R. L. Autoradiogrphic methods and principles for study of the nervous system with thymidine-H^3. In S. O. E. Ebbesson & W. J. H. Nauta (Eds.), *Contemporary research methods in neuroanatomy*. Berlin & New York: Springer-Verlag, 1970.
Sperry, R. W. Chemoaffinity in the orderly growth of nerve fiber patterns and connections.

Proceedings of the National Academy of Sciences, U.S., 1963, **50**, 703–710.
Stebbins, A. L. *Processes of organic evolution.* Englewood Cliffs, N. J. Prentice-Hall, 1966.
Valverde, F. Apical dendritic spines of the visual cortex and light deprivation in the mouse. *Experimental Brain Research*, 1967, **3**, 337–352.
Zamenhof, S., Mosley, J., & Schuller, E. Stimulation of the proliferation of cortical neurons by prenatal treatment with growth hormone. *Science*, 1966, **152**, 1396–1397.

Section 2

FETAL BRAIN FUNCTION: SENSORY AND MOTOR ASPECTS

INTRODUCTION

In order for sensory stimulation to have any significance whatsoever for the immature animal, its sensory systems must be capable of integrating the stimulation. As reviewed in the first article of Volume 1, all the different sensory systems do not become functional at the same time—in fact they seem to become functional in a certain sequence (tactile, vestibular, auditory, visual) which holds across a number of species, both in birds and in mammals. The connections which the sense organs make directly in one cerebral hemisphere of the brain and the cross connections between the two hemispheres of the brain also seem to proceed in a set sequence, the direct (contralateral) connections first and the interhemispheric connections second.

In order to study the very early development of sensory or afferent processes in the brain itself, it is necessary to work at the electrophysiological level, an arduous task described for us in this section by Dr. B. A. Meyerson and Dr. H. E. Persson. Since they wish to understand the development of cortical sensory function in placental mammals, Meyerson and Persson have chosen the relatively large, slow-growing sheep fetus as an experimental animal. It is only by pushing such analyses to the very earliest stages of cerebral development, as Meyerson and Persson are doing, that we will be able to come to a correct understanding of mammalian brain development, including such provocative problems as the maturation of excitatory and inhibitory circuits and the ontogeny of receptive fields in the cortex. Much of what we now know about these two problems in mammals comes from studies of *neonates* (specifically, newborn kittens), in which neural development is fairly advanced at birth, even in an altricial species such as the domestic cat. Thus, the studies of Meyerson and Persson on early fetal stages hold exceptional promise for increasing our knowledge of afferent processes in the brain.

In the second article in this section, Dr. R. M. Bergström makes a preliminary application of communication theory to the developing brain–behavior relationship in guinea pig fetuses—the first time that a communication-theoretical viewpoint has been applied to development. The inverted-U function (Fig. 2) in Dr. Bergström's article will be familiar to many readers of the psychological literature, particularly those who are acquainted with the many fruitful derivatives of Donald Hebb's neuropsychological perspective. Dr. Bergström's inverted-U function represents the notion that, developmentally speaking, as neural excitation increases (either through a growing number of efferent synapses or an increase in central or peripheral stimulation, or both), overt motor activity becomes more "organized" or "ordered" up to a certain point, beyond which organization falls off. The notion itself is of course not new—the novel aspect is in its application to prenatal brain–behavior relations. At the moment the formal aspect of the mathematical model does not yet accommodate the important development of inhibitory circuits which seem to come in around two-thirds of the way through gestation in the guinea pig and which cause a transitory age-related diminution in fetal activity upon central or peripheral stimulation. Dr. Bergström's future work on the model will involve the behavior of lower organisms with more primitive neural networks, and that should facilitate the working out and inclusion of further parameters into the model which are distinctive to developmental phenomena. Theoretical exposition and model building are not easy or trivial tasks, and when successful they can order a great deal of information and predict novel experimental outcomes; so one appreciates Dr. Bergström's efforts in this direction.

EARLY EPIGENESIS OF RECIPIENT FUNCTIONS IN THE NEOCORTEX

B. A. MEYERSON AND H. E. PERSSON*

Department of Physiology
Karolinska Institutet
Stockholm, Sweden

I. Introduction

One of the basic problems within the field of embryonic physiology is the question of the possible prenatal influence of sensory stimuli upon the functional development of the central nervous system. A prerequisite for

*Present address: Department of Neurosurgery, Karolinska Sjukhuset, Stockholm 60, Sweden.

attacking this problem is the availability of data concerning neurogenesis obtained by a descriptive-correlative approach. For instance, it is of prime interest to know when in ontogenesis an external signal is effective for the first time as a stimulus which induces a response in the central nervous system sufficient to produce a change in behavior (e.g., generalized or local muscular activation, or any other demonstrable changes such as electrical or chemical events). For the study of the complex phases of behavior in the immature postnatal animal, the probabilistic conception of development directs attention to the role of the developing cerebral neocortex as a "final site" for the processing of sensory information. This raises the question of when in ontogenesis signs of activation within the central nervous system may be traced up to a cortical level for the first time.

When considering an afferent system comprising direct pathways to the neocortical projection area, one may picture a developmental stage when the cortex has not yet been reached by the growing corticopetal fibers and when no functional contacts are present between the subcortical portion of the system and the cortical neurons. One may inquire into the properties of such an incomplete afferent system, capable of transmitting signals from the body surface to subcortical structures, and also ask whether its functional characteristics are in any way altered by the establishment of terminal-cortical contacts which may introduce a cortical feedback mechanism (like that serving sensory motor integration, cf. Conway, Wright, & Bradley, 1969).

In maturity, behavior is a result of the processing of a multiplicity of extra- and interoceptive signals. On a cortical level this integration is made possible, both in phylogenesis and ontogenesis, by the evolution of association areas, that is to say, fields with nonspecific sensory projections but with the function of providing a complicated interplay among influences from various sensory systems. However, it is not known how this differentiation into various cortical fields occurs. Applying general theories of development, one may assume the development of the cortex to occur *in toto* or *in partes.*

According to the *in toto* view, the species-specific relationship in adults between the primary projection fields and those denoted as associative is already present as functional and structural *anlagen* in the immature brain. This would imply that integrative processes take place in the cortex once the receptive functions are established, though on a comparatively primitive level. Hence, one would also expect the different sensory systems to develop uniformly with regard to the organization of their specific cortical projections.

Following the *in partes* conception, the epigenesis of each projective system at the cortical level proceeds independently of the others and functions as an isolated unit. One might assume the cortical fields destined for an integrative role at this initial stage to be nonfunctional, and the mutual interdependence of the different sensory systems consequently would not occur until later in development. With such a view the developmental hierarchy of the various sensory systems, known to be present in neonatal behavior, is also likely to occur in cortical development (for further discussion, see Gottlieb 1970, and in Volume 1 in this serial publication.

It is evident from this general outline that the study of cortical functions during early life demands the utilization of a variety of experimental methods. However, for obvious reasons, many of the very sophisticated techniques used in the study of central nervous function in the adult animal are not applicable to the embryo. Consequently, when electrophysiological methods are employed, one often has to draw conclusions from insufficient data obtained with comparatively crude methods. Furthermore, it should be emphasized that the questions raised above often cannot be answered by studies restricted to the postnatal period of development. That is, observations in various species during the *neonatal* period show that cortical potentials can already be evoked in the somesthetic, visual, and acoustic systems, that the callosal system is excitable, and that spontaneous cortical activity occurs sporadically (references in Bernhard & Meyerson, 1968; Gottlieb, 1971). This means that one must delve back into prenatal life in order to explore the *initial* stages of functional epigenesis of the cortex.

II. Choice of Experimental Animal

For the functional study of the central nervous system during early stages of development, we chose a species of animal with a relatively large fetus, which is easily accessible, and is comparatively resistent to technical manipulations. The classical investigations by Barcroft in the 1930's of prenatal circulation were performed on sheep fetuses which were externalized and kept in umbilical contact with the ewe. This indicated that the sheep fetus might also be a convenient preparation for an electrophysiological exploration of the immature central nervous system. A firm physiological basis has also been provided by the extensive studies published during the last decade by Dawes and his group on circulation and metabolism in the fetal sheep (reviewed in Dawes, 1968).

The sheep's gestational period comprises about 145 days, and the weight of the fetus at full-term is about 3 kg. Like other herd animals, the sheep is relatively mature at birth from a neurophysiological and behavioral point of view (cf. Ruckebusch, 1971). As shown by a morphological study of the developing cortex in the fetal sheep, each phase of cortical epigenesis seems to be more protracted than in animals with a shorter gestation period

(Åström, 1967). Furthermore, the fact that the process of maturation is almost completed before birth implies that various nervous functions can be conveniently studied under the same physiological and technical conditions during the entire cycle of development before the transition takes place from intrauterine to extrauterine life. Because of the anatomical arrangement of placental vessels, the sheep fetus is also relatively easily accessible from the surgical point of view. In this connection it should also be mentioned that in the sheep the pO_2 gradient between the maternal and fetal blood is comparatively high (Barron, 1951). Due to this fact, fetal hypoxia in the sheep does not occur until after drastic reduction of the maternal blood pO_2 (Comline & Silver, 1968) and changes in maternal pO_2 during the experiment are less likely to affect the fetus.

III. Surgical Preparation and Recording Technique

The ewe was decerebrated while under a short-acting barbiturate which was then withdrawn, and the actual experiment on the fetus did not start until several hours later. In this way the fetus was considered not to be under the influence of any general anesthetic during the time of the recording. In order to avoid distention of the rumen, ventriculotomy was performed and the ewe connected to a respirator. In later experiments the efficiency of artificial respiration was checked by a continuous monitoring of the expired CO_2 concentration. The fetus was externalized by caesarian section and kept in umbilical contact with the placenta *in situ*. The fetus was placed on a plastic cushion containing circulating water at a constant temperature and covered with cotton wool soaked in warm paraffin oil. The surgical procedure consisted of a wide craniotomy with removal of the dura from the dorsal aspect of the hemispheres, leaving the sagittal sinus intact. The physiological condition of the preparation was assessed by continuous EKG monitoring, microscopic inspection of the cortical microcirculation, measurement of the cortical steady potential, and the character of the spontaneous cortical activity. If care was taken to avoid spasm in the umbilical vessels and to maintain the temperature of the fetus, and if the surgical trauma was kept to a minimum, even fetuses at an early stage of development could be used for up to about 5 hours.

Evoked surface potentials were recorded in a monopolar arrangement with calomel electrodes with a recording area of .5 mm^2; DC coupling was used. Recordings of evoked unitary and gross potentials from the depth of the cortex were performed with glass micropipettes filled with 5.5 M NaCl or 2.8 M KCl. Impedance ranged from 1 to 50 $M\Omega$. Stimulation of the cortical surface was administered through a pair of ball-tipped silver electrodes separated by a distance of about .5 mm. For tactile stimulation of the nose, a ball-tipped probe with a diameter of .5 mm was used. The probe was regulated electromagnetically. (For further details concerning the surgical and recording techniques, see Meyerson, 1968; Persson, 1973.)

IV. On the Properties of the Neocortex in Newborn Animals

In a large number of studies performed on perinatal or postnatal animals (carnivores, rodents, and primates), it has been demonstrated repeatedly that stimulation of the somesthetic, visual, or acoustic system evokes a gross response in the appropriate projection area of the neocortex (e.g., Delhaye-Bouchaud, 1964; Ellingson, 1964; Marty, 1962; Rose, 1967; Rose & Lindsley, 1968; Scherrer & Occonomos, 1954). Stimulation of different thalamic nuclei as well as of the callosal system is also effective in producing cortical responses (Grafstein, 1963; Purpura, 1961a). Since such responses are actually generated *within* the cortex, a receptive cortical function regarding these afferent systems is present at birth. Correlative morphological studies show that the cortical cytoarchitectonics at this stage are already relatively differentiated with well-separated layers containing neurons in different phases of development. A gross somesthetic or visual evoked cortical response in the neonatal animal consists of a long-latency, monophasic surface-negative deflection. This has been ascribed to corticopetal activation of apical dendrites of perikarya located in the superficial pyramidal layers (II–III) (Marty & Scherrer, 1964; Purpura, Shofer, Houspian, & Noback, 1964). These dendrites are fairly well developed with spines and distal branching which intermingle with the marginal layer. Conversely, the basal dendrites of these pyramidal cells have more primitive appearance, being short and having few ramifications. On the basis of indirect morphological evidence, it has been assumed that excitatory synaptic mechanisms mature before inhibitory ones (Voeller, Pappas, & Purpura, 1963). Therefore, the neonatal, negative, evoked potential has been regarded as a sign of EPSP (excitatory postsynaptic potential) in the superficial layers of the cortex. However, this notion cannot be regarded as settled because the precocious maturation of the excitatory synapses has recently been questioned. This matter will be further dealt with later.

One of the most conspicuous morphological features of the neonatal cortex is the elaboration of a dense dendritic net in the fifth stratum. This contains comparatively extensive basal dendrites of pyramidal cells as well as fairly well-developed stellate and Martinotti cells. A functional correlate of the relatively complex cytoarchitectonic picture found in the newborn cortex has been demonstrated, for instance, in the visual area. Thus, it was shown by Hubel and Wiesel (1963; see also Wiesel & Hubel, 1963) that a few days after birth receptive cortical fields are already established in principle in kittens. However, in view of the previously postulated structural-functional relation, it seems likely that corticopetal influences above the deepest strata of the cortex are present even earlier. To provide a firm basis for understanding how the sensory functions are built up, we focused the study upon initial stages of development from the time that corticopetal activation is possible.

V. Results

A. Neonatal Type of the Evoked Somesthetic Response in Fetal Sheep

For reasons already stated we chose the fetal sheep for elucidating the early epigenesis of the neocortex, and the following presentation reviews a number of studies devoted to this problem. The sheep has a comparatively long gestation period, about 145 days, and at birth it is considerably more mature than, for example, the dog, the cat, and the rabbit (Adolph, 1970). This difference in the rate of relative pre- and postnatal development also affects the cerebral cortex (Åström, 1967).

The characteristics of the changing form of evoked cortical potentials are relevant as criteria for comparing different stages of functional cortical development. For example, the somesthetic evoked response changes from a monophasic negativity to the positive-negative configuration observed in postnatal animals. This change occurs in fetal sheep during the last trimester of gestation (Molliver, 1967). Thus, at the age of about 90 days, an evoked cortical response to tactile stimulation of the trigeminal nose area is predominantly surface negative as shown in Fig. 1A (upper trace). When this response is recorded with the aid of a semimicroelectrode which is advanced through the cortex in steps of 250 μ, a depth profile of the response can be constructed (Persson, 1973). The conventional interpretation of such a curve (see Fig. 1B, left) implies that the cortical depth at which negativity is recorded with maximal amplitude represents the "sink" of the response. Thus, in the case illustrated, the focus of activity is located at a depth of about 500 μ. However, this interpretation of a laminar potential distribution has been questioned by, for instance, Humphrey (1968) who advocates, instead, the use of the second derivation of the depth potential profile to obtain a more precise estimation of the locus of "sources" and "sinks." When applied to the records obtained in the present study, Humphrey's method provides results which do not differ significantly from those achieved with the more common method.

Extracellular unitary recordings have been performed to obtain a more thorough picture of the mode in which evoked cortical activation takes place. At the stage when the surface response was predominantly negative, evoked unitary activity was encountered throughout the entire depth of the cortex. However, as shown in the histogram in Fig. 1B, right, this activity was present most commonly in the deeper layers with a maximum at about 800–1000 μ. As a rule, evoked units were discharging with a single spike only, a feature considered to be a sign of immaturity (Fig. 1A, lower trace) (cf. Verley, Garma, & Scherrer, 1969). The spike generally occurred during the initial phase of the surface negativity, and there was no apparent correlation between the latency of the spikes and the cortical depth at which they were recorded.

An important recent study of the spatial distribution of synapses in the somethetic cortex of the newborn dog (Molliver & van der Loos, 1970) is relevant to the discussion of possible mechanisms generating the neonatal surface negative response. It was demonstrated that in this developmental stage there was a high density of synapses in the superficial layer I, that is to say, down to a depth of about 100 μ beneath the pia, and also in layers IV and V, at about 600 and 800 μ. Layer I contains Retzius-Cajal cells which are numerous and well developed at this stage. This stratum is also reached by branched apical dendrites from the superficial pyramidal cells. Layers IV and V are made up of a large pyramidal neurons which have extensive basal dendrites richly supplied with gemmules. It is striking that these deeper strata of a high synaptic density correspond approximately to the depths in which evoked unitary activity was most frequently found in the fetal sheep at a stage when the somesthetic response had a "neonatal" (negative) form. On the other hand, the fact that few units were found in the superficial layers does not necessarily invalidate the supposition that activation in these layers contributes to the surface negative potential. Molliver and van der Loos actually consider activation in the superficial stratum to be the main source of the negative response. The reason for this apparent lack of structure-function correlation may be a technical one, since unitary recording is subject to a substantial bias as recently emphasized by Towe and Harding (1970). This bias may be of even more importance in the case of immature neurons which are small and exceptionally fragile.

The evoked cortical response to trigeminal stimulation in a fetal sheep of about 90 days of age displays the same configuration and seems to reflect the same pattern of neuronal activation as, for example, in the newborn cat or dog. However, there are morphological features of the fetal sheep cortex at this stage which may suggest a more advanced maturation in this animal. Thus, in the sheep the brain is gyrencephalic (see Fig. 1A), whereas the dog and the cat have only a few shallow sulci. Furthermore, as illustrated in Fig. 1C, Golgi preparations of the cortex of a sheep fetus 80–90 days old offer a comparatively mature cytoarchitecture, and most of the primitive characteristics seem to have been lost (Åström, 1967). Despite the apparent mature features of the cortex in a 90-day-old sheep fetus, the formative phase of the somesthetic system in this animal is not completed as judged by the changes in the form of the evoked potential which occur during subsequent development. It is then obvious that the morphological parameters referred to above are insufficient as a basis for comparing developmental stages between different species; they illustrate the difficulty of establishing reliable structure-function relationships.

Although partly outside the scope of the present review, which is focused upon the initial ontogenesis, a few comments on the later phase of the developing evoked cortical potential should be made. Around an age of 100 days in the sheep fetus, the negative response is preceded by a successively increasing positive transient, similar to that seen in the 5- to 7-day-old kitten. The appearance of a positive component of the evoked potential as demonstrated in postnatal animals has been considered to reflect a further elaboration of activated, deep-seated, basal dendrites together with the development of axosomatic synapses (e.g., Marty, 1962; Purpura, 1961 b). The development of a neuropil in layer IV has also been assumed to contribute to the appearance of a surface positive deflection (Scheibel & Scheibel, 1964). However, as indicated above, well-developed basal dendrites can be seen in conjunction with the pyramidal cells of the fifth layer at an earlier stage. It does not seem likely that the growth of a dendritic

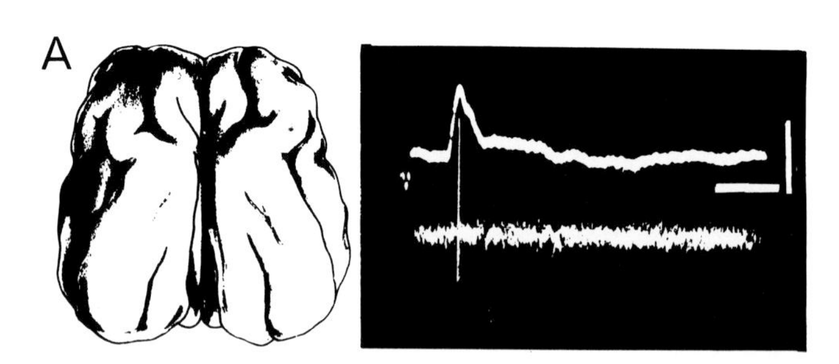

FIG. 1. A. (Left). Gyrencephalic brain of a 95-day fetus. (Right). Evoked somesthetic gross (upper trace) and unitary (lower trace) response in a 96-day fetus (spike retouched). Calibration: 100 μV, 100 msec. In this, as in following figures, negativity is an upward deflection. B. Laminar potential distribution (left) in the somesthetic cortex of a 94-day fetus corresponding to the latency of the peak of the surface negativity. All depth potential profiles were constructed from measurement of voltage values of the laminar records at a fixed latency. Cortical depth distribution of evoked unitary responses (right). Horizontal broken line in both graphs denotes the approximate lower border of the cortex. C. Camera lucida drawing of the neocortex from a 90-day fetus. Golgi preparation. Note the presence of well-developed deep and superficial pyramidal neurons. La ma, lamina marginalis; La py, lamina pyramidalis; ax, axon (from Åström, 1967).

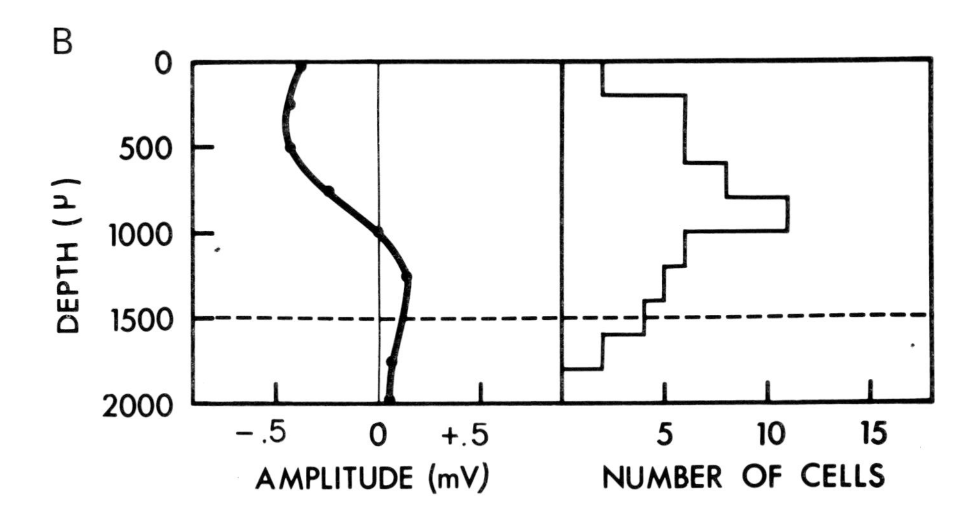

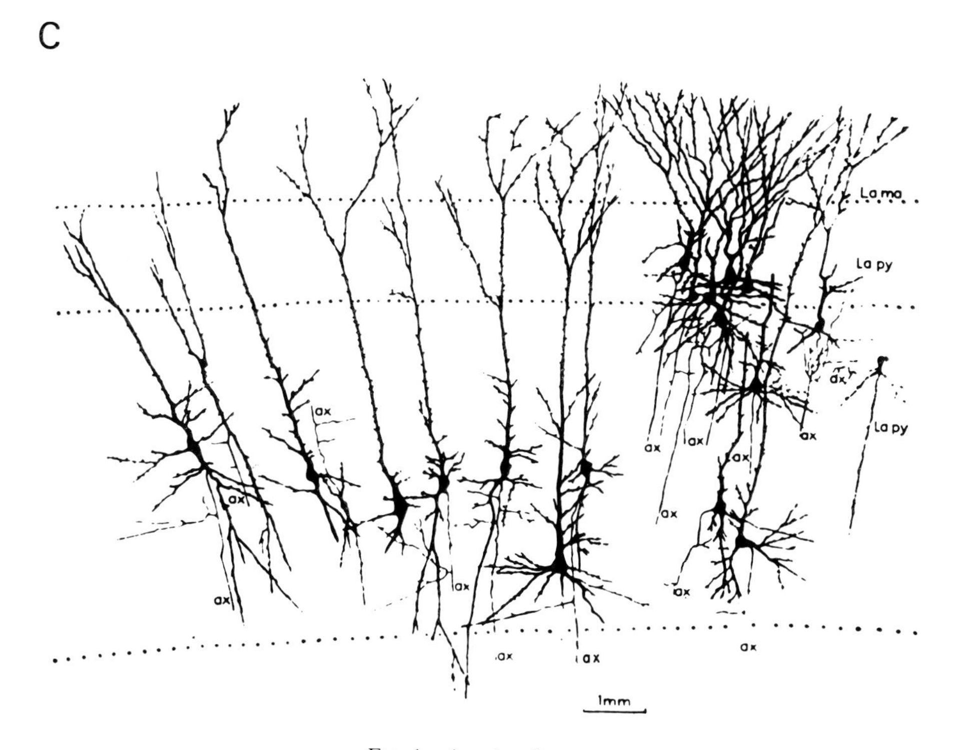

FIG. 1. *(continued)*.

net in the layer of the more superficial pyramids in layers II or III, which show a relatively delayed maturation, could be the sole cause of the changing surface pattern. On the other hand, there is the possibility that the involvement of IPSP's (inhibitory postsynaptic potentials) in superficial cortical strata may be of importance.

When interpreting the changing form of the developing evoked potentials in terms of alterations in the relative intracortical location of excitatory and inhibitory postsynaptic events, some recent findings in the dynamics of the developing neocortex presented by Fuentes and Marty (1969) should be taken into consideration. They demonstrated that the increasing thickness of the growing cortex occurs in a corticofugal direction. This implies that the deeper layers of the cortex, containing among other things, somata of pyramids with well-developed basal dendrites, are successively pushed to relatively deeper positions by the elaboration of cellular elements located closer to the surface. It is evident that the increasing distance between the activated basal dendrites of the deep pyramidal neurons, which presumably constitute an active "sink," and the surface should be considered when the changing form of developing evoked potential is interpreted in terms of volume conduction.

B. *Early Development of the Somesthetic Evoked Response*

Thanks to the classical studies by Barcroft and Barron (1939), it is well known that in the fetal sheep tactile stimulation of the nose elicits generalized motor responses as early as 40–45 days. From a functional point of view, this early age represents a far more primitive stage of cortical development than that described above (80–90 days). The effectiveness of inducing behavioral responses by trigeminal stimulation at a very early stage of development has been observed in a number of other mammals (e.g., Carmichael, 1954; Windle, 1940), and such stimulation is therefore appropriate to use in a study of the early epigenesis of corticoafferent systems.

The general motor "startle" reaction following a tap on the nose can easily be observed while a sheep embryo is still floating inside the transparent and intact fetal membranes. The primitive brain of such an embryo weighing 15 gm is shown in Fig. 2A. The cerebral hemispheres consist of two thin-walled vesicles, and the brain is dominated by the diencephalon and mesencephalon. There is a small anlage of the cerebellum. In Fig. 2B a similar fetal brain is reproduced in sagittal section to illustrate the very thin pallial wall and the wide lateral ventricle (Åström, 1967). It is very difficult indeed to maintain such immature embryos for a long period of experimentation, and advanced electrophysiological techniques can hardly be applied. However, some data have been obtained which may help to define the stage of

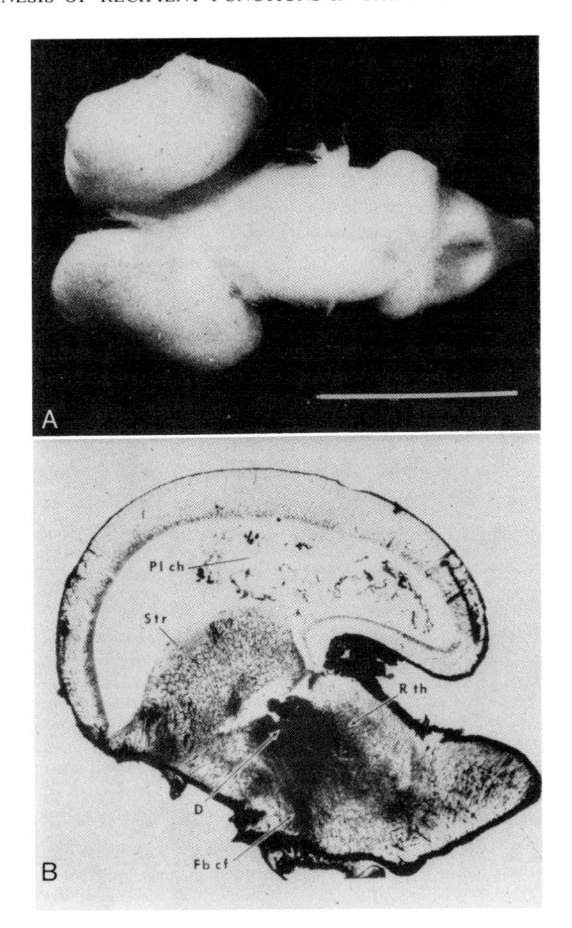

FIG. 2. A. Brain specimen from a 50-day fetus (from Kolmodin & Meyerson, 1966). B. sagittal section of a similar brain (from Åström, 1967). Decussation (D) of corticofugal, Fb cf, and thalamocortical, R th, fibers. Striatum, Str; Pl ch, choroid plexus. Horizontal bar in A, 1 cm.

functional cerebral development. It is fairly certain that in fetuses younger than about 50 days there are no signs of spontaneous activity as recorded with gross electrodes from the exposed surface of the cortex (Bernhard, Kaiser, & Kolmodin, 1959; Bernhard & Meyerson, 1968). Furthermore, the cortex is not excitable with direct electrical stimulation (Eidelberg, Kolmodin, & Meyerson, 1965). On the other hand, there is a so-called steady potential, i.e., the cortical surface generally being positive by some millivolts in relation to the calvarium. Topical application of KCl causes a rapid decrease of this potential which then becomes negative (Eidelberg,

Kolmodin, & Meyerson, 1967). This phenomenon has been thought to reflect the presence of membrane potentials of cortical neurons. In addition, it has been demonstrated that huge doses of Metrazol may cause the appearance of intermittent, "paroxysmal" activity which can be recorded from the cortical surface (Kolmodin & Meyerson, 1966). At present the functional significance of this observation can not be evaluated, since the cortex is very thin, and subcortical electrical events may be recorded from the cortical surface.

Against the background of these signs of cerebral immaturity, it is an unexpected finding that tactile stimulation of the trigeminal nose area evokes a response which can be recorded from the cortical surface. This observation was first made by Molliver (1967), who also described the subsequent development of this response in the fetal sheep. It was found that the somesthetic response in the smallest fetuses which could be experimentally handled (10 gm) (40 days), up to an age of about 65 days, consists of a long-latency surface *positive* transient (Fig. 3A). Later in development the response changes to a positive-negative form (Fig. 5A) and subsequently the positive component decreases in amplitude, whereas the negative increases and dominates the response. Eventually, at an age of about 90 days, the response is purely negative as described above. This sequence of changes of an evoked cortical potential had previously not been described and apparently represents a period of development preceding that found in postnatal animals.

These observations demanded a more detailed analysis (Bernhard, Meyerson, & Persson, 1972; Meyerson & Persson, 1969; Persson, 1971; Persson, 1973). The positive response of fetuses below 65 days of age can be obtained most easily when the ipsilateral upper lip is stimulated. The response is of a fairly high amplitude and is constant in form provided stimuli are given at intervals of at least 30 seconds. More frequent stimulation inevitably results in a considerable diminution of the response. A salient characteristic of the somesthetic trigeminal response is its wide cortical distribution; that is to say, the stimulation of one point on the lip may evoke a response which can be recorded from the entire anterior third of the exposed dorsal aspect of the still lissencephalic cortex (see Fig. 12A).

The results obtained when the surface positive response was recorded from the depths of the cortex are illustrated as a depth profile in Fig. 3B (cf. Persson, 1973). A comparison with the corresponding graph for the surface negative ("neonatal") response (Fig. 1B) clearly shows that in the youngest fetuses the response is generated in relatively deeper cortical layers, or subcortically. The estimated approximate cortical thickness has been marked with a horizontal dashed line on the depth profile, and it shows that the induced activity is actually located *beneath* the cortical plate.

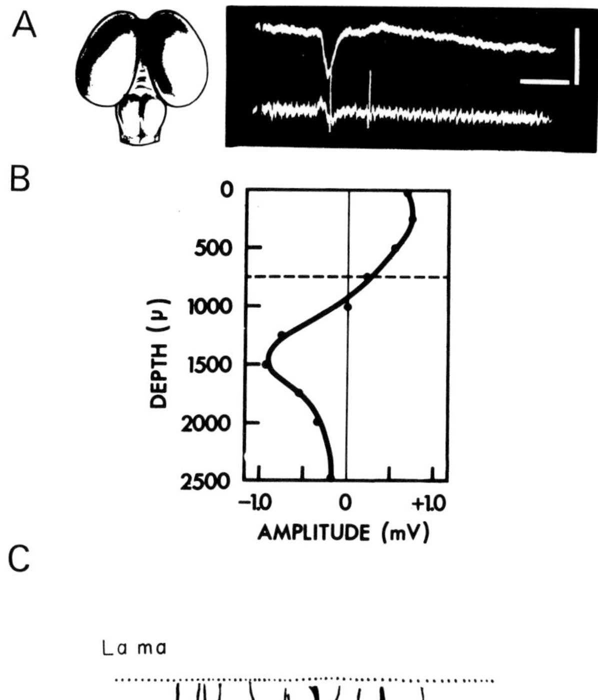

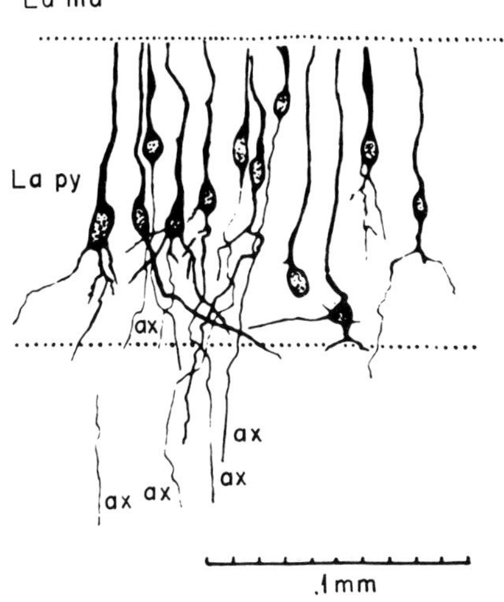

FIG. 3. A. Left. Lissencephalic brain of a 65-day fetus. Right. Evoked somesthetic gross (upper trace) and unitary (lower trace) response in a 64-day fetus (spikes retouched). Calibration; 200 μV, 100 msec. B. Laminar potential distribution of the response in A. Measurements made at a latency corresponding to the peak of the surface positivity. C. Camera lucida drawing of the neocortex from a 45-day fetus. Golgi preparation. Note immature bipolar cells in superficial layers and deep pyramidal neurons with short basal dendrites. La ma, lamina marginalis; La py, lamina pyramidalis; ax, axon (from Åström, 1967).

A number of experiments were performed aiming at extracellular recording of evoked unit activity. In fetuses of the youngest age group we found very few spontaneously discharging units. The firing rate was extremely low, and stable recordings were difficult to obtain. No evoked units were found at depths estimated to be within the cortex. At deeper locations, however, evoked units could be recorded in a few experiments. Discharges were generally repetitive, consisting of two to four spikes (Fig. 3A, lower trace). As a rule, such activated units were encountered at depths of about 1300–2800 μ, which should be compared with an estimated thickness of the cortex of approximately 750 μ in fetuses of this age group. The finding of a subcortical activation manifested as a surface positive transient is of considerable interest and will be discussed further.

The salient morphological features of the cortex during this developmental phase as given by Åström (1967) are shown in Fig. 3C and Fig. 4. The pyramidal cells have a primitive bipolar form with rudimentary basal dendrites. In the uppermost part of the subcortex, stellate cells are seen. Afferent fibers, presumably of thalamic and/or callosal origin, are present in the intermediate zone. They are directed toward the stellate cell layer but do not penetrate into the primitive cortex.

In the next developmental phase, when the surface responses are positive-negative (Fig. 5A), laminar recordings showed that the "sink" of the response had been displaced from subcortical to deep cortical regions as

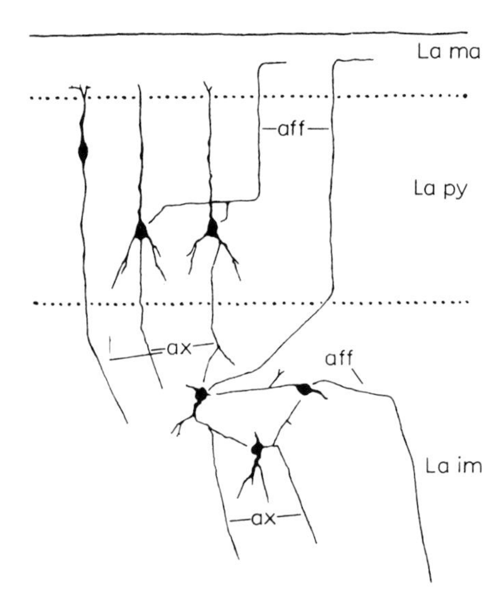

FIG. 4. Diagrammatic drawing showing the principal features of cortical organization in a 50-day fetus. Note that the ascending afferent fiber terminates in the subcortex (La im), which contains stellate cells. La ma, lamina marginalis; lamina pyramidalis; aff, afferent fiber; ax, axon (modified from Åström, 1967).

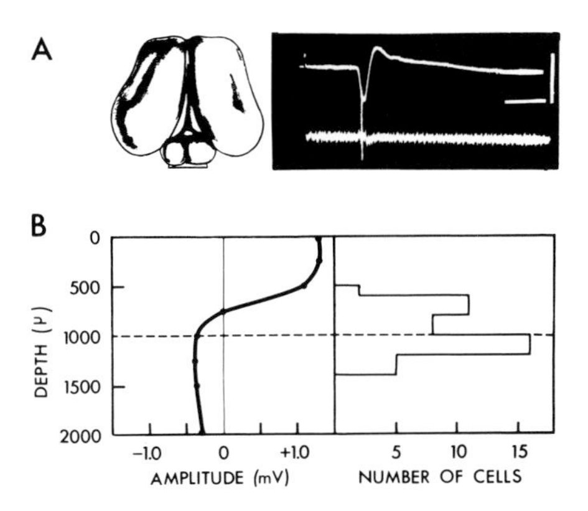

FIG. 5. A. (Left). Brain from a 70-day fetus. (Right). Evoked somesthetic gross (upper trace) and unitary (lower trace) response in a 72-day fetus (spike retouched). Calibration: 1mV, 100 msec. B. Laminar potential distribution (left) of the response in A. Measurements made at a latency corresponding to the peak of the surface positivity. Cortical depth distribution of evoked unitary responses (right).

shown by the depth profile for the surface positive component depicted in Fig. 5B, left. Similarly, evoked unitary activity is present with a frequency maximum at a depth corresponding to the junction between the cortex and the subcortex as shown in the histogram (Fig. 5B, right). It is noteworthy that evoked unitary activity in these fetuses could not be made to discharge repetitively regardless of the strength of the stimulus. In fetuses around 65 days of age, the appearance of a surface-negative deflection following the initial positivity obviously denotes a developmental stage during which activation *within* the cortex is possible. The possible morphological correlates of the changing functional properties of the cortex are summarized in the camera lucida drawing in Fig. 6 (Åström, 1967). It should be noted that the afferent fibers penetrate into the cortical plate and send collaterals to the midcortex. The deep pyramidal cells have reached a high degree of differentiation, and stellate cells are seen within the cortex for the first time. Collaterals from these cells provide for intracortical connections in the deep layers. These features are schematically summarized in the drawing from Åström in Fig. 7.

In fetuses in the youngest age group (from 40 days) and in those exhibiting a positive-negative somesthetic response (between 70 and 85 days old), an extensive area of the anterior portion of the cortex could be activated by nose stimulation. In addition, the amplitude of the response was often amazingly high, amounting to 1.5–2 mV compared to the corresponding adult value of approximately .2–.4mV (cf. Nougier, 1963). Furthermore, the responses generally appeared with a high degree of consistency, both in form and amplitude, which contrasts with the variable pattern of responses often observed in mature animals.

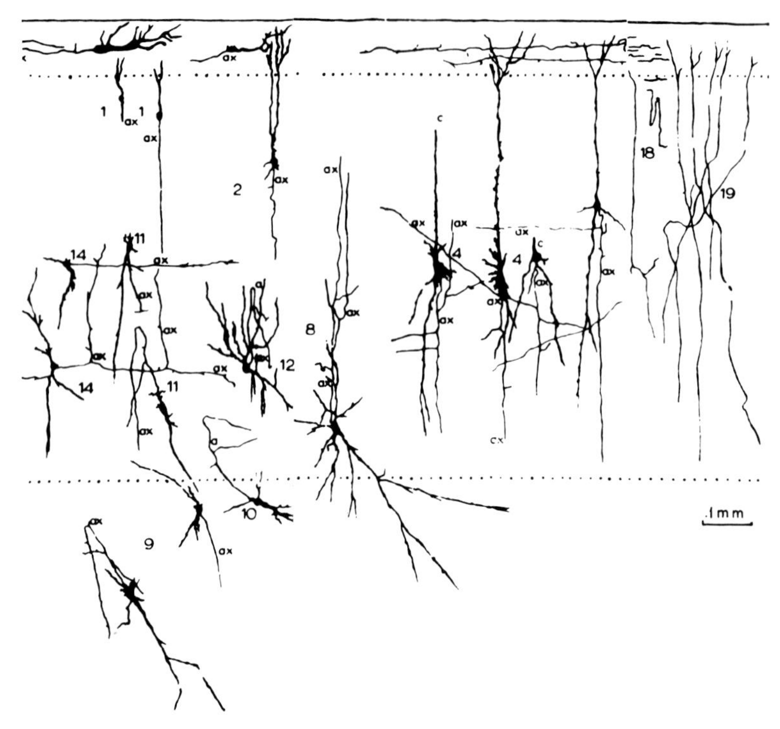

FIG. 6. Camera lucida drawing of the neocortex from a 67-day fetus. Golgi preparation. Note the elaboration of stellate cells (11, 12, 14) within the pyramidal layer; subpyramidal stellate cells (9, 10) of the type seen in younger specimens; Martinotti cells (8) with ascending axons. The superficial pyramidal cells (1,2) are less mature than those in deeper strata (4) which have axon collaterals. Ascending afferent fibers (19) reach the superficial zone (modified from Åström, 1967).

In a study of the organization of neocortical sensory projections in various species, Adrian (1943) presented some attractive theories concerning the correlation between the pattern of somesthetic projection areas and feeding behavior. In sheep, for example, the extensive cortical representation of the upper lip, which protrudes above the lower one, was considered to be important for grazing. Furthermore, it has been shown by Nougier (1963) and by Hatton and Rubel (1967) that in sheep there is a preponderance of the *ipsilateral* lip projection, and that this is also the case in the thalamus (Richard, Auffray, & Albe-Fessard, 1967). This organization seems to be a particular characteristic in sheep and is not found in other animals so far studied (Cabral & Johnson, 1971). Therefore, one may ask whether the monophasic positive form of the evoked somesthetic response during the early ontogenesis of sheep is a unique finding related to the

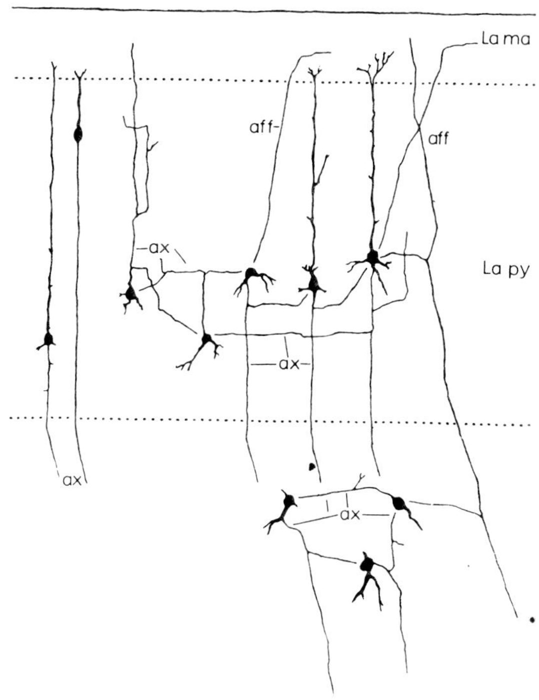

FIG. 7. Diagrammatic drawing showing the principal features of cortical organization in a 70-day fetus. Note ascending afferent fiber which at this stage penetrates into the cortical plate. Labels as in Fig. 4 (from Åström, 1967).

specific arrangement of the trigeminal sensory projection in this animal. However, this is probably not the case, since similar developmental features apparently exist in the dog (Molliver & van der Loos, 1970), suggesting that this is a general principle of development which may apply to other corticopetal systems as well. In order to further substantiate this point, we will present some data on the developing callosal system; and a recent investigation of the development of the visual evoked response will also be considered.

C. *Early Development of Interhemispheric Responses*

Whereas the trigeminal somesthetic system shows evidence of function at a comparatively early stage of ontogenesis, the neocommissural callosal system matures late. The callosal fibers display a delayed maturation both in terms of growth and myelination, of which the latter is actually not completed until a late postnatal stage. In phylogenesis, the appearance of a neocommissural system is closely bound to the evolution of the neocortex. In addition, the morphological characteristics of the corpus callosum reflect the relative development in a given species of the different areas of the neocortex. Thus, for example, the presence of a genu and of a splenium corporis callosi is considered to be associated with the existence of extensive frontal and occipital neocortical areas. It is notable that ungulates compare favorably with both carnivores and nonhuman primates as regards the relative size and gross morphology of the corpus callosum. In sheep, as in rabbits, there is a rich supply of neocommissural connections between the motor areas, whereas in most other animals these connections are predominantly directed toward associative cortical fields. On the other hand, the sheep resembles other animals in that callosal connections seem to be fairly well developed within the somatosensory face area (for references, see Meyerson, 1968).

Despite the interest shown in the phylogenesis of the commissural system and its relatively simple structural design, little is known about its functional ontogenesis. Interhemispheric transcallosal responses (TCR) mediated via the corpus callosum have been studied in the developing cat only during the postnatal period (Grafstein, 1963). As the response is already present at birth in that animal, it seemed reasonable to investigate the interhemispheric electrocortical function in the prenatal sheep (Meyerson, 1967, 1968). There is no need to repeat these findings in detail, and only those relevant to the present discussion are recapitulated.

A surface cortical response to stimulation of the contralateral, homotopic region can be evoked for the first time in fetuses about 70 days old. It is at about the same age that a cortical response to surface stimulation of the cortex can first be elicited, and this event may be considered as a sign of cortical excitability (Eidelberg *et al.*, 1965). At its first appearance the interhemispheric response is present only within a limited area in the anteromedial part of the still lissencephalic brain (see Fig. 12A). The response in fetuses up to an age of about 85 days generally consists of a positive deflection, sometimes followed by a low amplitude, slow negativity. The callosal origin of the response is shown by the fact that it is abolished by section of the corpus callosum. It should be recalled that the somesthetic evoked response during this same period displays a positive-negative form. In the following period (85–95 days old), the transcallosal response is altered in form by the appearance of a dominating negative transient. In fetuses over 95–100 days old the response may be purely negative. The developmental changes of the TCR are illustrated by the records in Fig. 8 A, B which were obtained from two different cortical areas. In fetuses over 90 days old the TCR is generally succeeded by a second response of variable configuration. This late response, which may be seen in some of the records in Fig. 8, is mediated

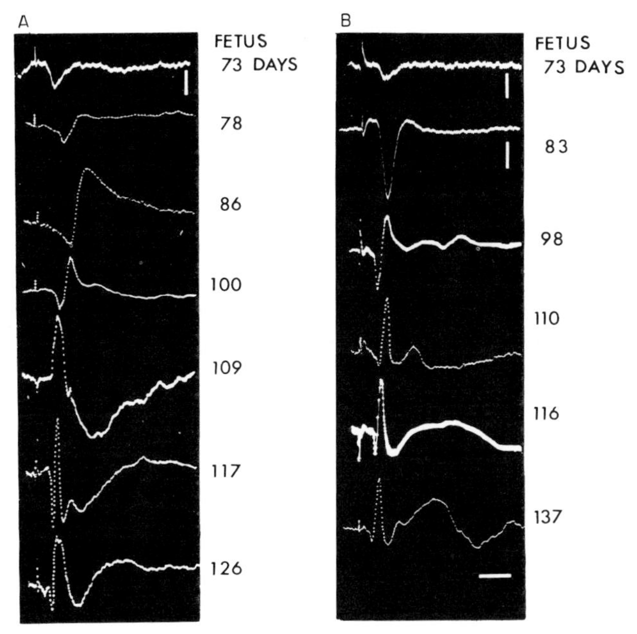

FIG. 8. Development of interhemispheric responses obtained from two different areas (A, g. frontalis medialis; B, g. frontalis superior). Delayed interhemispheric responses may be seen in some of the records from the older fetuses and appear as long-lasting negative or positive deflections following the primary complex. All but the two first responses in A and the first in B are averaged. Calibration: first record in A and B, 50 μV; second record in B, 100 μV; 100 msec.

via extracallosal pathways in the brainstem and is comparable to the interhemispheric delayed response (IDR) described in adult animals (Rutledge & Kennedy, 1960).

The changing form of the TCR during development is not as regular as that of the evoked somesthetic response, though in essence the same pattern is present. The transition from positivity to a dominating negativity of both, occurring at different fetal ages, indicates the heterochronous development of the two corticopetal systems. Nevertheless, the similarity in other respects suggests that the evolution of cortical recipient functions may follow the same pattern for the somesthetic and callosal afferent systems. In order to test this hypothesis, experiments have been designed to record subsurface unitary and gross activity in response to contralateral surface stimulation, but as yet only preliminary results can be presented (Meyerson & Persson, unpublished data).

In a few fetuses younger than 100 days, laminar depth recordings of the TCR were made. For instance, the records obtained from an 82-day fetus showed that the surface positive component reversed at the depth of about 1200μ and attained a maximal negative value at about 1500μ. At still greater depths a triphasic positive-negative-positive response was obtained. Histological examination of the brain, in which the track could be identified, disclosed that the electrode had been advanced in a direction parallel to the radiating callosal fibers, and that the thickness of the cortex amounted to about 1200μ. This experiment appears to favor the view that the surface positive deflection of the TCR is generated in strata just below the cortex or in the deepest cortical layers.

It appeared to be far more difficult to evoke unitary activity by transcallosal than by tactile trigeminal stimulation, which was also tried during the same experiments. It was immaterial whether transcallosal units were looked for in the sensory or in the motor area, though the latter was more liable to give consistent surface TCR's. The reason why comparatively few transcallosal units were encountered could be that cells responding to such activation may be smaller than those responding to sensory stimulation (cf. Hossmann, 1969). This is suggested by the remarkable discrepancy between the number of spontaneously active units and units responding to trigeminal stimulation on one hand, and the number of transcallosal units on the other.

Transcallosal units were not found until the age of about 85 days. These units were predominantly encountered at cortical depths of more than 500μ. As a rule, the surface TCR was still predominantly positive, and the unitary discharge always appears concomitant with this positivity. Although the material is far too limited to permit a statistical analysis of the depth distribution of unitary activity, the fact remains that quite a number of activated units were recorded at depths corresponding to strata *beneath* the cortex or at the junction between the cortex and the subcortex, that is to say, at a depth of 1200–1500μ. In Fig. 9, two examples of transcallosally activated units are shown which were encountered along the same track, that in A at a depth of 500μ and that in B at 1500μ. It should be noted that they were both discharging concomitantly with the surface positivity but with somewhat different latencies. The majority of the units discharged with a single spike, but occasionally two or three spikes could be seen. In a few fetuses of about 100 days, transcallosal units could be found exhibiting a postexcitatory silent period followed by a repetitive discharge (cf. Fig. 10 D). Intracellular recordings in adult cats have shown that the silent period preceding the initial discharge corresponds to an IPSP (Hossmann, 1969), and in preliminary experiments performed on sheep fetuses of about 130 days, similar results were obtained. Intracellular recordings have hitherto not been successful in younger fetuses.

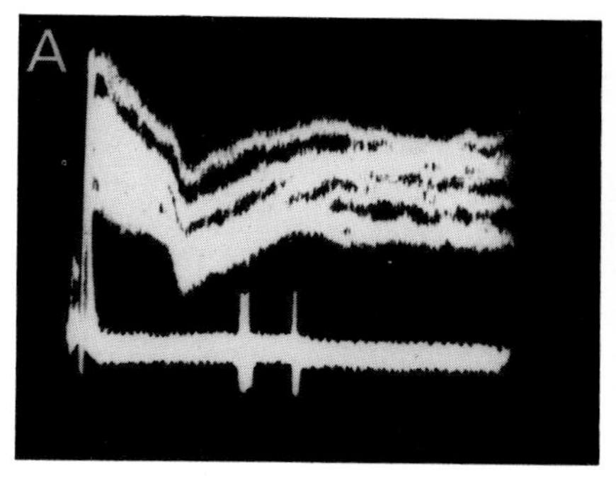

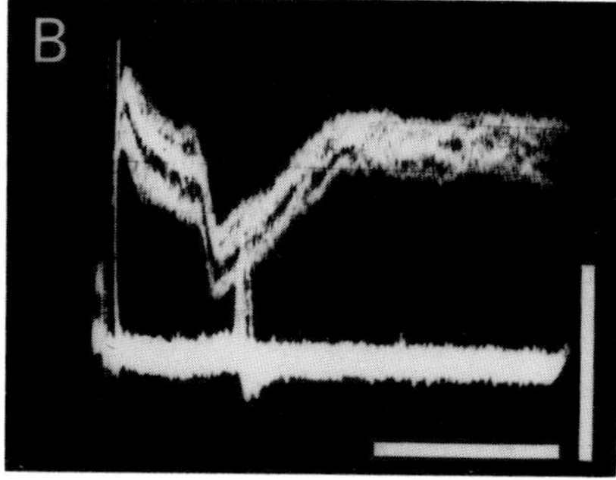

FIG. 9. Transcallosal gross and unitary responses obtained from an 82-day fetus. Gross responses were recorded from the cortical surface, and unitary activity was recorded in the same penetration, in A at a depth of 500 μ, in B at 1500 μ. Calibration: 100 μV, 100 msec.

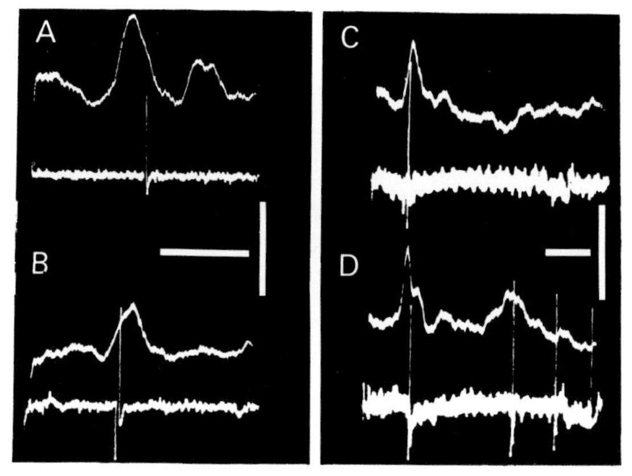

FIG. 10. Somesthetic (A and C) and transcallosal (B and D) gross and unitary responses obtained from a 100-day fetus. Convergent activation in A and B, and in C and D. Calibration: 100 μV, 100 msec.

Activation by means of trigeminal nose stimulation was attempted when recording transcallosal units from the somesthetic area. However, this was not possible until an age of about 100 days, and even in these and older fetuses there were few units which could be activated by both a callosal and a somesthetic input. A typical example is shown in Fig. 10A and B in which there is a remarkable similarity in the form of the transcallosal and trigeminal evoked surface potentials as well as in the concomitant unitary activity. This finding suggests a similar mode of activation for the two responses which would not be unreasonable if one supposed that they both reflect similar developmental cortical dynamics. But the records illustrated in Fig.

10C and D show that the mode of somesthetic and callosal activation may differ, as in this case the latter displays a more complex behavior as described previously.

The fact that convergent inputs from the two corticopetal systems are not seen in younger fetuses may be taken as a further illustration of their heterochronous development. More specifically, this means that the cortical neurons which, from an early age, have funtional contacts with sensory afferent fibers, are not reached by callosal elements until a later stage.

D. *Early Development of the Visual Evoked Response*

To pursue the discussion on cortical functions during early ontogenesis, it is of interest to report on some of the salient findings collected in a recent study of the developing visual evoked response (Persson & Stenberg, 1972). As in the somesthetic and transcallosal responses, the *initial* development of the visual response in mammals has hitherto only been examined in fetal sheep. Responses in the visual cortex were evoked by electrical stimulation of the optic nerve. Such stimulation could evoke a surface cortical response even in the youngest fetus tested, which was only 55 days old. As illustrated in Fig. 11 (upper records), the visual response in this fetus consisted of a predominantly positive deflection. For comparison, somesthetic evoked responses are also depicted in the figure (lower records), and it appears that during subsequent development the changes in the visual evoked response are remarkably like those observed in the somesthetic response. The visual response has hitherto only been recorded from the cortical surface, but there

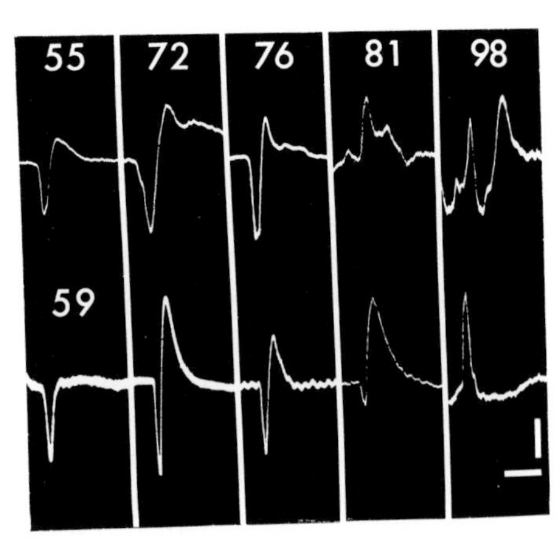

FIG. 11. Comparison between visual (upper row) and somesthetic (lower row) responses. Both responses in each age group are from the same animal except the first two responses. Gestational age in days is marked. Calibration: 100 μV, 100 msec (from Persson & Stenberg, 1972).

is good reason to assume that the developmental changes of its gross configuration reflect the same pattern of functional maturation within the cortex as has been shown to account for the developing somesthetic and transcallosal responses (cf. Bernhard *et al.*, 1972).

VI. Comments

A. Developmental Pattern of Intracortical Organization

The similarity of developmental changes in the form of the somesthetic, transcallosal, and visual responses suggests that the generative neuronal mechanisms within the cortex and subcortex are alike. On the basis of laminar depth recordings of evoked gross and unitary activity, it has been claimed that the mainly monophasic, surface-positive deflection seen during the initial phases of development is a sign of subcortical activation (Bernhard, Kolmodin, & Meyerson, 1967; Meyerson & Persson, 1969; Persson, 1973). Whether postsynaptic mechanisms are involved or whether the activity is only or partially evoked in the afferent terminals can not be stated definitely at present. The possibility that the activity is predominantly presynaptic seems more likely, since in neonatal kittens spontaneous spike activity, thought to be generated in corticopetal terminals, has been demonstrated in the subcortex, whereas intracortical unitary discharges were not found until later (Huttenlocher, 1967). At least in the very early stage of development, nonsynaptic terminal activation appears more probable than postsynaptic activity in the basal dendrites of the deep pyramidal neurons, as was assumed recently by Molliver and van der Loos (1970). This latter mechanism is certainly involved at a somewhat later stage, although the surface positivity remains unchanged. Alternatively, it may be suggested that postsynaptic activity is actually present in subcortical strata, since they have been shown to contain migrating pyramidal and stellate cells which appear fairly mature. As pointed out by Holmes and Short (1970), it is unlikely that activation of stellate cells with their irregular dendritic arrangement would be a major source of surface gross potentials. Whether the subcortical cells have well-developed gemmules or other signs of synaptic membrane specialization is not known. One has as yet no idea of the significance of the finding that subcortical units discharge with repetitive spikes.

In recent publications by Purpura (1969) and Crain (1969), it has been claimed emphatically that inhibitory synapses mature earlier than excitatory ones, both in the hippocampus and neocortex. The long-lasting IPSP's found in kittens older then 3–5 days have been assumed to account for the extreme "fatiguability" of immature evoked responses. (Purpura, Shofer, & Scarff, 1965). Instead, in earlier studies, Purpura and other investigators have considered the delayed appearance of axosomatic synaptic structures, compared to that of synapses in conjunction with dendrites, to be a sign of a precocious maturation of excitatory synapses (Purpura, 1961b; see also Huttenlocher, 1967; Meller, Breipohl, & Glees, 1968). Although the recent results presented by Purpura *et al.* (1965) seem convincing, it is of some importance from a general developmental point of view that the perinatal period was not included. The reason for this was the extreme difficulty in obtaining intracellular records from immature animals. As already described, there are reasons for equating the newborn kitten with the sheep fetus of about 85 days. This might imply that the preparations studied by Purpura did not represent a sufficiently immature stage of development to justify a generalized statement about the relative rate of functional development of the excitatory and inhibitory synaptic mechanisms. It seems highly improbable that the positive surface response in the youngest fetuses is a sign of inhibitory postsynaptic events in the most superficial layers, since at this age no corticopetal fibers, thalamic or callosal, can be seen to penetrate the cortical plate (Åström, 1967). Furthermore, it is not likely that the first functional contacts to be established between a corticopetal fiber and a cortical neuron would be inhibitory, since even in the adult the existence of inhibitory monosynaptic thalamocortical connections has been questioned (Creutzfeldt & Sakmann, 1969). The present discussion deals only with indirect evidence about the relative development of inhibitory and excitatory mechanisms. For obvious reasons, it has not been possible to obtain any reliable intracellular records in sheep fetuses during the initial developmental period. Thus, only extracellular recordings have been made, and even these have provided only a limited number of stable records by comparison with those which can be obtained in mature animals. Despite these limitations, some of the results are relevant. Thus, it has been repeatedly observed that not until the age of about 95–100 days in the sheep fetus is it possible to obtain an arrest (inhibition) of spontaneously discharging units by peripheral or transcallosal stimulation (Persson, 1973). Similarly, only during later stages can such stimuli result in a postexcitatory silent period.

When examining the data from depth recordings, obtained with somesthetic or transcallosal stimulation, it emerges that the changing pattern of the developing surface response reflects the progressive activation of cortical neurons from deeper to more superficial layers. Thus, generally speaking, the early phases of the intracortical functional development seems to proceed along a corticopetal gradient. In a somewhat later stage of cortical epigenesis, when activation is possible throughout the whole cortex, the picture becomes more complex as the formative processes involve an intracortical rebalancing of excitatory and inhibitory influences in various cortical strata. In this context some specific features of the TCR may have significance for maintaining the concepts of a corticopetal developmental gradient.

There is substantial evidence that the positive component of the adult TCR, as well as of the TCR in the postnatal kitten, is generated by a separate set of fibers which connect the deeper cortical layers of the two hemispheres (Grafstein, 1959; 1963). In a thorough morphological study of the development of the neocommissural connections, Auroux (1964) found that callosal fibers could first be seen when there was differentiation of the fifth layer of the cortex. In developing sheep, the configuration of the first appearing positive TCR can not be influenced by a change of the stimulus voltage which suggests a fairly simple neuronal arrangement involving few or no synapses. These findings, together with the results obtained from depth recording, substantiate the view that at an early stage deep-seated fibers are the only transcallosal connections present. In addition, it has been shown that there is a heterochronous development of functioning interhemispheric connections in different cortical areas. The immature positive form of the TCR is lost earlier in areas where the response appears first. Thus, later developing areas seem to repeat the sequence of potential changes formed in more precocious areas.

The conception of a corticopetal gradient of functional development must conform with the principles of structural neurogenesis of the cortex. This has recently been discussed by Molliver and van der Loos (1970), who scrutinized older theories favoring either the precocity of superficial or of deep intracortical neuronal elements. On the basis of their own electron microscopic study, it was concluded that the earliest synapses are established deep in the cortex in fetal life. A delayed maturation of superficial cortical neurons relative to those in deeper strata was originally described by Vignal (1888) and has recently been further demonstrated in various animals by a number of authors (e.g., Berry & Rogers, 1965; Caley & Maxwell, 1968; Marty & Pujol, 1966; see also Berry, this volume). These morphological findings seem to confirm the postulated corticopetal developmental gradient.

B. *Some Evidence for Lack of Integration in the Immature Neocortex*

Certain features common to the development of the three different kinds of evoked responses dealt with in this review may serve to elucidate some general problems in the neurogenesis of the corticopetal systems.

There is a striking difference between the relative extent of the projection areas in the immature and the mature brain. In the right hemisphere of the brain shown in Fig. 12 A, the approximate areas are marked within which a response can be evoked by stimulation of the ipsilateral upper lip (triangles)

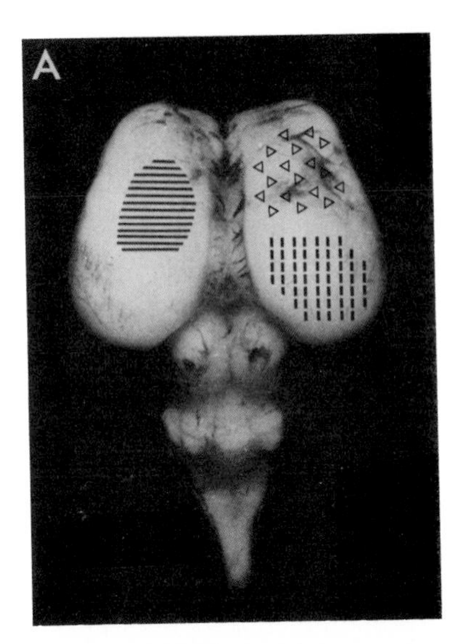

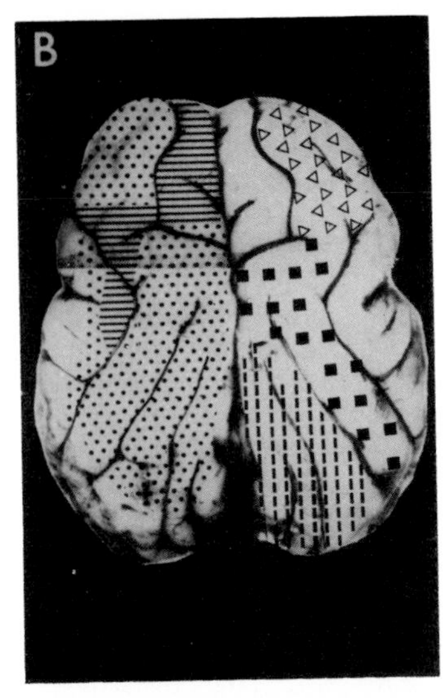

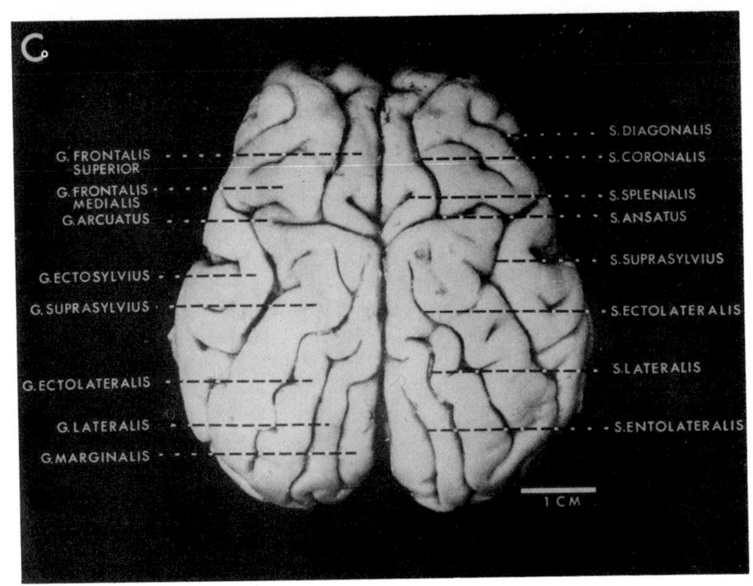

FIG. 12. Brain specimens from a 77-day (A), 104-day (B) fetus and from an adult sheep (C). On the left hemispheres in A and B are marked the areas from which TCR's were readily obtained (hatched) and areas displaying inconsistent responses (dotted). On the right hemispheres in A and B are marked the distribution of somesthetic (triangles) and visual responses (broken lines). The region considered to be associative is marked with squares.

and by stimuli of the optic nerve (broken lines). The relative extent of those areas contrasts with the corresponding ones in the brain of a more mature fetus (Fig. 12B). The area considered to be "associative" is marked with squares. On the left cerebral hemispheres in Fig. 12 A and B, the regions have been marked in which TCR's can be obtained. In the brain of the younger fetus, responses could be evoked within a limited frontoparietal area, although with a high threshold (hatched). A comparison with the brain in Fig. 12B shows that there is considerable change of the relative extent and location of the areas in which TCR's were obtained. In Fig. 12B, the areas characterized by a relatively low TCR threshold are hatched, and those in which the responses were less prominent and which had a high threshold are dotted. The motor area which readily displays TCR's is located frontomedially in the brain in Fig. 12B and is both functionally and structurally well demarcated from the nearby sensory area. For general orientation a brain from an adult sheep is shown in the Fig. 12C with the nomenclature for the different gyri and sulci. It appears from the illustrations that the primary somesthetic and visual areas occupy the major part of the immature neocortex, and that those denoted as associative become more prominent with advancing maturation. This parallels a recent finding that polysensory unit responses in the associative region are not present in the kitten until 8 days after birth, whereas primary responses can be evoked in the neonate (Mayers, Robertson, Rubel, & Thompson, 1971). It is also known that the relative extent and location of various cortical areas is altered during development (Kahle, 1966), and it has been assumed on the basis of morphological studies that projection fields mature before other areas (cf. Poliakov, 1966). The assumption of a heterochronous functional development of primary and nonprimary cortical fields is most obvious when the somatosensory system is considered. As regards the visual system, on the other hand, the nature of the first appearing responses has been much discussed (cf. Mysliveček, 1967; Rose, 1967) and on the basis of the present investigations no conclusion can be reached. However, the controversy seems to be partly a matter of semantics due to the lack of uniform use of the concepts of primary and secondary, specific, nonspecific, and associative cortical areas (Persson, 1973).

As pointed out previously, evoked potentials are obtained with an amazingly reproducible configuration in fetuses of up to an age of about 100 days and generally, moreover, with a higher amplitude than in the mature animal. This phenomenon was first observed by Scherrer and Oeconomos (1954) and later by Marty (1962), but this sign of high excitability in immature nervous tissue has not been further discussed. It is true that the consistent appearance of evoked potentials is favored by the fact that they are not obscured by spontaneous activity, which during this period is discontinuous and of low amplitude (Bernhard *et al.*, 1959; Bernhard & Meyerson, 1968). However, this does not account for the relatively high amplitudes which are often observed in younger fetuses. The consistency and high amplitude of an immature evoked potential is perhaps most conspicuous in the case of the interhemispheric delayed response (IDR). In adult animals this response is difficult to study unless chloralose anesthesia is employed, and even so it is rather variable in form and appearance. In Fig. 13 is shown a number of such responses superimposed to illustrate this developmental feature. Typical responses have been chosen comprising both a TCR and an IDR obtained from different cortical regions in fetuses of 85 (A) and 100 (B) days. In contrast to these consistent responses are those obtained from a lamb (E and F) and from an adult sheep (C and D), which have a more variable form. The records shown in Figs. 13 E and F illustrate the "unmasking" of the IDR brought about by a combination of chloralose and barbiturate. In the latter case the corpus callosum had been sectioned to prove the

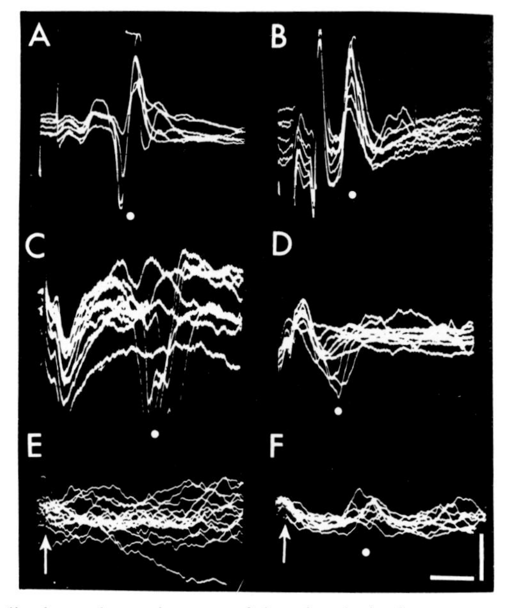

FIG. 13. Amplitude and consistency of interhemispheric responses in immature and mature stages of development. White spots denote the interhemispheric delayed response (IDR). Records in A and C from association areas, in B and D from the motor area, and in E and F from g. ectosylvius. A, from an 85-day and B, from a 100-day fetus. C and D from an adult sheep. E, before and F, after administration of α-chloralose and barbiturate in a lamb in which the corpus callosum had been sectioned. Arrows in E and F denote stimulus. Calibration: A, B, D, F, 200 μV. C and E, 100 μV; 100 msec.

extracallosal origin of the IDR. The effect of chloralose is of interest since this drug is generally considered to be an inhibition-blocking agent (cf. Bava, Fadiga, & Manzoni, 1966). In view of the extensive cortical area which can be occupied by a somesthetic or visual response in immature fetuses, it may be of relevance that in adult animals the postulated disinhibiting effect of chloralose cause an enlargement of the focal area from which a somesthetic response can be recorded (Malcolm & Smith, 1958). As yet there is no direct experimental evidence available to explain the two phenomena described: the wide spatial distribution and the consistency and high amplitude of evoked potentials in the immature brain. The "all-or-none," stereotyped feature of these responses may possibly be to a result of a lack of modifying influences from the lower centers, notably the brain stem. This notion is of course highly speculative and is based on indirect evidence only. It is known, however, that in adult animals the amplitude and form of evoked potentials are to a great extent parallel to the type of prevailing EEG pattern (Favale, Loeb, & Manfredi, 1964), and it has also been shown that the form of the responses may be directly influenced by brain stem stimulation (Purpura, Girado, & Grundfest, 1960). In the fetus up to about 90–100 days old, there is a discontinuous EEG of a very characteristic type. The activity consists of burst, sometimes spindle-shaped, consisting of rhythmic waves and appearing in scattered areas of the cortex. In between these bursts there is electrical silence. Possible thalamic driving of this type of activity has previously been discussed (Bernhard *et al.*, 1972). During subsequent development, the activity progressively reverses to a more adult pattern, that is to say, continuous and consisting of various frequencies and amplitudes. These changes occur during the period when evoked responses lose their consistency in form, appear with a lower amplitude, and furthermore show variations which sometimes seem to be related to the EEG pattern present at the moment of stimulation. Moreover, arousal EEG reactions, which cause striking changes in the evoked responses, cannot be induced until late in ontogenesis (Bernhard *et al.*, 1959). The supposedly increasing influence from lower centers upon the neocortex may then be taken as a sign of the development of integration within the brain. The relatively late appearance in development of the brain stem mediated IDR, known to be related to nonspecific afferent influences and to polysensory integration (Rutledge, 1963), fits into such a developmental scheme. An indication of a relatively delayed maturation of integrative functions, and of intracortical organization as well, is given by the finding that convergent, somesthetic and transcallosal, unitary activation could not be produced until about 100 days of fetal age. This is true despite the fact that in younger fetuses, units activated by either input were frequently found in the same penetration.

These observations lead to the tentative formulation of a generalized principle of central nervous development, according to which the function of a particular system during an initial phase of maturation is manifested rather rigidly and in isolation. Not until the function of each system has reached a fairly advanced stage of maturation does it become integrated with, and subordinated to, other systems capable of modifying its functions.

VII. Summary

With the aim of exploring how the recipient functions of the neocortex are organized during early ontogenesis, three types of cortical evoked responses were studied: somesthetic, interhemispheric, and visual. Experiments were performed on sheep fetuses, externalized and kept in umbilical contact with the placenta *in situ*. Specimens from the age of 40 days to full-term were used. The gross morphology of evoked surface of intra- and subcortical responses, as well as the concomitant extracellular unitary activity, are described.

Using developmental changes in the form of the somesthetic and visual responses as a basis for comparison, it is concluded that the phase of functional cortical development in sheep fetuses older than 85–90 days corresponds to that in the neonatal period described in other species. The predominantly negative surface somesthetic response in the 85-day sheep fetus is shown to represent a developmental stage at which activation throughout the entire depth of the cortex is already possible. Long before this "neonatal" phase of cortical ontogenesis, signs of corticopetal function can be demonstrated.

Somesthetic responses may be evoked at about 40 days, while transcallosal responses are found from 70 days. Visual responses have been studied from an age of 55 days. At their first appearance, all these responses are predominantly surface-positive. During subsequent development there is a transition from a surface-positive to a positive-negative form of the evoked potential, which subsequently attains a monophasic negative shape. Depth recordings indicate that during the earliest stage, evoked corticopetal activity is not present above the lower limit of the primitive cortex. This subcortical activity may be the result of postsynaptic events or of the depolarization of the afferent terminals. It is highly unlikely that inhibitory postsynaptic mechanisms are involved. When intracortical activation is first possible, it is confined to the deepest layers and with advancing maturation activity appears also in more superficial strata. This developmental gradient of corticorecipient functions is correlated with a similar gradient of structural changes during maturation.

During a limited period around 85 days of fetal age, responses appear with a higher amplitude and a more consistent form than in older fetuses or in adult animals. This characteristic of immature evoked responses becomes less prominent as the developing EEG patterns increase in complexity, suggesting the possibility of a causal relationship. In the lissencephalic stage, the cortical areas from which evoked responses can be recorded occupy an extensive part of the neocortex, and with advancing maturity the relative extent of these areas becomes markedly reduced. A principle of cortical development is presented, according to which each corticopetal system in early epigenesis functions as an isolated unit, suggesting that integration between the different systems does not emerge until later in development.

Acknowledgment

This study has been supported by grants to the Department of Physiology II from The Association for the Aid of Crippled Children and from the Swedish Medical Research Council, by personal grants from Karolinska Institutet, Tidningen Expressens Prenatalforskningsfond, and from Hierta-Retzius' Scientific Fund.

References

Adolph, E. F. Physiological stages in the development of mammals. *Growth*, 1970, **34**, 113–124.

Adrian, E. D. Afferent areas in the brain of ungulates. *Brain*, 1943, **66**, 89–103.

Åström, K. E. On the early development of isocortex in fetal sheep. *Progress in Brain Research*, 1967, **26**, 1–59.

Auroux, M. Apport de l'embryologie à la physiologie du corps calleux. Thèse. Laboratoire d'Embryologie, Faculté Médicine, Paris, 1964. (Mimeo.)

Barcroft, J., & Barron, D. H. Movement in the mammalian foetus. *Ergebnisse der Physiologie, Biologischen Chemie und Experimentellen Pharmakologie*, 1939, **42**, 107–152.

Barron, D. H. Some aspects of the transfer of oxygen across the syndesmochorial placenta of the sheep. *Yale Journal of Biology and Medicine*, 1951, **24**, 169–190.

Bava, A., Fadiga, E., & Manzoni, T. Interactive potentialities between thalamic relay nuclei through subcortical commissural pathways. *Archivio di Scienze Biologiche* (*Bologna*), 1966, **50**, 101–133.

Bernhard, C. G., & Meyerson, B. A. Early ontogenesis of electrocortical activity. With special reference to experimental studies on the fetal sheep. In P. Kellaway & I. Petersén (Eds.), *Clinical electroencephalography of children*. Stockholm: Almqvist & Wiksell, 1968 (New York: Grune & Stratton). Pp. 11–29.

Bernhard, C. G., Kaiser, I. H., & Kolmodin, G. M. On the development of cortical activity in fetal sheep. *Acta Physiologica Scandinavica*, 1959, **47**, 333–349.

Bernhard, C. G., Kolmodin, G. M., & Meyerson, B. A. On the prenatal development of function and structure in the somesthetic cortex of the sheep. *Progress in Brain Research*, 1967, **26**, 60–77.

Bernhard, C. G., Meyerson, B. A., & Persson, H. E. Etudes electrophysiologiques de l'ontogenèse précoce des fonctions réceptrices au sein du cortex sensorimoteur. *Actualités Neurophysiologiques*, 1972, **9**, 119–144.

Berry, M., & Rogers, A. W. The migration of neuroblast in the developing cerebral cortex. *Journal of Anatomy*, 1965, **99**, 691–709.

Cabral, R. J., & Johnson, J. I. The organization of mechanoreceptive projections in the ventrobasal thalamus of sheep. *Journal of Comparative Neurology*, 1971, **141**, 17–36.

Caley, D. W., & Maxwell, D. S. An electron microscopic study of neurons during postnatal development of thė rat cerebral cortex. *Journal of Comparative Neurology*, 1968, **133**, 17–44.

Carmichael, L. The onset and early development of behaviour. In L. Carmichael (Ed.), *Manual of child psychology*. New York: Wiley, 1954. Pp. 60–185.

Comline, R. S., & Silver, M. PO_2 levels in the placental circulation of the mare and ewe. *Nature* (*London*), 1968, **217**, 76–77.

Conway, C. J., Wright F. S., & Bradley, W. E. Electrophysiological maturation of the pyramidal tract in the post-natal rabbit. *Electroencephalography and Clinical Neurophysiology*, 1969, **26**, 565–577.

Crain, S. M. Discussion. In H. J. Jasper, A. A. Ward, & A. Pope (Eds.), *Basic mechanisms of the epilepsies*. Boston: Little, Brown, 1969. Pp. 506–516.

Creutzfeldt, O, & Sakmann, B. Neurophysiology of vision. *Annual Review of Physiology*, 1969, **31**, 499–544.

Dawes, G. S. *Foetal and neonatal physiology*. Chicago: Yearbook Publ. 1968.

Delhaye-Bouchaud, N. Étude de l'évolution du potential évoqué somesthésique chez le lapin pendant la periode néonatale. These. Faculté des Sciences, Paris, 1964. (Mineo.)

Eidelberg, E., Kolmodin, G. M., & Meyerson, B. A. Ontogenesis of steady potential and direct cortical response in fetal sheep brain. *Experimental Neurology*, 1965, **12**, 198–214.

Eidelberg, E., Kolmodin, G. M., & Meyerson, B. A. Effect of asphyxia on the cortical steady potential in adult and fetal sheep. *Acta Physiologica Scandinavica* 1967, **69**, 257–261.

Ellingson, R. J. Studies of the electrical activity of the developing human brain. *Progress in Brain Research*, 1964, **9**, 26–53.

Favale, E., Loeb, C., & Manfredi, M. Modifications of calloso-cortical response by sleep. *Archives Internationales de Physiologie et Biochemie*, 1964, **72**, 863–870.

Fuentes, C., & Marty, R. Maturation centripète du cortex cérébral. *Journal für Hirnforschung*, 1969, **11**, 67–78.

Gottlieb, G. Conceptions of prenatal behavior. In L. R. Aronson, E. Tobach, D. S. Lehrman & J. S. Rosenblatt (Eds.), *Development and evolution of behavior*. San Francisco: Freeman, 1970. Pp. 111–137.

Gottlieb, G. Ontogenesis of sensory function in birds and mammals. In E. Tobach, L. R. Aronson, & E. Shaw (Eds.), *The biopsychology of development*. New York: Academic Press, 1971. Pp. 67–128.

Grafstein, B. Organization of callosal connections in suprasylvian gyrus of cat. *Journal of Neurophysiology*, 1959, **22**, 504–515.

Grafstein, B. Postnatal development of the transcallosal evoked response in the cerebral cortex of the cat. *Journal of Neurophysiology*, 1963, **26**, 79–99.

Hatton, G. I., & Rubel, E. W. Somatic sensory projection to cerebral cortex of sheep. *Anatomical Record*, 1967, **157**, 256–257. (Abstract)

Holmes, O., & Short, A. D. Interaction of cortical evoked potentials in the rat. *Journal of Physiology* (*London*), 1970, **209**, 433–452.

Hossmann, K. A. Untersuchungen über transcallosale potentiale an der akuten Corpus Callosum-Katze. *Deutsche Zeitschrift für Nervenheilkunde*, 1969, **195**, 79–102.

Hubel, D. H., & Wiesel, T. N. Receptive fields of cells in striate cortex of very young visually inexperienced kittens. *Journal of Neurophysiology*, 1963, **26**, 994–1002.

Humphrey, D. R. Re-analysis of the antidromic cortical response. I. Potentials evoked by stimulation of the isolated pyramidal tract. *Electroencephalography and Clinical Neurophysiology*, 1968, **24**, 116–129.

Huttenlocher, P. R. Development of cortical neuronal activity in the neonatal cat. *Experimental Neurology*, 1967, **17**, 247–262.

Kahle, W. Zur ontogenetischen Entwicklung der Broddmannschen Rindenfelder. In R. Hassler & H. Stephan (Eds.), *Evolution of the forebrain.* Stuttgart: Thieme, 1966. Pp. 305–315.

Kolmodin, G. M., & Meyerson, B. A. Ontogenesis of paroxysmal cortical activity in foetal sheep. *Electroencephalography and Clinical Neurophysiology*, 1966, **21**, 589–600.

Malcolm, J. L., & Smith, J. D. Convergence within the pathways to cat's somatic sensory cortex activated by mechanical stimulation of the skin. *Journal of Physiology (London)*, 1958, **144**, 257–270.

Marty, R. Développement post-natal des réponses sensorielles du cortex cérébral chez le chat et le lapin. Aspects physiologiques et histologiques. *Archives d'Anatomie Microscopique et de Morphologie Expérimentale*, 1962, **51**, 129–264.

Marty, R., & Pujol, R. Maturation post-natale de l'aire visuelle du cortex cérébral chez le chat. In R. Hassler & H. Stephen (Eds.), *Evolution of the forebrain.* Stuttgart: Thieme, 1966. Pp. 405–418.

Marty, R., & Scherrer, J. Critères de maturation des systèmes afférents corticaux. *Progress in Brain Research*, 1964, **4**, 222–234.

Mayers, K. S., Robertson, R. T., Rubel, E. W., & Thompson, R. F. Development of poly-sensory responses in association cortex of kitten. *Science*, 1971, **171**, 1037–1038.

Meller, K., Breipohl, W., & Glees, P. Synaptic organization of the molecular and the outer granular layer in the motorcortex in the white mouse during postnatal development. A Golgi- and electronmicroscopical study. *Zeitschrift für Zellforschung und Mikroskopische Anatomie*, 1968, **92**, 217–231.

Meyerson, B. A. Electrophysiological signs of interhemispheric functions during development. In Jílek & S. Trojan (Eds.), *Ontogenesis of the brain.* Prague: Charles University Press, 1967. Pp. 73–83.

Meyerson, B. A. Ontogeny of interhemispheric functions. *Acta Physiologica Scandinavica, Supplementum*, 1968, **312**, 1–111.

Meyerson, B. A., & Persson, H. E. Evoked unitary and gross electric activity in the cerebral cortex in early ontogeny. *Nature (London)*, 1969, **221**, 1248–1249.

Molliver, M. E. An ontogenetic study of evoked somesthetic cortical responses in the sheep. *Progress in Brain Research*, 1967, **26**, 78–90.

Molliver, M. E., & van der Loos, H. The ontogenesis of cortical circuity: The spatial distribution of synapses in somesthetic cortex of newborn dog. *Ergebnisse der Anatomie und Entwicklungsgeschichte*, 1970, **42**, 1–54.

Mysliveček, J. Subcortical visual relays and specific cortical response in developing animals. In L. Jílek & S. Trojan (Eds.), *Ontogenesis of the brain.* Prague: Charles University Press, 1967. Pp. 359–366.

Nougier, M. Étude des projections des lèvres sur le cortex cérébral du mouton par la technique des potentiels évoqués. Diplome d'Études Supérieures, Laboratoire de Physiologie Générale, Faculté des Sciences, Marseille, 1963. (Mimeo.)

Persson, H. E. Electrophysiological studies on the functional development of the somatosensory cortex during early prenatal ontogenesis (in Russian). In *X scientific conference on age morphology, physiology and biochemistry.* Moscow: 1971.

Persson, H. E. Development of somatosensory cortical functions. *Acta Physiologica Scandinavica, Supplementum*, 1973, **394**, 1–64.

Persson, H. E., & Stenberg, D. Early prenatal development of cortical surface responses to visual stimuli in sheep. *Experimental Neurology*, 1972, **37**, 199–208.

Petersen, J., Di Perri, R., & Himwich, W. A. The comparative development of the EEG in rabbit, cat and dog. *Electroencephalography and Clinical Neurophysiology*, 1964, **17**, 557–563.

Poliakov, G. I. Embryonal and post-embryonal development of neurons of the human cerebral cortex. In R. Hassler & H. Stephan (Eds.), *Evolution of the forebrain*. Stuttgart: Thieme, 1966. Pp. 249–258.

Purpura, D. P. Analysis of axodendritic organization in immature cerebral cortex. *Annals of the New York Academy of Sciences*, 1961, **94**, 604–654. (a)

Purpura, D. P. Ontogenetic analysis of some evoked synaptic activities in superficial neocortical neuropil. In E. Florey (Ed.), *Nervous inhibition*. Oxford: Pergamon, 1961, Pp. 424–446. (b)

Purpura, D. P. Stability and seizure susceptibility of immature brain. In H. J. Jasper, A. A. Ward, & A. Pope (Eds.), *Basic mechanisms of the epilepsies*. Boston: Little, Brown, 1969. Pp. 481–505.

Purpura, D. P., Girado, M., & Grundfest, H. Components of evoked potentials. *Electroencephalography and Clinical Neurophysiology*, 1960, **12**, 95–110.

Purpura, D. P., Shofer, J., Houspian, E. M., & Noback, C. R. Comparative ontogenesis of structure-function relations in cerebral and cerebellar cortex. *Progress in Brain Research*, 1964, **4**, 187–221.

Purpura, D. P., Shofer, R. J., & Scarff, T. Properties of synaptic activities and spike potentials of neurons in immature neocortex. *Journal of Neurophysiology*, 1965, **28**, 925–942.

Richard, P., Auffray, P., & Albe-Fessard, D. Activités thalamiques évoquées par des stimulations somatiques chez le mouton anesthésié au chloralose. *Electroencephalography and Clinical Neurophysiology*, 1967, **23**, 401–410.

Rose, G. H. The comparative ontogenesis of visually evoked responses in rat and cat. In L. Jílek & S. Trojan (Eds.), *Ontogenesis of the brain*. Prague: Charles University Press, 1967. Pp. 347–358.

Rose, G. H., & Lindsley, D. B. Development of visually evoked potentials in kittens. Specific and unspecific responses. *Journal of Neurophysiology*, 1968, **31**, 606–623.

Ruckebusch, Y. Activité électro-corticale chez le foetus de la brebis (*Ovis aries*) et de la vache (*Bos taurus*). *Revue de Médicine Vétérinaire*, 1971, **34**, 483–510.

Rutledge, L. T. Interactions of peripherally and centrally originating input to association cortex. *Electroencephalography and Clinical Neurophysiology*, 1963, **15**, 958–968.

Rutledge, L. T., & Kennedy, T. T. Extracallosal delayed response to cortical stimulation in chloralosed cat. *Journal of Neurophysiology*, 1960, **23**, 188–196.

Scheibel, M., & Scheibel, A. 1964. Some neural substrates of postnatal development. In E. Hoffman (Ed.), *Annual review of child development*. New York: Russell Sage Foundation, 1964. Pp. 481–519.

Scherrer, J., & Oeconomos, D. Réponses corticales somesthésiques du mammifère nouveau-né comparées à celles de l'animal adulte. *Etudes Néo-natales*, 1954, **3**, 199–216.

Towe, A. L., & Harding, G. W. Extracellular microelectrode sampling bias. *Experimental Neurology*, 1970, **29**, 366–381.

Verley, R., Garma, L., & Scherrer, J. Conceptions récentes sur le développement du système nerveux des mammifères. *Année Psychologique*, 1969, **69**, 455–489.

Vignal, W. Recherches sur le développement des éléments des couches corticales du cerveau et du cervelet chez l'homme et les mammifères. *Archives de Physiologie Normale et Pathologique*, 1888, **2**, 228–254.

Voeller, K., Pappas, G. D., & Purpura, D. P. Electron microscope study of development of cat superficial neocortex. *Experimental Neurology*, 1963, **7**, 107–130.

Wiesel, T. N., & Hubel, D. H. Single-cell responses in striate cortex of kittens deprived of vision in one eye. *Journal of Neurophysiology*, 1963, **26**, 1003–1017.

Windle, W. F. *Physiology of the fetus: Origin and extent of function of prenatal life*, Philadelphia: Saunders, 1940.

ENTROPY AND INFORMATION IN FETAL BEHAVIOR

R. M. BERGSTRÖM

Institute of Physiology
University of Helsinki
Helsinki, Finland

I. Introduction

An increasing amount of evidence testifies to the importance of environmental factors in the ontogenetic development of the central nervous system (CNS) (see introductory chapter to Volume 1 by G. Gottlieb). This implies a need for consideration of the problem of fetal behavior as a problem of the change in communicative interaction of the fetus with its environment during development (R. M. Bergström, 1968, 1969b). However, if a communication-theoretical view of fetal behavior is to be applied, a need also arises for a definition of the appropriate concepts used in the description of the exchange of signals and information through specified channels between the fetal organism and its environment. This definition, moreover, has to rest upon an empirical foundation if it is to provide us with operational measures for the description of fetal behavioral patterns.

Concepts employed with a view to characterizing the change of patterns in fetal behavior, such as the degree of "organization," of "order," of "regularity," of "randomness," of "probability," and so on, do not provide us with quantitative measures, unless they are operationally defined. The possibility of these, and other corresponding concepts, being connected with information-theoretical concepts, such as entropy and information, was proposed in an earlier publication (R. M. Bergström, 1969c). According to this view, a high degree of order or organization is equivalent to a high information content and to a low entropy content (or high content of negative entropy = negentropy), a connection which is in accordance with Brillouin's (1962) interpretation of the concept of information. Thus, if a communication-theoretical view is to be applied to fetal behavior, an analysis is necessary of the entropic and informational properties of the changing behavioral patterns of the fetus during development.

An attempt is made below, in conjunction with computer-simulated modeling of a growing neural network, to show how certain features of fetal behavior are explicable by means of these communication-theoretical aspects.

II. Development of Order in Fetal Behavior

To insure a correct application of communication theory to fetal behavior, it would be necessary to possess a knowledge of the development of the structural and functional organization in different parts of the brain. Since relatively little adequate data are available to permit definition of brain organization at different developmental stages, it is appropriate to proceed in another way: if a model of the fetal brain can be developed on the foundation of empirical evidence, then the behavior of the model is comparable with the behavior of real fetal brains.

As was suggested earlier (R. M. Bergström, 1968, 1969b), sufficient morphological and functional evidence exists for the assumption that in the adult mammalian brain the core is built up of randomly connected networks, termed the reticular substance. It was also suggested that the term "random" could be used here in its strict physical sense (Brillouin, 1962): that a lack of measurable order exists in the geometrical structure of the network. The term is further applicable in the information-theoretical sense; that is, that the high entropy content is equal to the statement that we lack information on the structure in question. This latter statement is in conformity with the physical concept of entropy (Brillouin, 1962).

We know from studies of fetal brains (R. M. Bergström, 1969a) that the reticular core is the first of all the parts of the brain to mature functionally. The older concept (cf. Windle, 1944), that maturation proceeds from the medullary level to the caudal and oral direction, should be revised to the effect that it proceeds from the inner core outward, that is, toward the shells

Without detailed examination of the basic assumptions upon which the model network was founded (for this, cf. R. M. Bergström, 1967, 1969b, 1972; R. M. Bergström & Nevanlinna, 1972), it needs to be stated that, unlike most neural models, the present model includes the definition of a neural magnitude, here called "neural energy"

$$Q = N\nu, \tag{1}$$

where N is the number of efferent synaptic connections of a neuron, and ν the average impulse frequency that they mediate, a magnitude which shows the same conservative properties as the physical energy (for such properties of neural activity, see Griffith, 1971). This definition enables calculation of a main expression of neural entropy

$$H = U \ln P, \tag{2}$$

where P gives the amount and order content of the neural excitation, and U is dependent upon the number of neuronal units in the system.

For fulfillment of these preconditions, the total neural energy is calculated as the integrated sum of impulses in the units of the system, and the constancy of the energy is based upon the direct proportionality between the threshold of the neuron and the size of its soma (Henneman, Somjen, & Carpenter, 1965), and between soma size and the number of its efferent branches (Ramón y Cajal, 1909).

For the ideal neural system, in which no loss of neural energy owing to the synaptic transfers needs to be assumed (if it occurs in real systems, it can be handled in a analogous way to frictional energy loss in mechanical systems), an expression for the entropy (H) is derived as a function of the neural energy (E_n), the number of units (M), and the number of their efferent branches (N):

$$H(E_n, M, N) = 4E_n/MN\,[1 - (E_n/MN)]\,(M - 1)\log(N + 1). \tag{3}$$

Figure 2 illustrates the computer simulation of function for a network in which the random organization was derived with a program simulating the natural growth of the network. The function is approximately parabolic, and the entropy has a linear dependence upon the number of units in the system, a logarithmic dependence upon the number of efferent branches, and the entropy exhibits a maximum for a medium amount of energy.

In Eq. (3), the macrostate (entropy H) is described by means of structural (M, N) and neuroenergetic (E_n) microevents. It is also possible to calculate the capacity of information from the expression. This calculation shows that this capacity, that is, the range ΔH, is at a maximum with maximum entropy.

The result is of interest from the viewpoint of the behavior of individuals

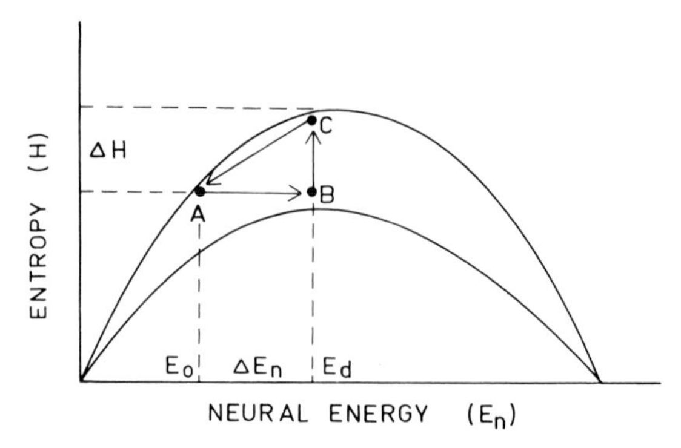

FIG. 2. The relation between entropy (H) and neural energy (E_n) in the model network of randomnly connected neurons. ΔH: Entropy shift of the system, caused by an increase in energization (ΔE_n). ABCA: subsequent changes in the internal state of the network.

with primitive neural systems (low value of M, N and E_n) to the extent that if the momentary information content is to be changed, the total energy of the system has to be changed. These organisms are consequently dependent upon the physical energy of the environment, a feature which is actually known from the behavior of lower forms of animals with primitive neural systems (Horridge, 1968). Nevertheless, the capacity to handle information is greatly dependent upon the number of units in the neural system. This result is in conformity with the finding (Rensch, 1964) that the greater the brain of an animal is, the more it is capable of sensorimotor performance. In the model of McCulloch and Pitts (1943), learning capacity is also said to be proportional to the number of (logical) units in the system.

The overall parabolic form of Eq. (3) shows that—from the aspect of information processing—a neural system works best with an optimum energy. This is analogous to functions of a similar form in adult human subjects, in which the "level of cue functions" is dependent on the level of arousal (Hebb, 1955), such magnitudes referring to information capacity and energization of the brain, respectively. The preference for an optimum energy in living systems is of course of advantage from the aspect of a stabilized behavioral performance of individuals in specified environmental energy levels, typical of each species, or each ontogenetic stage. With the help of its behavior, the individual is actively forced to seek this optimum level in order to survive.

At each developmental stage a given state of equilibrium thus appears between the individual and the environment, the driving force of which can be stated in physical terms: the neural system tends to move toward its most probable state, that is, to maximum entropy. Each disturbance from this state is followed by a behavioral act tending to move the system toward the entropy maximum. For this, an energetic input or output (increase or decrease of neural energy) to or from the neural system is needed, depending upon the direction of the disturbance (loss or gain of neural energy). This is achievable by behavior.

A preliminary investigation of the impulse-interval histograms of the units of the computer-simulated model of the primitive neural network resulted in histograms with long right-hand tails; so far as can be judged from the rather meager material, these are exponential or gamma-type histograms. Consequently, they also display the same features as histograms recorded from real, primitive networks.

IV. Dynamics of Fetal Behavior

From the viewpoint of the observed characteristics of fetal behavior, specifically, an increasing order content during development, the model reveals an interesting result. The model predicts that the increase in the number of neuronal units, and in their efferent branches during ontogeny, is followed by an increase in the order capacity of the behavioral output of the CNS. This, as has been observed in experiments on the fetal guinea pig, is how the order content of the behavioral pattern increases with fetal age. However, the model also predicts that the order content of the behavioral motor output depends upon the excitatory state of the CNS; that is to say, upon the excitatory afferent input: the greater the afferent input, the greater will be the order content of the motor output, until an optimum level of input is reached. Subsequently, the order content of the output decreases with further enhancement of the afferent input.

In a series of studies on the fetal guinea pig, a study was made of the dependence of the order content of the pattern of motor behavior on the excitatory state of the CNS, with a view to testing the model (L. Bergström, unpublished data). Alteration in the excitatory state of the CNS was brought about both by skin stimulation of the various parts of the body (reflexogenic activity), and by gross electrical stimulation of the mesencephalic brainstem. The unstimulated or "spontaneous" motor activity of the intact fetus in the amniotic sac served as a control for the stimulated activity. Figure 3 illustrates the overall results, which disclosed an enhancement of the total amount of motor activity by both central or peripheral stimulation, except around day 47 (central stimulation) and day 57 (reflexogenic activity) (gestation period: 65 days). The failure to obtain an increase in the motor output with central stimulation around the day 47 may be attributed to the maturation of powerful inhibitory subcortical centers in the forebrain at this age

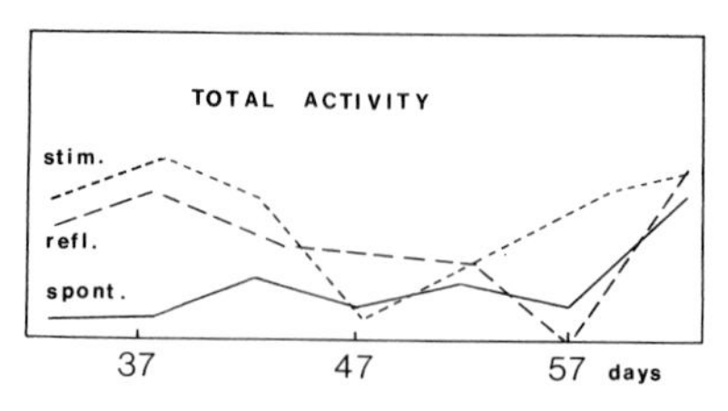

FIG. 3. Spontaneous (spont.) behavioral activity and activity aroused by skin stimulation (refl.) and by electrical stimulation of the mesencephalic brain stem (stim.) in the fetal guinea pig (gestation period 65 days). From L. Bergström (unpublished data).

(R. M. Bergström, 1968), and the same failure with peripheral stimulation around the day 57 to the maturation of inhibition in the reflex arcs (R. M. Bergström, 1962). An additional observation was that at each age, except as regards the very late fetus, a more organized pattern of motor behavior was obtained by stimulation (central and peripheral) than had been observed in spontaneous motor activity at the corresponding age. This implies that the fetus possesses a "latent capacity' of organized behavioral pattern, which can be released by energization of the CNS through afferent channels, or by means of artificial stimulation of the brain. As can be predicted by the model, the order content of the output increased with rising energization of the network. The fact that Sedláček (this volume) observes a significant increase of order in the guinea pig's brain and behavior during the later perinatal period—after the initiation of lung ventilation and the increased afference resulting from the onset of breathing—fits in very well with the present concept.

The model and the empirical findings suggest that the order content of fetal behavior is dependent not only upon the size of CNS, but also upon the degree of the excitatory input from afferent channels. This question of the dependence of the pattern of fetal motor activity upon the intensity of stimulation was also put forward by Gottlieb (1970) in a review of Coghill's theory of fetal behavior. The model also predicts that a maximum order content of motor behavior is obtained only by an optimal degree of afferent stimulation. This fact might also be of value in the treatment of human prematures (Parmelee, personal communication), since this optimal value of input varies with the age of the developing organism (that is, with the size of the CNS).

The sudden increase in the amount of motor activity of the guinea pig fetus several days before birth, together with the observation that stimulation did not increase the order content of the behavior in the late fetus in comparison with the order content of the "spontaneous" activity at the same age, indicates that the increase in motor activity at that time is attributable to external stimulation. The occurrence of such stimulation in the prehatching bird embryo is indicated by observations presented in Volume 1 of this serial publication by Gottlieb, Introduction to Section 4—Impekoven and Gold, and Vince. The resulting behavior, which exhibits a highly organized pattern and order content (phase, rhythm, coordination, etc.) might act as a drive for the birth process. (For a further discussion of the factors causing changes in the guinea pig fetus' behavior around the time of birth, see Sedláček's article in this volume.)

V. Conclusions

The empirical findings on fetal behavioral patterns, along with the application of a quantitative entropy model of the developing brain with respect to these findings, indicate that a communication-theoretical view might be of assistance in the solution of some problems in the ontogeny of behavior. The introduction of operational concepts of neuromuscular function, such as entropy and information, as a substitute for qualitative concepts, such as organization and order, may help us in the quantification of behavioral patterns at different developmental stages in the fetus. The quantitative entropy model of the developing brain, tested with observations on the guinea pig fetus, indicates that the information (order) content of fetal behavior depends not only upon the size of the maturing CNS (number of neuronal elements and the number of their efferent branches) but also upon the level of excitation of the CNS effected by the afferent input. The maximum information content of the behavioral output is obtained with an optimal amount of afferent input only. A lower degree of this input, or an excess of it, is followed by a diminution in the information content of the behavior. The optimal amount of input varies with the maturation age of the fetus.

Acknowledgment

This work was supported by a grant from the National Research Council for Medical Sciences, Finland.

References

Änggård, L., Bergström, R. M., & Bernhard, C. G. Analysis of prenatal reflex activity in sheep. *Acta Physiologica Scandinavica*, 1961, **53**, 128–136.

Bergström, L. Foetal development of mesencephal motor functions in the guinea pig. *Acta Physiologica Scandinavica, Supplementum*, **277**, 22.

Bergström, R. M. Prenatal development of motor functions. A study on the intrauterine guinea pig foetus in the conscious, pregnant animal. *Annales Chirurgiae et Gynaecologiae Fenniae, Supplementum*, 1962, **112**, 1–48.

Bergström, R. M. Neural macrostates. *Synthese*, 1967, **17**, 425–443.

Bergström, R. M. Development of EEG and unit electrical activity of the brain during ontogeny (with special reference to the development of entropy relations of the brain). In (L. Jílek & S. Trojan (Eds.), *Ontogenesis of the brain.* Prague: Charles University Press, 1968.

Bergström, R. M. Electrical parameters of the brain during ontogeny. In R. J. Robinson (Ed.), *Brain and early behaviour: Development in the fetus and infant.* London: Academic Press, 1969. (a)

Bergström, R. M. An entropy model of the developing brain. *Developmental Psychobiology*, 1969, **2**, 139–152. (b)

Bergström, R. M. Structure-function relationships: A classification of concepts. In R. J. Robinson (Ed.), *Brain and early behaviour: Development in the fetus and infant.* London: Academic Press, 1969. (c)

Bergström, R. M. Neural micro- and macrostates. In (G. Newton & A. Riesen (Eds.), *Advances in psychobiology.* New York: Wiley, 1972.

Bergström, R. M., & Bergström, L. Prenatal development of stretch reflex functions and brain stem activity in the human. *Annales Chirurgiae et Gynaecologiae Fenniae, Supplementum*, 1963, **117**, 1–12.

Bergström, R. M., Hällström, P. E., & Stenberg, D. E. Prenatal stretch reflex activity in the guinea pig. *Annales Chirurgiae et Gynaecologiae Fenniae*, 1961, **50**, 458–466.

Bergström, R. M., Hirvonen, J. I., & Karlsson, L. K. J. Respiratory changes during electrical stimulation of rhinencephalic structures in the foetal guinea pig. *Nature* (London), 1966, **21**, 1176–1178.

Bergström, R. M., & Nevanlinna, O. An entropy model of primitive neural systems. *International Journal of Neuroscience*, 1972, **4**, 171–173.

Brillouin, L. *Science and information theory*. New York: Academic Press, 1962.

Brooks, V. B., Kameda, K., & Nagel, R. Recurrent inhibition in the cat's cerebral cortex. In C. Von Euler, S. Skoglund, & U. Söderberg (Eds.), *Structure and function of inhibitory neuronal mechanisms*. Oxford: Pergamon, 1968.

Burns, D. *The uncertain nervous system.* London: Arnold, 1968.

Eccles, J. C. Postsynaptic inhibition in the central nervous system. In C. von Euler, S. Skoglund, & U. Söderberg (Eds.), *Structure and function of inhibitory neuronal mechanisms.* Oxford: Pergamon, 1968.

Gottlieb, G. Conceptions of prenatal behavior. In L. R. Aronson, E. Tobach, D. S. Lehrman, & J. S. Rosenblatt (Eds.), *Development and evolution of behavior.* San Francisco: Freeman, 1970. Pp. 111–137.

Griffith, J. S. *Mathematical neurobiology.* London: Academic Press, 1971.

Hamburger, V. Emergence of nervous coordination. Origins of integrated behavior. In M. Locke (Ed.), *The emergence of order in developing systems.* New York: Academic Press, 1969.

Hassler, R., & Riechert, T. Effects of stimulations and coagulations in the basal ganglia in stereotactic brain surgery. *Nervenarzt*, 1961, **32**, 97–109.

Hebb, D. O. Drives and the C.N.S. (Conceptual nervous system). *Psychological Review*, 1955, **62**, 243–254.

Henneman, F., Somjen, G., & Carpenter, D. O. Functional significance of cell size in spinal motoneurons. *Journal of Neurophysiology*, 1965, **28**, 560–580.

Horridge, G. A. *Interneurons.* London: Freeman, 1968.

Hyvärinen, J. Analysis of spontaneous spike potential activity in developing rabbit diencephalon. *Acta Physiologica Scandinavica, Supplementum*, 1966, **278**, 1–67.

Jung, R., & Hassler, R. The extrapyramidal motor system. In J. Field, H. W. Magoun, & V. E. Hall (Eds.), *Handbood of physiology.* Vol. 1, Sect. 2. Baltimore: Waverly, 1960.

McCulloch, W. S., & Pitts, W. H. A logical calculus of ideas immanent in nervous activity. *Bulletin of Mathematical Biophysics*, 1943, **5**, 115–133.

Monnier, M., & Lévy, A. Die physio-pathologischen Mechanismen der Dystonien und Dyskinesien. *Schweizer Archiv für Neurologie und Psychiatrie*, 1961, **85**, 109–139.

Needham, C. W., & Dila, C. J. Synchronizing and desynchronizing systems of the old brain. *Brain Research*, 1968, **11**, 285–293.

Ramón y Cajal, S. *Histologie du systéme nerveux de l'homme et des vertébrés.* Paris: Maloine, 1909.

Rensch, B. Memory and concepts of higher animals. *Proceedings of the Zoological Society of Calcutta*, 1964, **17**, 207–221.

Scheibel, M. E., & Scheibel, A. B. Neural correlates of psychophysiological development in the young organism. *Anatomical Record*, 1961, **139**, 319–320.

Scheibel, M. E., & Scheibel, A. B. Anatomical basis of attention mechanisms in vertebrate brains. In G. C. Quarton, T. Melnechik, & F. O. Schmitt (Eds.), *The neurosciences: A study program.* New York: Rockefeller University Press, 1967.

Stenberg, D. The ontogenesis of the spontaneous electrical activity of the lower brain stem. *Acta Physiologica Scandinavica, Supplementum*, 1967, **31**, 162.

Stenberg, D. 1968. Analysis of the EEG of the guinea pig foetus. *Acta Physiologica Scandinavica*, 1968, **74**, 509–510.

Stenberg, D., & Vehaskari, M. Development of gross electrical activity in the hippocampus of the guinea pig. *Developmental Psychobiology*, 1969, **2**, 29–33.

Tsukahara, N., & Brooks, V. B. Cortical recurrent inhibition of corticorubral cells. In C. von Euler, S. Skoglund, & U. Söderberg (Eds.), *Structure and function of inhibitory neuronal mechanisms.* Oxford: Pergamon, 1968.

Windle, W. F. Genesis of somatic motor function in mammalian embryos: a synthesizing article. *Physiological Zoology*, 1944, **17**, 247–260.

Section 3

METAMORPHOSIS AND BIRTH: HORMONAL AND PHYSIOLOGICAL ASPECTS

INTRODUCTION

There are two very important elements in common between the processes of metamorphosis and birth (and hatching, for that matter): the apparently crucial participation of biochemical and hormonal factors, and the fact that a successful outcome in each case leads to a rather different organism equipped for—and presented with—a new way of life.

The transformation is greatest in the case of amphibians. In fact, by way of emphasis, Dr. A. F. Hughes speaks of two nervous systems, one the "insect-like" premetamorphic nervous system and the other the postmetamorphic one. It is possible to overdraw this distinction, of course, such that one might erroneously conclude that there are *no* continuities between pre- and post-metamorphosis. As indicated in the introductory article in Volume 1 of this serial publication, there are continuities in *behavior* between pre- and postmetamorphosis in insects as well as in amphibia. Dr. Hughes also reminds us of the omnipresent diversity of species *and mechanisms*, important points which are often neglected or underemphasized.

The significant changes in brain function in mammals during the period around birth, described by Dr. Jindřich Sedláček in the guinea pig, certainly transform the behavioral abilities and cortical activity of the fetus toward those of the neonate. The rapidity with which these striking changes occur, once the fetus (or newborn) begins breathing, leads Dr. Sedláček to suppose that the neural basis for them is organized during previous prenatal development, and that the gaseous, biochemical, and endogenous sensory stimulative events connected with lung ventilation merely trigger the cortical changes (or allow their expression).

tially, and when cell death appears, the curve inflects. There is a peak at stage 57, after which numbers decrease, and then finally level out (Prestige, 1965). Thus, in the late larva there is continuous reconstruction within the nerve centers which innervate the limbs, a behavioral correlate of which in another species can perhaps be seen in the observations of Jacobson and Baker (1969) on the reactions of frogs to skin grafts reversed in position in early life so that a large area of flank skin originally from the ventral surface is placed in a dorsal position, and vice versa. As was first shown by Miner (1956), local stimulation in an adult bearing such grafts results in a "maladaptive response," as Sperry and Miner (1949) term it, whereby the frog wipes with fore or hindlimb an area of the body surface from which the stimulated area originally belonged. Jacobson and Baker showed that the first reactions of early postmetamorphic juveniles were normal and took no account of the reversed position of part of the body surface. Only later does the maladaptive response supervene. It may be that the modulation of sensory neurons by this peripheral change affects only relatively late generations of sensory cells, while their predecessors made contact with the periphery too early to be influenced by the ectopic positions where the first nerve endings terminate. Whether or not such functional explanations of cell death in the developing nervous system are valid, it is clear that not all instances, particularly at early stages of development, can be explained along these lines.

Cell death occurs in all phases of the development of the nervous system, from early formative stages onward (Glücksmann, 1951), though little is known about its incidence within the brain. In their recent work on brain DNA during the development of *Rana pipiens*, Hunt and Jacobson (1970) find that both normally and under hormonal treatment, their curves rise to a point of inflexion, reach a plateau, and then decline toward metamorphosis, a phase which is presumably due to cell death, though it has yet to be recognized histologically. It can be said that while some of the links can be recognized between hormones and the replacement of the larval by the postmetamorphic nervous system, and between these neural events and the related patterns of motility, we have little or no understanding of how these mechanisms originate. Study by molecular methods of other organ systems in tadpoles which undergo metamorphic changes at cell or organ level have shown that thyroxine molecules find the receptor sites on the target cells at stages well before structural alterations are recognizable microscopically (Tata, 1970).

While we are a long way from any understanding of how these events are programmed, it is clear that in larval Anura, thyroxine is the dominant hormone, and, as I hope to show here, occupies a unique importance among tetrapods in the control of early neural development. The question arises whether this condition represents a basic pattern in developing tetrapods or whether it is part of an evolutionary specialization concerned with the far-reaching changes which occur within the metamorphosing anuran tadpole. Certainly among living Anura, the duration of the larval stage varies considerably in different genera, as is the size attained by the full-grown tadpole. At one extreme is the bizarre example of the tropical *Pseudis paradoxa* where the larva grows to a foot in length and lives off its own tail during a protracted metamorphosis. Another curious fact is that one of the two most primitive Anura now extant, *Leiopelma*, has an embryonic period of unusual length.

I would now direct attention to an anuran whose entire ontogeny is embryonic. Caribbean species of the genus *Eleutherodactylus* lay their eggs on land and develop in about 2 weeks from cleavage stages to a miniature frog, smaller than a house fly, and already able to take jumps of half a meter or so. Nearly all larval features have been suppressed. There is no fishlike stage of the respiratory and vascular systems. All that is left is the loss of the tail, which within the egg capsule serves as a breathing organ mimicking an allantois. Comparison with larval Anura with respect to endocrine factors in the development of the nervous system provides a fascinating field for study. My friend, Dr. W. Gardner Lynn, is the pioneer here (Lynn, 1942; Lynn & Peadon, 1955), and I have attempted in recent years to follow his lead. All too little has yet been done, but the general conclusion seems to emerge that in *Eleutherodactylus* the role of thyroxine in the development of the nervous system is less than in larval Anura. In the first place, the limb buds appear at an early stage of ontogeny as in other embryonic tetrapods, and their development seems wholly independent of the thyroid. Neither hypophysectomy nor thyroidectomy affect either their differentiation (Hughes, 1966b) or their development of motility. However, as in larval Anura, the latter is accompanied by cell loss within the lateral motor column, which is thus freed from indirect thyroid control through any influence on limb development, although the column seems specially dependent on the pituitary.

In hypophysectomized *Eleutherodactylus* embryos, motor cells lose their normal affinity for silver in standard histological procedures, which presumably depends on the presence of microtubules in the neurocytoplasm (Gray & Guillery, 1966). These argyophobic neurons then die, and their total number falls to levels below those of the normal embryo. Again, unlike the larval anuran, thyroidectomy has no effect on numbers in the column, which decrease at a normal rate as development proceeds. We have recently found that in embryos treated early enough with prolactin, the ventral horn is unusually large, and it seems likely that maintenance of these cells is dependent upon a prolactinlike hormone secreted by the pituitary (Hughes & Reier, 1972). Exogenous thyroxine has the same effect in promoting the differentiation of the individual motor neuron as in larval Anura.

In embryos later than the early digit stages of the limbs, i. e. at 7–7½ days, no effect results either from treatment with prolactin or from thyroidectomy. The main effect of thyroidectomy performed before this stage is the retention of the tail. Within the nervous system, the only effects observable under the light microscope are in a slower loss of Rohon-Beard cells than normal, and in a slight lag in maturation of cells of the ventral horn.

The development of the nervous system and of embryonic behavior show features which *Eleutherodactylus* shares with amniote embryos. The spinal cord from the first has a thick mantle layer in marked contrast with that of the early Anuran larva where the number of cells is reduced to the essential minimum. Study of the development of motility in *Eleutherodactylus* necessitates freeing the embryo from its tough capsule, after which normal development can continue *in vitro*. Limb motility develops in the standard fashion, with flexion and passive relaxion preceding the appearance of an extensor thrust. As with reptile and bird embryos, there are spontaneous movements of the unstimulated embryo, at first uncoordinated, but building up into a clear pattern of diagonal ambulation, in contrast to the bilateral thrusts which follow tactile stimulation (Hughes, 1966a).

III. Urodela

The urodeles are a more diversified group of animals than are the Anura. In them we find resemblances with and differences from the Anura relating to the three aspects of development with which we are here concerned. The primary metamorphosis of newts and salamanders is known to be under thyroid control (Schwartzenbach & Uhlenhuth, 1928), and prolactin has been shown to antagonize the action of thyroxine at this period (Gona & Etkin, 1970). Though hypophysectomy of larval *Ambystoma punctatum* retards general growth, no differences are seen between such operated larvae and controls with respect to limb development until near the time of metamorphosis, when the growth rate slows in the normal animal, but paradoxically not in the absence of the pituitary (Blount, 1935). At a later phase of urodele life history, the first observations on the activity of prolactin were described over 40 years ago. One of the fascinating facts about North American Amphibia is the double metamorphosis of the urodele *Triturus* (*Notophthalmus*) *viridescens*. The larva emerges from water at first metamorphosis and begins the terrestial phase of the "red eft," which after a variable interval of weeks or months again seeks water. It then changes color and spends the rest of life in a second aquatic existence. In 1939, Reinke and Chadwick showed that implantation of adult pituitaries into muscles of the red eft would cause a premature return to water (Reinke & Chadwick, 1939). Two years later, Chadwick (1941) tried the effect of injecting what hormones had then been isolated and found that prolactin, then known to occur among nonmammalian vertebrates, could reproduce the effect of pituitary implants. Yet nothing is known of the nervous mechanisms induced by prolactin which govern the "water drive" of the red eft.

More recently, Gona, Pearlman, and Etkin (1970) have shown that there is a complex interaction between thyroxine and prolactin at this period, when a balance between the two hormones shifts in favor of prolactin, though a second metamorphosis requires an optimal level of thyroxin for its initiation. In the adult crested newt, exogenous prolactin enhances the uptake of iodine by the thyroid (Peyrot, Vellano, Andreoletti, Pons, & Biciotti, 1971), whereas the opposite effect is seen in the anuran tadpole at prometamorphosis (Gona, 1968).

Nothing is yet known what influence prolactin exerts on those Urodeles which do not undergo any metamorphosis, the absence of which may be due either to insufficient production of TSH by the pituitary (Blount 1950), as in the axolotl, or to unresponsiveness of tissues to thyroxine (Necturus, Lynn & Wachowski, 1951), or to the absence of any trace of the thyroid gland (*Typhlomolge*, Emerson, 1905). Nothing is known of the development of the median eminence in urodeles, or whether thyroxine exerts any influence. A difference between the endocrine systems of the two groups of Amphibia after metamorphosis is that in the urodeles the rate of thyroxine release does not fall after metamorphosis.

The Urodele nervous system differs profoundly from that of the Anura. In the spinal cord, there is no recognizable distinction either in size or morphology between motor neurons and cells of the mantle layer, nor does the cord enlarge at the levels of the limbs. Székely (1968) has shown by stimulation experiments that the motor cells innervating the forelimb extend over a considerable length of the spinal cord, with no clear relationships in position to the individual limb segments. The limbs of urodeles develop well before primary metamorphosis, though with considerable differences between species, both in their time of appearance and the development of patterns of behavior (Faber, 1956). Coghill (1929a) described how in *Ambystoma punctatum* the limbs first move only during periods of axial swimming, and later acquire independence of trunk movement, a sequence to which all other tetrapods were expected to conform. Faber (1956) subsequently showed that in the more slowly growing *A. mexicanum*, limb action was independent from the beginning.

No abrupt changes within the spinal cord such as we find in the Anura have been described at primary metamorphosis. Burkhardt (1889) found that Rohon-Beard cells were still present in postlarval stages of *Triton*, apparently undergoing reduction in number, for they were more abundant at caudal levels and were highly variable in form throughout the cord (Beard, 1896). The primary motor cells of urodeles persist into adult life (Youngstrom,

1941). No effects have here been described of any differences caused by deprivation of endocrine organs. Thus, while pituitary-thyroid interaction has as much control as in Anura in regard to the loss at primary metamorphosis of larval respiratory organs and in the histological structure of the skin, little or no influence is exerted on basic nervous mechanisms in the spinal cord. The retraction of the eyeball on touching the cornea is a response which appears toward the end of the larval period in both groups of Amphibia. Hypophysectomy has no effect on the development of the reflex in urodeles but inhibits its development in Anura, when it can then be induced by exogenous thyroxine (Kollros, 1968).

Further comparison of the two groups of Amphibia awaits further investigation, mainly with regard to the urodeles. Though so much of the classical experimental embryology of the earlier years in this century concentrated on this group, there is still much to learn concerning their interrelationships of endocrine and neural development.

IV. Mammals

There is an extensive literature belonging largely to the 1930's on the behavior of the mammalian fetus; this literature calls for some review. It concentrates on five species of laboratory animals (rat: Angulo y González, 1932; East, 1931; Windle & Baxter, 1936; Windle, Minear, Austin, & Orr, 1935; cat: Coronios, 1933; Windle & Griffin, 1931; Windle, Orr, & Minear, 1934; guinea pig: Bridgeman & Carmichael, 1935; Carmichael, 1934; rabbit: Pankratz, 1939; sheep: Barcroft & Barron, 1939; Barcroft, Barron, & Windle, 1936). The origin of behavior in the mouse has not yet received attention. The human fetus has been studied in a long series of papers by Hooker (e.g., 1952) and by Humphrey (e.g., 1964). In the placental mammal the study of motility is attended by peculiar difficulties. The random spontaneous movements which in other amniotes precede reflex activity demand observation on embryos subjected to minimal disturbance over extended periods. Only recently has this been achieved for a mammalian fetus in the studies of Narayanan, Fox, and Hamburger (1971) on the rat.

The study of early reflex activity has been marked by controversy. Coghill (1929b) interpreted the observations of Minkowski on the genesis of human fetal movement in terms of an initial "total pattern" gradually giving place to clearly demarcated individual reflexes. In the cat, Windle and Griffin (1931) stated that "the movements of embryos and young fetuses are, to a large degree, massive and generalised [p. 186]." Within a few years, however, improvements in techniques of opening the uterus which minimized disturbance to the placental circulations led Windle *et al.* (1934) to the conclusion that at 24–26 days of gestation "reactions have the characteristics of local reflexes. Each seems to occur for the first time unassociated with the others, and can be elicited only by applying the adequate stimulus locally [p. 615]." Studies by Barcroft and his associates under equally favorable physiological conditions showed that the type of early response was not uniform for all areas of the body and depended on the amount of musculature involved. Thus, stimulation of trigeminal branches at about 38 days evoked extensive movements in head, forelimb, and axial musculature as far distant as the tail, whereas at much the same period, reactions of the limbs were entirely local. For these authors, the controversy whether early movements are generalized or restricted "contains an element of unreality." Indeed, they regarded the "whole issue as artificial (Barcroft & Barron, 1939, pp. 477–478)."

In the human fetus, the observations of Hooker and of Humphrey show that generalized responses to cutaneous stimulation over trigeminal branches are seen at a menstrual age of $7\frac{1}{2}$ weeks, while not until 3 weeks later does the forelimb react to such stimuli. While study of the human fetus at abortion necessarily involved interruption of the placental circulations, it seems that in these observations the antecedence of the total pattern type of reflex is a human characteristic related to early development of the trigeminal system and owes little to anoxia. Bodian's (1966b) observations on the origin of behavior in monkeys show that the onset of cutaneous reflexes the macaque fetus "showed greater reflexogenic activity to hand stimulation than to perioral stimulation [p. 117]" to which, moreover, responses were usually limited only in the forelimb.

Hitherto it has been tacitly assumed that the appearance of motility signaled the completion of a neural circuit, along which impulses could at once be transmitted. Recently, however, Robbins and Yomezawa (1971) have shown in cultures of rat embryonic tissues where outgrowing axons were juxtaposed with developing muscle fibers, and functional contacts were established between them *in vitro*, that transmission across such nerve-muscle junctions may not at once follow stimulation, for the amount of acetylcholine liberated in the first place may be insufficient to evoke an action potential. To apply this result to the whole embryo is to suggest that the first appearance of motility depends not only on the completion of neural circuits through the outgrowth of axons and the formation of synapses, but also on the release of adequate amounts of transmitter substances, a consideration which suggests that patterns of early movement may not bear the significance and importance with which they have hitherto been regarded.

Where anatomical and behavioral studies have been combined, following Coghill's lead, workers have been concerned with establishing correlations between structure and function with the aim of implicating particular aspects of neural development as limiting factors in the first appearance of motility. Myelination was early eliminated from this role (Angulo y González, 1929; East, 1931; Langworthy, 1928). Windle and Baxter (1936) correlated the development of reflex pathways as seen in silvered preparations with the appearance of forelimb reflexes. It is now realized, however, such techniques provide only a partial view of embryonic nerve tracts, and that a large number of fibers escape notice because they are smaller than the light microscope can resolve.

The most successful endeavors of this nature have been the studies of Bodian (1966a, 1966b) on the distribution and type of synaptic endings which appear in the monkey cord at successive stages of fetal behavior. Bodian described three stages in the development of *Macacus*. First, a premotile stage period ending at 42 days(CR lengths up to 17–22 mm) and before synaptic bulbs can be recognized in the ventral horn; secondly, a short period of early local reflexes (24–28 mm CR length) when on the dendrites of motor neurons synapses are present, containing circular vesicles (Type S), and a third stage of more vigorous activity, with long intersegmental and crossed reflexes, when axosomatic end bulbs are found, in some of which flattened vesicles are found (Type F). These, he suggests, contain an inhibitory transmitter. The proportion of those with Type F increases during the subsequent stages of fetal life. Later observations have shown that confusion between these two types of vesicles may arise if the second stage of fixation with osmic acid is delayed (Bodian, 1970). Attention has been given to the development of inhibitory mechanisms in several contexts. Barron (1941) has studied the effect of brain transections at various levels in the sheep fetus. Reciprocal inhibition at spinal levels appears later than the establishment of proprioceptive circuits (Änggård, Bergström, & Bernhard, 1961) and in the cat not before birth (Malcom, 1955). Twenty years ago it was thought that the quiescence of the later fetus was largely due to anoxia of the brain (Barron, 1950), for which the increase in pressure and in oxygen tension of arterial blood and in activity of the newborn seemed ample evidence. In recent years, however, Crenshaw, Meschia, and Barron (1966) found that placental progesterone is also a factor in maintaining the passive condition of the late fetus. While in late chick embryos there is a largely parallel situation with respect to arterial pressure and oxygenation, nevertheless a great deal of behavioral development is in progress at that time (Hamburger & Oppenheim, 1967).

Only a few authors have compared the histogenesis of the spinal cord with the development of motility, though the studies on the development of the ventral horn of the rat by Angulo y González (1927) and of Romanes (1941b) on the rabbit are of detailed importance. The only quantitative study on numbers of motor cells is due to Flanagan (1969) who studied the mouse.

The first stage in the development of the ventral horn is a lateral migration of neuroblasts from the mantle layer. In the mouse, rat, and rabbit, a compact ventral horn is thus formed. In the mouse, Flanagan's counts show that from 11 to 15 days there is a marked decrease in numbers by cell death. This period precedes the appearance of motility in the limbs. Later the compact ventral horn is subdivided into parallel axial columns of motoneurons, each of which is concerned with the innervation of a group of muscles of similar function (Romanes, 1964).

In such infraprimate mammals as have been investigated, the time of segregation of the compact ventral horn into separate columns (rat: Angulo y González, 1940; rabbit: Romanes, 1941 (b); sheep: Barron, 1941) corresponds with early stages of motility of the limbs (rat: Swenson, cited in East, 1931; rabbit: Pankratz, 1939; sheep: Barron, 1941). In primates, however, it appears that early limb motlilty may precede this stage in ventral horn development, for Bodian (1966b) found that while the macaque fetus at 44–47 days showed "faint twitches in response to hand and forelimb prick," the ventral horn is still then made up of closely packed cells, though his observations at the light microscope level, which were only incidental to his electron micrograph studies, need to be extended in this regard. In the human fetus, the first spinal reflex arcs which involve the forelimb are completed during the eighth week (Humphrey, 1964). In a sectioned fetus in our collection of 9 weeks (31 mm CR length), groups of motor cells can be seen migrating laterally through the mantle layer, with pycnotic nuclei trailing in their wake. Cell degeneration in the mantle layer of the human cord is also seen at stages which precede motility. Further observations are needed between 9 and the 14-week fetus described by Romanes (1941a) in which the cell columns had all assumed their adult arrangement.

The question whether there is any endocrine control during the formative stages of the eutherian nervous system is more easily asked than answered. Colloid is seen in the thyroid follicles of the human fetus by 80 days (Shephard, 1968), while motility begins in the second month. In the rat, the two events stand in a similar relationship. Geloso (1967) found that thyroxine in the blood stream of the rat fetus can be traced from both maternal and fetal sources. In the sheep, evidence whether thyroxine crosses the placental barrier is at present contradictory (Comline, Nathaniels, & Silver, 1970; Hopkins & Thorburn, 1971). Furthermore a lactogenic hormone of placental origin has been identified in rat, mouse, rhesus monkey, and human (Simmer, 1968). In the latter, the hormone does not appear until the fourth week of gestation, and then rises steadily in concentration to a sharp cutoff at parturition. High levels of a growth hormone are known to be present in human fetal blood (references in Simmer, 1968). What effect any of these hormones exercise on the growth of the nervous system is entirely unknown.

Such questions gain in interest now that some data is available on the growth of the mammalian brain in terms of increase in total DNA, and hence with some qualification, of total cell number (Dobbing & Sands, 1970a, 1970b). It seems likely that there are considerable diversities in this respect between various species. While the curve for the guinea pig is sigmoid, inflecting toward the end of the fetal period, that for the human brain is more complex and consists of two exponential segments, the first ending at the twentieth week of gestation. The second is still rising at parturtion. These authors suggest that the first phase relates to neuroblast multiplication, and the second to glial multiplication. We can only guess what part endocrines play in the control of these sequences. At relatively late stages of development, deficiences in the nervous system of neonatally thyroidectomized rats have been studied behaviorally (Eayrs, 1959, 1964; Eayrs & Levine, 1963) and parallel the clinical symptoms of human cretinism. At fine structural levels, some disturbance of axonal growth has been observed in laboratory animals. My colleague, Dr. Paul Reier, has recently shown a clear-cut effect in the peripheral nervous system of neonatally thyroidectomized mice (Reier & Hughes, 1971). Bundles of unmyelinated axons show a clear retardation in the penetration of cytoplasmic processes of Schwann cells between them. Finally, each axon is separately wrapped by a Schwann process, a stage which is much delayed in the hypothyroid animal. Mutants lacking various components of endocrinal mechanisms provide much scope for investigation of the effects of hormonal deficiency in the fetus. The homozygous recessive of Snell's dwarf strain (Wegelius, 1959), where the causative abnormality is a failure of TSH production, shares in the effect on unmyelinated fibers seen after neonatal thyroidectomy.

With marsupials we find a simpler situation than in the Eutheria. The only apposition of maternal and fetal epithelia is transitorily with the yolk sac, and uterine development comes to an end with much of the organization of the newborn still at an embryonic level. In the opossum at birth, the thyroid is still epithelial, and has lost contact with the lining of the mouth cavity only 2 days earlier. The muscle fibers throughout the newborn are all at the myotube stage of histogenesis, a level of organization which Love, Stoddard, and Grasso (1969) have shown in chicks decapitated *in ovo* required thyroxine for further differentiation.

The opossum is, moreover, of particular interest for our present field of inquiry with regard to the development and behavior of the limbs. A day and a half before birth the embryo is apparently immobile. A day later it is active and can execute crawling movements like those of the newborn (McCrady, 1938). Hartmann (1920) discovered that the transfer of the newborn to the pouch was due entirely to its own efforts-thanks to an overarm action of the forelimbs, it climbs from the birth canal to the pouch along a tract prepared by maternal licking. The premature development of motility in the forearms is rivaled in interest by its extremely tardy appearance in the hindmost pair. Not until after some 50 days in the pouch do they show any coordinated control. When the 60-day pouched young animal was placed on a level surface with the fore part of the body supported, it walked backward more readily than forward (Langworthy, 1925). Clearly there is much here for neurological investigation. I have recently had the opportunity to study some features of the cord and spinal ganglia before and after birth.

In the 10-day embryo at stage 28 of McCrady's invaluable monograph on opossum embryology, the mantle layer of the cord resembles that of a 2–3 day chick in general appearance. Yet already axons can be traced laterally from some cells to emerge from the cord as ventral roots, though their perikarya show no signs of differentiation from surrounding cells. A day before birth, at stage 33, the mantle layer contains two types of cell, the nuclei in one small and dark, and in the other larger and less dense. Degenerating cells are common at cervical and anterior thoracic levels. The newborn cells with the larger nuclei of the mantle layer have now all migrated to the surface of the gray matter, forming a compact ventral horn. Their distribution exactly corresponds with that of the degenerating cells of the mantle layer seen a day or so earlier (Hughes, in press). Degeneration accompanying lateral migration of motor neuroblasts seems widespread among developing mammals. No signs of these changes are yet visible at the levels of the hindlimbs, which are still at the paddle stage of development. The neurons of the opossum cord and ganglia are large, and their numbers are lower than one would expect among amniotes. Their large size apparently extends to their axons, as far as one can judge with the light microscope, and may well be associated with the fact that limb motility in the newborn depends wholly on unmyelinated fibers, a fact discovered by Langworthy in 1928.

At stage 33, counts of cells in the dorsal root ganglia, both in interphase and mitosis, show peaks at both fore- and hindlimb levels. Some cells are already ahead of others in differentiation, with an evident margin of cytoplasm surrounding the nucleus. They are more abundant toward the distal pole of each ganglion. In the newborn these are surrounded by satellite cells. At the level of origin of the main forelimb nerves, C_7, C_8, and T_1 (Voris, 1928), the dorsal root ganglia show an extensive degeneration among the more advanced cells. The distal pole of C_8 is largely empty, with pycnotic satellite cells round the spaces which mark the sites of degenerated perikarya, traces of cell debris from which still remains. Whatever the cellular mechanism which governs this large-scale destruction of these particular neurons, it seems that their function was solely related to the action of the forelimb at birth. They were most likely exteroceptive, for there are no signs of the presence of muscle spindles among the muscles with their embryonic level of histogenesis.

A week later, much has happened within the spinal cord of the pouched young. At the levels of both fore- and hindlimbs, groups of large neurons at the margin of the gray matter foreshadow the adult columns of motor cells as described by Voris (1928). Counts of groups related to the forelimbs, both lateral and ventrolateral, are well below those of the compact ventral horn of the newborn, and their number continues to fall in later stages. At hindlimb level the motor columns show no decrease in cell number until the onset of motility. Here the pouched young marsupial is unique in the development of motor columns composed of neurons of mature aspect at non-motile stages of a limb, yet which in external form is well advanced. A remarkable feature of these neurons is that they show the signs of chromatolysis usually associated with the regrowth of axons after damage, with the nucleus at the margin of a swollen cytoplasm, and the sparse Nissl substance confined to the periphery.

In the dorsal root ganglia there is also a decrease in cell numbers at brachial levels in the pouched young, with the cervical and first thoracic members of the series well in advance of the lumbosacral in this respect. So here again there is a correlation between loss of neurons and functional development of the related limb.

What factors stand in the way of motility of the early hindlimb cannot be discerned in sections stained with haematoxylin and eosin; anatomically, large nerves can be traced in their adult relationships, and the histology of the muscles is then mature at all levels. These observations, it is hardly necessary to say, do not exhaust the interest of neuromuscular development in the opossum. There is wide scope for further research; hormones could be injected into the newborn as readily as Rowlands and Dudley (1969) have shown possible with antigens in their study of immunological development. The techniques of limb amputation have already been worked out (McCrady, 1938). A high priority in biology, one may suggest, should be given to the provision of a nationally sponsored experimental colony of opossums.

Though our survey of the three aspects of tetrapod development is incomplete, we can say that the anuran tadpole stands apart in the degree to which events toward metamorphosis are governed by the endocrine system. Although much more is known about control of nervous development by hormones in Anura than in other vertebrates, it is unlikely that our generalization will be displaced by further work.

In mammals, and possibly in all amniotes, it seems that endocrines play little or no part in the early formative stages of the nervous system. Yet in the late fetus and in the newborn, it is probable that a wide range of hormonal influences remain to be discovered. While the role of thyroxine in the development of the higher functions of the mammalian nervous system is recognized, and a beginning has been made in the study of its effects at fine structural levels, the question of how far growth and lactogenic hormones are also concerned is at present a completely unexplored field.

V. Summary

1. It is suggested that endocrine control of nervous development and the neural basis of the ontogeny of behavior should be considered together wherever possible.

2. Most is known about the anuran Amphibia concerning both these topics. In the spinal cord of the tadpole, a larval nervous system, consisting of sensory Rohon-Beard cells and primary motor cells, is superseded toward metamorphosis by the permanent dorsal root ganglia, and at limb levels, the ventral motor horns. These changes are largely or wholly under thyroid control.

3. The thyroid exerts less influence on nervous development in the embryonic anuran *Eleutherodactylus*, and among the Urodela.

4. Among amniotes, only in the marsupials is there clear evidence that the primary stages of functional neural differentiation proceed independently of hormonal control.

5. In placental mammals, labeling studies have shown that the neuroblastic precursors of large neurons cease mitosis much earlier than do those of microneurous, which in rodents are still being produced in postnatal stages. Endocrine control affects mainly the later stages of neural development.

6. Even with our present incomplete data, it is clear that patterns of neural development vary widely, even within each group of vertebrates. The correlation of these differences with developing patterns of behavior affords much scope for future work.

References

Änggård, L., Bergström, R. M., & Bernhard, C. G. Analysis of prenatal reflex activity in sheep. *Acta Physiologica Scandinavica*, 1961, **53**, 128–136.

Angulo y González, A. W. The motor nuclei in the cervical cord of the albino rat at birth. *Journal of Comparative Neurology*, 1927, **43**, 115–142.

Angulo y González, A. W. Is myelinogeny an absolute index of behavioral capability? *Journal of Comparative Neurology*, 1929, **48**, 459–464.

Angulo y González, A. W. The prenatal development of behavior in the albino rat. *Journal of Comparative Neurology*, 1932, **55**, 395–442.

Angulo y González, A. W. The differentiation of the motor cell columns of albino rat fetuses. *Journal of Comparative Neurology*, 1940, **73**, 469–488.

Barcroft, J., & Barron, D. H. The development of behavior in foetal sheep. *Journal of*

Comparative Neurology, 1939, **70**, 477–502.

Barcroft, J., Barron, D. H., & Windle, W. F. Some observations on genesis of somatic movements in sheep embryos. *Journal of Physiology* (*London*), 1936, **87**, 73–78.

Barron, D. H. The functional development of some mammalian neuro-muscular mechanisms. *Biological Reviews of the Cambridge Philosophical Society*, 1941, **16**, 1–33.

Barron, D. H. Genetic neurology and the behavior problem. In P. Weiss (Ed.), *Genetic neurology*. Chicago: University of Chicago Press, 1950. Pp. 223–231.

Beard, J. The history of a transient nervous apparatus in certain Ichthyopsida. *Zoologischer Jahrbuch*, 1896, **9**, 319–426.

Beaudoin, A. R. The development of lateral motor columns in the lumbo-sacral cord in *Rana pipiens*. II. Development under the influence of thyroxine. *Anatomical Record*, 1956, **125**, 247–260.

Bern, H. A., Nicoll, C. S., & Strohman, R. G. Prolactin and tadpole growth. *Proceedings of the Society for Experimental Biology and Medicine*, 1967, **126**, 518–520.

Blount, R. F. Size relationships as influenced by pituitary rudiment implantation and extirpation in the Urodele embryo. *Journal of Experimental Zoology*, 1935, **70**, 131–185.

Blount, R. F. The effects of heteroplastic grafts upon the Axolotl, *Ambystoma mexicanum*. *Journal of Experimental Zoology*, 1950, **113**, 717–739.

Bodian, D. Development of fine structure of spinal cord in monkey fetuses. I. The Motoneuron neuropil at the time of onset of reflex activity. *Bulletin of the Johns Hopkins Hospital*, 1966, **119**, 129–149. (a)

Bodian, D. Development of fine structure of spinal cord in monkey fetuses. II. Pre-reflex period to period of long intersegmental reflexes. *Journal of Comparative Neurology*, 1966, **133**, 113–166. (b)

Bodian, D. An electron microscopic characterization of classes of synaptic vesicles by means of controlled aldehyde fixation. *Journal of Cell Biology*, 1970, **44**, 115–124.

Bridgeman, C. S., & Carmichael, L. An experimental study of the onset of behavior in the fetal guinea pig. *Journal of Genetic Psychology*, 1935, **47**, 247–267.

Brown, P. S., & Frye, B. E. Effects of prolactin and growth hormone on growth and metamorphosis of tadpoles of the frog, *Rana pipiens*. *General and Comparative Endocrinology*, 1969, **13**, 126–138.

Burkhardt, K. R. Histologische Untersuchungen am Rückenmark der Tritonen. *Archiv für Mikroskopische Anatomie*, 1889, **34**, 131–156.

Carmichael, L. An experimental study in the prenatal guinea pig of the origin and development of reflexes and patterns of behavior in relation to the stimulation of specific receptor areas during the period of active fetal life. *Genetic Psychology Monographs*, 1934, **16**, 337–491.

Chadwick, C. S. Further observations on the water drive in *Triturus viridescens*. II. Induction of the water drive with the lactogenic hormone. *Journal of Experimental Zoology*, 1941, **86**, 175–187.

Coghill, G. E. *Anatomy and the problem of behavior*. Cambridge, Eng.: Cambridge University Press, 1929. (a)

Coghill, G. E. The early development of behavior in *Ambystoma* and in man. *Archives of Neurology and Psychiatry*, 1929, **21**, 989–1009. (b)

Comline, R. S., Nathaniels, P. W., & Silver, M. Passage of thyroxine across the placenta in the foetal sheep. *Journal of Physiology* (*London*), 1970, **207**, P3–P4.

Coronios, J. D. Development of behavior in the fetal cat. *Genetic Psychology Monographs*, 1933, **14**, 283–386.

Crenshaw, M. C., Meschia, G., & Barron, D. H. Role of progesterone in inhibition of muscle tone and respiratory rhythm in foetal lambs. *Nature* (*London*), 1966, **212**, 842.

Dobbing, J., & Sands, J. Growth and development of the brain and spinal cord of the guinea pig. *Brain Research*, 1970, **17**, 115–123. (a)

Dobbing, J., & Sands, J. Timing of neuroblast multiplication in the human. *Nature* (*London*), 1970, **226**, 639–940. (b)

East, E. W. An anatomical study in rat embryos of the initiation of movement. *Anatomical Record*, 1931, **50**, 201–219.

Eayrs, J. T. The status of the thyroid gland in relation to the development of the nervous system. *Animal Behaviour*, 1959, **7**, 1–17.

Eayrs, J. T. Endocrine influence on cerebral development. *Archives de Biologie*, 1964, **75**, 529–565.

Eayrs, J. T., & Levine, S. Influence of thyroidectomy and subsequent replacement therapy upon conditioned avoidance learning in the rat. *Journal of Endocrinology*, 1963, **25**, 505–513.

Emerson, E. T. General anatomy of *Typhlomolge rathbuni*. *Proceedings of the Boston Society of Natural History*, 1905, **32**, 43–74.

Etkin, W. The metamorphosis activating system in the frog. *Science*, 1963, **139**, 810–814.

Etkin, W. Hormonal control of amphibian metamorphosis. In W. Etkin & L. Gilbert (Eds.), *Metamorphosis: A problem in developmental biology*. New York: Appleton, 1968. Pp. 313–348.

Faber, J. The development and co-ordination of larval limb movements in *Triturus taeniatus* and *Ambystoma mexicanum*. *Archives Néerlandaises de Zoologie*, 1956, **11**, 498–517.

Flanagan, A. E. H. Differentiation and degeneration in the motor horn of the foetal mouse. *Journal of Morphology*, 1969, **129**, 281–306.

Geloso, J.-P. Fonctionnement de la thyroide et correlations thyreohypophysaires chez le foetus de rat. *Annales d'Endocrinologie*, 1967, **28**(Suppl.), 1–80.

Glücksmann, A. Cell deaths in normal vertebrate ontogeny. *Biological Reviews of the Cambridge Philosophical Society*, 1951, **26**, 59–86.

Gona, A. G. Radioiodine studies on prolactin action in tadpoles. *General and Comparative Endocrinology*, 1968, **11**, 278–283.

Gona, A. G., & Etkin, W. Inhibition of metamorphosis in *Ambystoma tigrinum* by prolactin. *General and Comparative Endocrinology*, 1970, **14**, 589–603.

Gona, A. G., Pearlman, T., & Etkin, W. Prolactin-thyroid interaction in the newt, *Diemictylus viridescens*. *Journal of Endocrinology*, 1970, **48**, 585–590.

Gray, E. G., & Guillery, R. W. Synaptic morphology in the normal and degenerating nervous system. *International Review of Cytology*, 1966, **19**, 111–182.

Gudernatsch, J. F. Feeding experiments on tadpoles. I. The influence of specific organs given as food on growth and differentiation. A contribution to the knowledge of organs with internal secretion. *Archiv für Entwicklungsmeckanik der Organismen*, 1912, **53**, 457–483.

Hamburger, V., & Oppenheim, R. Pre-hatching motility and hatching behavior in the chick *Journal of Experimental Zoology*, 1967, **166**, 171–204.

Hartmann, C. G. Studies in the development of the opossum *Didelphys virginiana*. V. The phenomenon of parturition. *Anatomical Record*. 1920, **19**, 1–11.

Hooker, D. *The prenatal origin of behavior*. Lawrence, Kan.: University of Kansas Press, 1952.

Hopkins, P. S., & Thorburn, G. D. Placental permeability to maternal thyroxine in the sheep. *Journal of Endocrinology*, 1971, **49**, 549–550.

Hughes, A. The blood pressure of the chick embryo during development. *Journal of Experimental Biology*, 1942, **19**, 232–237.

Hughes, A. The development of the primary sensory system in *Xenopus laevis* (Daudin). *Journal of Anatomy*, 1957, **91**, 323–328.

Hughes, A. Cell degeneration in the larval ventral horn of *Xenopus laevis* (Daudin). *Journal of Embryology and Experimental Morphology*, 1961, **9**, 269–284.

Hughes, A. The development of behavior in *Eleutherodactylus martinicensis* (Amphibia Anura). *Proceedings of the Zoological Society of London*, 1965, **144**, 253–161. (a)

Hughes, A. A quantitative study of the relationships between limb and spinal cord in the embryo of *Eleutherodactylus martinicensis. Journal of Embryology and Experimental Morphology*, 1965, **13**, 9–34. (b)

Hughes, A. Spontaneous movements in the embryo of *Eleutherodactylus martinicensis. Nature* (*London*), 1966, **211**, 51–53. (a)

Hughes, A. The thyroid and the development of the nervous system in *Eleutherodactylus* martinicensis. An experimental study. *Journal of Embryology and Experimental Morphology*, 1966, **16**, 401–430. (b)

Hughes, A. *Aspects of neural ontogeny*. London: Logos, 1968.

Hughes, A., & Prestige, M. C. Development of behaviour in the hind limb of *Xenopus laevis. Journal of Zoology*, 1967, **152**, 347–359.

Hughes, A., & Reier, P. Some effects of bovine prolactin on embryos of *Eleutherodactylus ricordii. Journal of General and Comparative Endocrinology*, 1972, **19**, 304–312.

Humphrey, T. Some correlations between the appearance of human fetal reflexes and the development of the nervous system. *Progress in Brain Research*, 1964, **4**, 93–133.

Hunt, R. K., & Jacobson, M. Brain enhancement in tadpoles; increased DNA concentration after somatotropin or prolactin. *Science*, 1970, **170**, 342–344.

Hunt, R. K., & Jacobson, M. Neurogenesis in frogs after early larval treatment with somatotropin or prolactin. *Developmental Biology*, 1971, **26**, 100–124.

Jacobson, M. Development of specific neuronal connections. *Science*, 1969, **163**, 543–547.

Jacobson, M., & Baker, R. E. Development of neuronal connections with skin grafts in frogs: behavioral and electrophysiological studies. *Journal of Comparative Neurology*, 1969, **137**, 121–142.

Kollros, J. J. Endocrine influences on neural development. In G. E. W. Wolstenholme & M. O'Connor (Eds.), *Ciba Foundation symposium on growth of the nervous system*. London: Churchill, 1968, Pp. 179–192.

Langworthy, O. R. The development of progression and posture in young opossums. *American Journal of Physiology*, 1925, **74**, 1–13.

Langworthy, O. R. The behavior of pouch young opossums correlated with myelinization of tracts. *Journal of Comparative Neurology*, **1928**, **46**, 201–240.

Love, D. S., Stoddard, F. J., & Grasso, J. A. Endocrine regulation of embryonic muscle development. Hormonal control of DNA accumulation, pentose cycle activity and myoblast proliferation. *Developmental biology*, 1969, **20**, 563–582.

Lynn, W. G. The embryology of *Eleutherodactylus nubicola*, an Anuran which has no tadpole stage. *Carnegie Institution Contributions to Embryology*, 1942, **190**, 27–62.

Lynn, W. G., & Peadon, A. M. The role of the thyroid gland in direct development in the Anuran *Eleutherodactylus martinicensis. Growth*, 1955, **19**, 263–286.

Lynn, W. G., & Wachowski, H. E. The thyroid in cold-blooded vertebrates. *Quarterly Review of Biology*, 1951, **26**, 123–168.

McCrady, E. The embryology of the opposum. American Anatomical Memoirs: 1938.

Malcom, J. L. The appearance of inhibition in the developing spinal cord of kittens. In H. Waelsch (Ed.), *Biochemistry of the developing nervous system*. New York: Academic Press, 1955, Pp. 104–109.

Miner, N. Integumental specification of sensory fibers in the development of cutaneous local sign. *Journal of Comparative Neurology*, 1956, **105**, 161–170.

Narayanan, C. H., Fox, M. W., and Hamburger, V. Prenatal development of spontaneous and evoked activity in the rat. (*Rattus norvegicus albinus*). *Behavior*, 1971, **40**, 100–134.

Nicoll, C. S., Bern, H. A., Dunlop, D., & Strohman, R. C. Prolactin, growth hormone, thyroxine, and growth of tadpoles of *Rana catesbiana. American Zoologist*, 1965, **7**, 738–739.

Nieuwkoop, P. D., & Faber, J. *Normal table of Xenopus laevis (Daudin)*. Amsterdam: North-Holland Publ., 1956.

Pankratz, D. S. (1939) Motion pictures of fetal movements in the rabbit. *Anatomical Record*, 1939, **73** (Suppl.), 72.

Pesetsky, I. The thyroid-stimulated enlargement of Mauthner's neuron in Anurans. *General and Comparative Endocrinology*, 1962, **2**, 229–235.

Peyrot, A., Vellano, C., Andreoletti, G. E., Pons, G., & Biciotti, M. On the activating effect of prolactin on thyroid metabolism in the crested newt. Comparison between the effect of prolactin and methylthiouracil. *General and Comparative Endocrinology*, 1971, **16**, 524–534.

Prestige, M. C. Cell turnover in the spinal ganglia of *Xenopus laevis* tadpoles. *Journal of Embryology and Experimental Morphology*, 1965, **13**, 63–72.

Prestige, M. C. The control of cell number in the lumbar ventral horns of *Xenopus laevis* tadpoles. *Journal of Embryology and Experimental Morphology*, 1967, **18**, 359–387.

Prestige, M. C. Differentiation, degeneration, and the role of the periphery. Quantitative considerations. In F. O. Schmitt (Ed.), *The neurosciences: Second study program*. New York: Rockefeller University Press, 1970. Pp. 73–82.

Reier, P., & Hughes, A. The effect of neonatal thyroidectomy upon peripheral nerve development in the mouse. *Anatomical Record*, 1971, **169**, 409–410.

Reinke, E. E., & Chadwick, C. S. Inducing land stage of *Triturus* to assume water habitat by pituitary implantations. *Proceedings of the Society for Experimental Biology and Medicine*, 1939, **40**, 691–693.

Reynolds, W. A. The effects of thyroxine upon the initial differentiation of the lateral motor column and differentiation and motor neurons in *Rana pipiens*. *Journal of Experimental Zoology*, 1963, **153**, 237–249.

Reynolds, W. A. Mitotic activity in the lumbosacral spinal cord of *Rana pipiens* larvae after thyroxine or thiourea treatment. *General and Comparative Endocrinology*, 1966, **4**, 453–465.

Robbins, N., & Yomezawa, T. Physiological studies during formation and development of rat neuromuscular junctions in tissue culture. *Journal of General Physiology*, 1971, **58**, 467–481.

Romanes, G. J. Cell columns in the spinal cord of a human fetus of fourteen weeks. *Journal of Anatomy*, 1941, **75**, 145–152. (a)

Romanes, G. J. The development and significance of the cell columns in the ventral horn in the cervical and upper thoracic spinal cord of the rabbit. *Journal of Anatomy*, 1941, **76**, 112–130. (b)

Romanes, G. T. The motor pools of the spinal cord. *Progress in Brain Research*, 1964, **11**, 93–119.

Rowlands, D. T., & Dudley, M. A. The development of serum proteins and humoral immunity in opossum "embryos." *Immunology*, 1969, **17**, 696–675.

Scharrer, B., & Scharrer, E. *Neuroendocrinology*. New York: Columbia University Press, 1963.

Schwartzenbach, S. S., & Uhlenhuth, E. Anterior lobe substance, the thyroid stimulator. IV. Effect of the absence of thyroid gland. *Proceedings of the Society of Experimental Biology and Medicine*, 1928, **26**, 253–254.

Shephard, T. H. Development of the human fetal thyroid. *General and Comparative Endocrinology*, 1968, **10**, 174–181.

Sherrington, C. S. Experiments in examination of the peripheral distribution of the fibres of the posterior roots of some spinal nerves. *Philosophical Transactions of the Royal Society of London, Series B*, 1893, **184**, 641–763.

Simmer, H. H. Placental hormones. In N. S. Assali (Ed.), *Biology of gestation*. Pp. 290–354, Vol. 1 New York: Academic Press, 1968.

Sperry, R., & Miner, N. Formation within sensory nucleus of V of synaptic associations mediating cutaneous localization. *Journal of Comparative Neurology*, 1949, **90**, 403–423.

Stephenson, N. G. Observations on the development of the amphicoelous frogs, *Leiopelma* and *Ascaphus*. *Journal of the Linnean Society, Zoology*, 1950, **52**, 18–28.

Székely, G. Development of limb movements. Embryological, physiological and model studies. In G. E. W. Wolstenholme & M. O'Connor (Eds.), *Ciba Foundation symposium on growth of the nervous system*. (*London*) Churchill, 1968. Pp. 77–93.

Tata, J. R. Simultaneous acquisition of metamorphic response and hormone binding in *Xenopus* larvae *Nature* (*London*), 1970, **227**, 686–689.

Voris, H. C. The morphology of the spinal cord of the Virginian opossum (*Didelphis virginiana*). *Journal of Comparative Neurology*, 1928, **46**, 407–459.

Wegelius, O. The dwarf mouse—an animal with secondary myxedema. *Proceedings of the Society for Experimental Biology and Medicine*, 1959, **101**, 225–227.

Windle, W. F., & Baxter, R. E. The first neurofibrillar development in albino rat embryos. *Journal of Comparative Neurology*, 1936, **63**, 173–209.

Windle, W. F. & Griffin, A. M. Observations on embryonic and fetal movements of the cat. *Journal of comparative Neurology*, 1931, 149–188.

Windle, W. F., Minear, W. L., Austin, M. F., & Orr, D. W. The origin and early development of somatic behavior in the albino rat. *Physiological zoology*, 1935, **8**, 156–185.

Windle, W. F., Orr, D. W., & Minear, W. L. The origin and development of reflex in the cat during the third fetal week. *Physiological Zoology*, 1934, **7**, 600–607.

Youngstrom, K. E. Studies on the developing behavior of Anura. *Journal of Comparative Neurology*, 1938, **68**, 351–379.

Youngstrom, K. E. A primary and a secondary somatic innervation in *Ambystoma*. *Journal of Comparative Neurology*, 1941, **73**, 139–151.

THE SIGNIFICANCE OF THE PERINATAL PERIOD IN THE NEURAL AND BEHAVIORAL DEVELOPMENT OF PRECOCIAL MAMMALS

JINDŘICH SEDLÁČEK

Laboratory of Embryophysiology
Institute of Physiology
Charles University
Prague, Czechoslovakia

I. Introduction

The perinatal phase represents a relatively short but very important interval in the individual development of mammals, especially of their central nervous system. During this stage all functional systems of mammalian organisms are subjected to the essential reorganization of physicochemical, biochemical, and morphological bases of their physiological activity.

The success of this stage is very important for further postnatal development of the central nervous system (CNS) and for behavioral relations of the newborn animal to its extrauterine environment. Any abnormalities appearing during this developmental course, summarized as "perinatal encephalopathy" in clinical terminology, have far-reaching consequences for postnatal ontogeny (Holub, 1963; Lesný, 1957).

It is important to accept C. A. Smith's (1959) thesis that "to understand the fundamentals of its [i.e. the newborn organism's] life is the first step in helping it to survive [p. 4]." For this particular reason we have aimed our research (started in 1957) at the descriptive and analytical study of the complex changes which occur in the CNS during the sudden passage from the fetal to the neonatal condition of life.

A. Perinatal Period

We speak about sudden changes during the passage from the intrauterine to the external environment in contrast to the relatively long duration of prenatal and postnatal development.

The term "perinatal period" has different connotations in different fields of the medical literature (in pediatrics, obstetrics, or medical statistics). The main differences regard the length of time included in this stage by each of these fields. For example: The perinatal period is defined as the beginning of labor or time of rupture of the amniotic membrane, whichever is first, through the first day of life (Nelson, 1966). The perinatal period, according to the description by Berfenstam (1967), includes the time interval from parturition to the first week of postnatal life. Shaffer (1966) delimits the perinatal period from the onset of labor to the delivery of the infant.

With regard to such discrepancies in the definition of this period, it is more important to define the distinctive *features* of the physiological changes during this developmental stage. This postulate is of particular significance for the construction of experimental work in this research field.

During the perinatal stage the fetus is suddenly removed from complete dependence on the maternal organism in an aqueous environment to a relatively independent status in air. The crucial changes in the perinatal period of development involve the morphological and functional transformation of the circulatory system into the adult-type and the establishment of pulmonary respiration (Dawes, 1968; Stave, 1970b).

From this point of view—reflected in the introductory remarks in Smith's book on developmental physiology (Smith, 1959)—we shall discuss here some problems of perinatal changes in the CNS of the guinea pig.

It is necessary to understand the perinatal changes in relation to each of the functional systems (Ranck & Windle, 1959). Most importantly, while the extrauterine circumstances activate other functional systems (digestive, excretory, endocrine, etc.) quantitatively, the changes in the pulmonary and circulatory systems are of a qualitative kind. We shall try to demonstrate that this fact also refers to the perinatal changes in the central nervous system, which must insure the behavioral relations to the extrauterine environment.

B. Experimental Animals

There are two main possibilities for perinatal research with mammals: altricial or precocial species.

1. Altricial Species

If one studies this problem with an altricial mammal, the nutritive and behavioral dependence on the mother continues in full fashion after birth, the period of dependence varying between species. During the postnatal period the gradual reduction of the importance of the maternal organism for the survival of the newborn organism is accomplished by the changes in the regulatory and adaptive mechanisms of the developing neonate (Fig. 1). The immaturity of behavioral functions in the altricial neonate at birth and during the first days of postnatal life is compensated for by the behavior of the mother.

One of the excellent examples of maternal compensation is observed in the development of micturition and defecation in altricial mammals. The realization of these acts in infant rats and puppies is insured during the first postnatal days only by means of stimulation of the perineal region of the offspring by the mother's tongue. If the mother fails to stimulate that region by licking it, the infant animal dies from rupture of the urinary bladder (Čapek & Jelínek, 1956a, 1956b).

A similar situation is seen regarding thermoregulation. The infant rat cannot maintain its body temperature till day 14 without the help of its mother and siblings in the nest. Thus, at this age the mechanisms of thermoregulation are not sufficiently developed in the infant rat, and they must be supplied by external sources. During the first 2 weeks of life, the infant rat is not able to produce sufficient heat to reduce effectively its heat losses to the external environment (Hahn, 1953; Hahn, Křeček, & Křečková, 1956).

The immature brain tissue passes through critical developmental periods (birth and weaning) under different influences of the external environment, which may have positive or negative effects on the process of maturation [e.g. effect of undernutrition (Mourek, Himwich, Mysliveček, & Callison, 1967), premature weaning [Křeček, 1971], effects of enriched environment

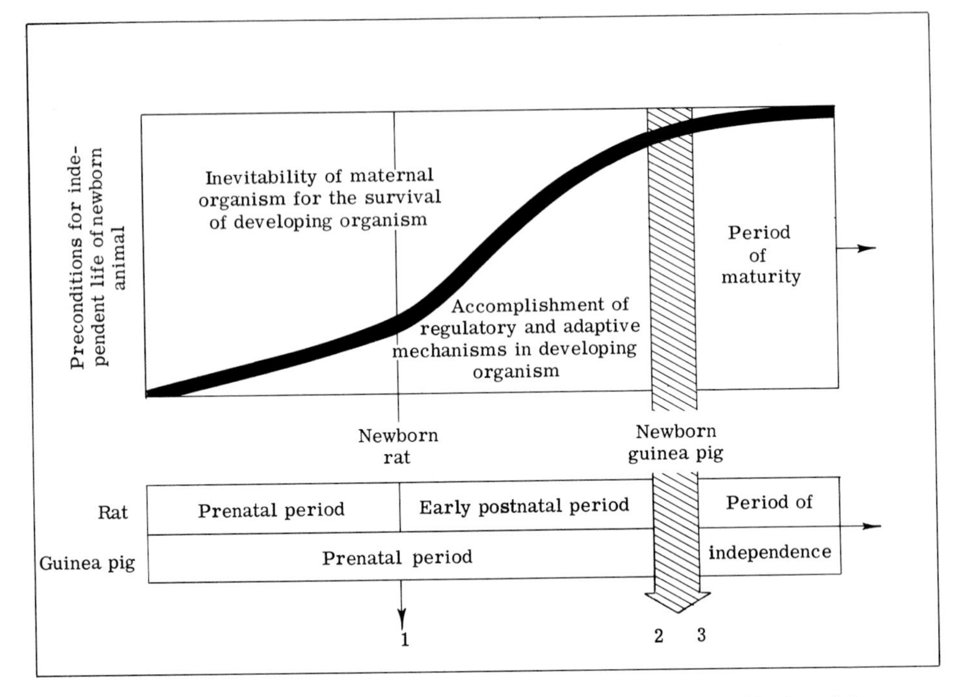

FIG. 1. Scheme of the developing relationships between mother and offspring of the rat and guinea pig. The upper part illustrates (in arbitrary units) the relationship between the stage of maturation in the developing organism and the inevitable contribution of the maternal organism in the survival of the offspring. The vertical arrows show the different relationship in immature newborn rat and mature newborn guinea pig. The lower part shows the relationship between developmental phases of the rat and guinea pig. (1) The perinatal period of the rat; (2) the weaning period of the rat; (3) the perinatal period of the guinea pig.

or of different degrees of sensory deprivation (Scherrer & Fourment, 1964)].

It must be taken into consideration during the study of perinatal changes that the master plan of maturation is not yet finished at the moment of birth in newborn altricial animals.

2. Precocial Species

The second possibility is to study this problem in an animal which at the time of birth has reached a very high stage of development (precocial). The guinea pig is such an animal. The advantage lies in the fact that the decisive part of ontogeny in this organism, including the CNS, is realized during the fetal period. In the case of precocial mammals, the newborn organism is already practically mature for independent life soon after birth.

C. Prenatal Environment

The master plan of maturation in (precocial) newborns is accomplished during the fetal period within the intrauterine environment. With respect to this fact it is important to take into consideration the following consequences.

Fetal maturation takes place under relatively stable conditions in comparison with the variability of the external environment which may strongly intervene in the process of maturation in altricial infants. Factors of the external environment in guinea pig fetuses are mediated instead by the maternal organism throughout the entire prenatal developmental period. Moreover, within the fetal guinea pig itself, which develops in a homeostatically regulated maternal organism, there occurs a maturation of its own mechanisms of fetal homeostasis. During gestation the fetus creates its own homeostasis and is able to maintain internal stability, although supported and buffered by the placental barrier and maternal metabolism (Stave, 1970b).

In this situation the development of neuronal sensory function arises first of all from endogenous developmental patterns and mechanisms, which are part of the master plan of fetal maturation. The insulation of the fetus by means of the maternal organism and its homeostatic mechanisms brings about special conditions which are characterized by different degrees of physiological sensory deprivation. By the term "relative fetal sensory deprivation" we would like to emphasize the difference in environmental conditions for the process of maturation in fetal guinea pigs (precocial) and for newborn altricial mammals.

The degree of this deprivation in the fetal condition is quite different for different sensory systems. It is low for those systems that require the fetus itself to generate stimulation, e.g., proprioception. It is high for those systems which are insulated by the intrauterine conditions from natural sources of adequate stimulation, e.g., vision.

There are many significant facts about the possibility of activating the sensory systems in *externalized fetuses in experimental conditions*. Tactile sensitivity of guinea pigs manifests itself first on day 31–32 of gestation (Carmichael, 1934). There are many findings on the vestibular functions (Avery, 1928; Carmichael, 1934). Acoustic sensitivity is evidently present around day 60–62 (Avery, 1928), and visual electrophysiological responses are present on day 60 (Jasper, Bridgman, & Carmichael, 1937). From these facts follows the primary developmental pattern of the onset of sensory functions in guinea pig fetuses and other mammals, altricial as well as precocial (Gottlieb, 1971).

But the fact that it is possible to activate a sensory system in externalized fetuses does not necessarily mean that sensory stimulation influences the maturation of the sensory systems under normal conditions of intrauterine existence.

With regard to these circumstances, which characterize the prenatal environment, birth for the guinea pig means a sudden passage from a relatively isolated fetomaternal symbiosis into an independent style of life in an external environment with an abundance of stimulative features.

II. Subjects and Methods

In light of the above mentioned factors, we chose the second possibility for our study, namely the precocial guinea pig. Furthermore, this choice was made with other practical considerations in mind.

The guinea pig has a long gestation period (about 67–68 days—Draper, 1920; Ibsen, 1929) in comparison with the rat (21 days) and the rabbit (32 days). The number of animals in one litter is rather standard (2 or 3), and the fetuses, which are relatively large in the second half of gestation, allow various methodological techniques to be transferred from adult research with only small adaptations. The guinea pig belongs to the same animal species as the rat and rabbit (*Rodentia*), so that many useful comparisons can be made about the dynamics of ontogenetic development and its critical phases.

The economic aspect should also not be neglected. The expenses in the case of guinea pigs are much more moderate than in the case of fetuses of larger precocial animals (sheep, pigs).

Certain problems for the continuity of work follow from the tendency of the guinea pig to breed seasonally (spring, autumn); however, this problem may be overcome in a sufficiently large colony of females.

Some problems are connected with the evaluation of fetal age, which has been determined in our experiments from the comparison of gestation-age and weight-age of fetuses according to Draper (1920). The determination is very exact in such cases if fertilization occurs during the first day after parturition (Asdell, 1946).

There are many different methods of preparation of both the pregnant female and the fetus, especially when using anesthetics or drugs for immobilization, which may influence, in a different way, the reactivity of fetuses and therefore the final experimental results. The different procedures have been summarized by Schwartze, Schwartze, and Schönfelder (1971). A very important consideration is whether one uses a centrally acting general anesthetic to immobilize the pregnant dam (Basmajian & Ranney, 1961; Bergström, 1962c; Carmichael, 1934; Schwartze *et al.*, 1971), or whether one uses drugs which merely inhibit peripheral neuromuscular transmission. In all our experiments we have used the latter method, with Tubocurarine or Flaxedil as the peripherally acting agent, since these drugs do not penetrate the placental barrier. All surgical manipulations (incising the jugular vein to administer the Tubocurarine or Flaxedil, incising the trachea for insertion of the artificial respiratory tube, and the caesarian section) were accomplished under local anesthesia. Under these conditions the fetus is not affected by any pharmacological influences connected with the surgical preparation of the pregnant female. This fact is most important, especially in experiments with the natural onset of pulmonary respiration in full-term fetuses after the ligature of the umbilical cord. In other respects our preparation is the same as the one commonly used (thermoregulated bath with saline, etc.).

The head of the fetus is fixed in a special stereotaxic stand (Sedláček, 1967), which minimizes the transfer of trunk movements to the head, but does not alter the onset and development of respiratory movements, especially of the first initial gasps.

The newborn guinea pigs were prepared for the experimental investigations under local anesthesia, usually accompanied by peripheral Tubocurarine blockade and artificial intratracheal respiration.

We risked the possibility of painful stimulation because of the advantage of such investigations on animals without any influence of anesthetic or narcotic substances upon the neuronal elements.

Content of Developmental Research

One of the keys to understanding ontogenetic development is the initial description of its critical moments or phases. From the physiological point of view, the first one is the onset of functional activity.

If we follow the fetal development of the cerebral cortex in guinea pig fetuses, we may observe changes in many electrophysiological and functional parameters during the second half of the gestation period. The first critical point of the fetal development of the cerebral cortex appears to occur about days 41–46 of gestation (Flexner, 1954; Flexner, Tyler, & Gallant, 1950). The maturation of neuroblasts into neurons is completed at about this time, cell processes and Nissl bodies first appear, and the nucleus ceases to increase in volume. Also during this critical phase of cortical development many biochemical systems also increase their activity which, in guinea pig fetuses, develop long before the perinatal period (Stave, 1970b). Also, spontaneous electrical activity (Bergström, 1962a; Bergström, Hellström, & Stenberg, 1962; Flexner *et al.*, 1950; Jasper *et al.*, 1937) and sensitivity of cortical neurons to direct stimulation occur at around 41–50 days (Stenberg, 1968). Powerful cortical inhibitory circuits also seem to be maturing around this time (Bergström, this volume).

These signs of functional activity during days 41–50 give evidence for the maturation not only of neuronal excitability, but also of the development of synaptic interconnections among the population of cortical neurons, which is important for the complex electrical activity of neuronal structure (Crain, Peterson, & Bornstein, 1968).

At this stage it is also possible to evoke the responses of respiratory muscles by the compression of umbilical vessels (Bergström, 1962b). At the same time the electrical properties of cortical tissue begin to show a sensitivity to cortical hypoxia after the clamping of the umbilical cord (Sedláček, 1967).

Therefore, Bergström's (1968) suggestion of a critical period of cortical fetal development between day 40 and 50, when the EEG develops from discontinuous to regular waveform activity, would seem to be correct.

After the cortical structures reach this stage, there remains a period of nearly 3 weeks before development approaches the second critical point, i.e., the perinatal period. During this period many quantitative changes occur in the properties of the cortical tissue.

It is possible to distribute the process of functional maturation into three groups of developmental characteristics:

1. The first group includes the steady electrical properties. In this group we investigated the following electrical parameters. (*a*) The steady potential differences between normal and damaged (by thermocoagulation) points on the cortical surface. According to comparative study (Bureš, 1957), this kind of injury potential, compared with the anoxic depolarization of brain tissue, is a significant expression of cortical steady potential. (*b*) The average membrane potential of cortical cell elements derived from single spike deflections developed during the slow passage of the tip of a glass microelectrode through the cortical layer. The value of an average membrane potential includes the membrane potentials of all cortical cell elements (Bureš, Fifková, & Mareš, 1964; Deza & Eidelberg, 1967). (*c*) The impedance of cortical tissue, measured by the bridge method at the frequency range up to 1 kc, indicating the extracellular conductivity as a function of extracellular compartment of cortical tissue (Schwan 1957; Van Harreveld & Schadé, 1959).

2. The second group of developmental characteristics contains the phasic spontaneous and evoked cortical activities. We have centered our investigations on EEG activity and on cortical infraslow potential oscillations (ISPO's) on one hand and the primary evoked responses in cortical projection areas to visual stimulation and to electric stimulation of the sciatic nerve on the other hand (Sedláček, 1971a).

3. In the third group of our investigations on developing guinea pigs are some findings concerning the development of reflex activity, especially the reactions of full-term fetuses and newborn guinea pigs to acoustic stimulation (Sedláček, 1968; Sedláček, Hlaváčková, & Švehlová, 1964).

These investigations on guinea pigs have been included as one part of a complex study of prenatal development of the CNS with the comparative aspects performed on rat and rabbit fetuses (Sedláček, 1961, 1963, 1967) and especially on chick embryos (Sedláček, 1971b; Sedláček & Macek, 1968).

III. Results

A. Fetal Development until Term

We determined the cortical steady potential differences first in fetuses on day 42 of gestation. The value at this stage amounted to 3.66 ± 0.16 mV. During the rest of the fetal period this value increased by more than by 3 mV and in full-term fetuses reached 6.93 ± 0.30 mV (Sedláček & Macek, 1965).

The average of the membrane potentials of cortical cell elements increased from 7.6 ± 0.86 mV on day 47 by more than 12 mV up to 19.3 ± 2.03 mV in full-term fetuses before clamping of the umbilical cord.

This developmental progress was well manifested in histograms of single values of membrane potentials, which shifted from 30 to 60 mV (Sedláček, 1969).

The impedance (i.e., the inverse value of tissue conductivity) increased from day 47 until term by more than by 3 kΩ from 1.0 ± 0.24 kΩ up to 4.73 ± 0.43 kΩ (Sedláček, 1967).

The stage of maturation of steady electrical properties was also described by their changes during brain hypoxia evoked by artificial clamping of the umbilical cord. The size of hypoxic changes, i.e., the depression of cortical steady and average membrane potentials and the increase of tissue impedance, progressively developed with the developmental increase of the resting values of all three electrical parameters. All values are given as final values after 10 minutes of brain hypoxia. The hypoxic depression of steady potential increased from day 42 until term by 3.60 mV, the depression of average membrane potential by 9.1 mV, and the depression of tissue conductivity by 31%.

All these steady electrical parameters are derived from the state of cell membranes and their permeability, which play a very important part in the developing compartmentalization of cortical tissue. It is possible to evaluate the progressive development of all investigated steady electrical properties as illustrating the maturation of the structural and enzymic bases of active transport and polarization in cortical tissue.

The development of phasic spontaneous and evoked cortical activities is characterized by typical quantitative improvement of temporal and voltage parameters (Bergström, 1962a; Sedláček, 1971a; Stenberg, 1968). The EEG activity of full-term fetuses is characterized by the mean frequency of 2.5 Hz and by the mean voltage of 45 uV. This activity is superimposed on very slow waves with a frequency of 7.28 (3.8–10.8) cycles per minute and a voltage of 0.48 (.05–2.0) mV (Fig. 2). We registered the cortical infraslow potential oscillations (ISPO's) first in fetuses on day 55–56, but both the voltage and frequency show that this age is already past the time of onset of this very slow activity.

The cortical primary evoked response to peripheral flash stimulation was first recorded in fetuses on day 56–57 of gestation (Fig. 3). The eyelids were fused at this age, but they could be gently pulled apart. The further development until term is characterized by increased consistency of the cortical responses, not only to single flashes, but also to higher frequencies of visual stimulation—from .1 Hz to .2 Hz. The latency of the cortical responses decreased by more than 60 msec, and the voltage of the dominant negative spike increased by more than 200 uV.

The morphology of superficial evoked responses remained unchanged from the fetal period until term.

In full-term fetuses the primary cortical response to electric stimulation of the sciatic nerve is also well developed (Fig. 4).

In the third group we investigated the general motor reaction of full-term fetuses to acoustic stimulation (a loud bell), and the possibility of formation of a simple conditioned reaction on the basis of a connection between acoustic (a bell, the intensity of which did not evoke an unconditioned reaction) and electric stimulation of the neck skin. The incidence of the first reaction was registered in about 8% of unconditioned acoustic stimulations, but the test of the formation of conditioned reaction was negative in all cases (Sedláček, 1967; Sedláček *et al.*, 1964).

This then summarizes the situation of certain cortical electrical properties, of functional activities, and of some behavioral manifestations in guinea pig fetuses until term, during which the fetoplacental connections with the maternal organism are still intact. We emphasize this circumstance because in the following part our attention will be concentrated on changes evoked by natural or artificial interruption of the umbilical circulation.

B. *General Situation in Full-Term Fetuses of Guinea Pig*

Just before birth of the guinea pig fetus there are many signs of insufficiency of placental functions. For that reason the general situation of the full-term fetus is extremely strained, as may be derived from the following facts.

There are, first of all, apparent conflicts in metabolic relations, including blood gases exchanged through the placental barrier. The regression of the weight of placenta (not only the growth retardation as in other mammals) occurs simultaneously with the progressive growth of the guinea pig fetus.

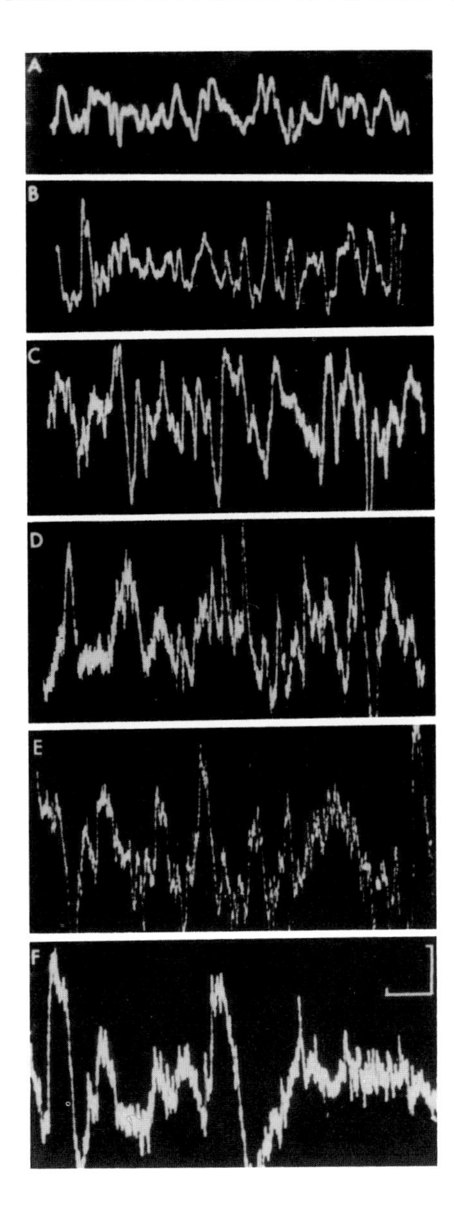

FIG. 2. The development of cortical infraslow potential oscillations (ISPO's) in fetal and newborn guinea pigs. (A) Day 55–56 of gestation; (B) day 58–59; (C) day 62–63; (D) day 65–66; (E) full-term fetus; (F) newborn animal. Calibrations: vertical: .5 mV, horizontal: 10 sec.

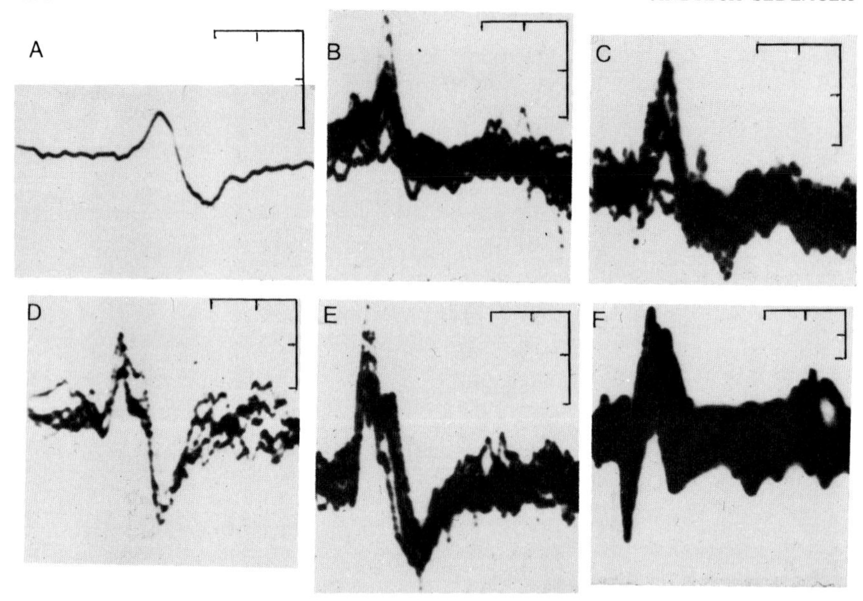

FIG. 3. Developmental patterns of cortical optic evoked responses in fetal and newborn guinea pigs. (A) Day 56–57 of gestation, single record; (B) day 58–59, superimposed records, .1 Hz; (C) day 60–61, .1 Hz; (D) day 62–63, .1 Hz; (E) full-term fetus, .2 Hz; (F) newborn, 1 Hz. Calibrations: vertical, 50 uV per division (note a different voltage range in record F); horizontal, 50 msec per division. Negativity upward.

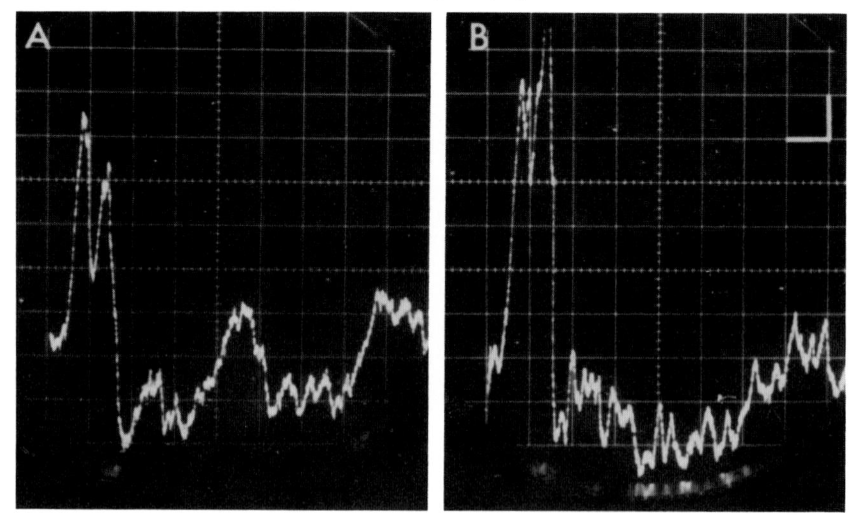

FIG. 4. Primary cortical responses evoked by electrical stimulation of sciatic nerve in full-term fetus (A) and in newborn guinea pig (B). The beam was triggered by the electrical impulse to the left sciatic nerve (2.5 msec, 5 V, rectangular pulse). The responses were recorded from the surface of right parietal cortex just before the bregma in the angle between sagital and coronary sutures. Calibrations: vertical, 50 uV; horizontal, 50 msec. Negativity upward.

These two antagonistic processes must result in extremely unfavorable ratios between the weight of the fetus and its placenta. The weight of the placenta, even when it is of hemoendothelial type (Amoroso, 1952; Swenson, 1970) at the end of gestation comprises only 5% of the fetal weight, whereas in the rat it is 11%, and in the cat, 15%, etc. (Ibsen, 1929).

The central nervous system of a full-term guinea pig fetus displays in this situation a very high sensitivity to disturbances of its oxygen supply. The time interval up to the last evoked gasp during ischemia of the uterus takes only 5.4 minutes in full-term guinea pig fetuses, as compared to about 20 minutes in the rat fetus (Becher, King, Marsh, & Wyrick, 1964). The EEG activity disappeared within 40 seconds after the cord was clamped 3 minutes and the amplitude of cortical ISPO's decreased to 25% of the initial resting value (Sedláček, unpublished data).

The critical situation at the end of the fetal period may also be derived from low metabolic reserves, indicated, e.g., by extremely low content of cardiac glycogen, which in term fetuses of the guinea pig is six times smaller than in the rat (Shelley, 1961). In contrast, oxygen consumption is relatively high (Becher *et al.*, 1964). The tightness of this situation in full-term guinea pig fetuses may be compared to a certain extent with the situation in artificially delivered rabbit fetuses (Barcroft & Young, 1943). A strong decrease of oxygen saturation of cerebral blood develops during artificial delivery, evoked by application of exogenous progesterone to the pregnant female. When artificial delivery exceeds 3 days (from the normal 32–35 days of gestation in the rabbit), the oxygen blood saturation decreases from 43–53% to only 15%. It is evident that the placental mechanisms for oxygen supply appear unable, in this situation, to keep up with fetal growth.

The CNS of the full-term guinea pig fetus is exposed, among other things, to two important factors which may influence fetal maturation: (*a*) A relatively high degree of physiological fetal hypoxia resulting from the low oxygen saturation of cerebral blood, which amounts to about only 62% of saturation, as compared to 95–97% in newborn animals. This relation is perhaps a typical feature of the mature fetus (Born, Dawes, Mott, & Widdicombe, 1954). (*b*) A degree of sensory deprivation resulting from the intrauterine homeostatic environment which may be the cause of the dormant state of the fetal CNS.

C. *Neonatal State of the Central Nervous System*

In order to appreciate the nature of the perinatal changes, it is useful to characterize the functional and electrophysiological parameters of the cerebral cortex in newborn guinea pigs based on a comparison between the full-term mature fetus and the newborn animal.

There are, in some cases, only quantitative differences and changes, but these may be greater than the differences within the whole fetal period. The difference between the term and the neonatal values of cortical steady potential, amounting to about 6 mV, results from the increase of the full-term fetal value of 6.93 mV up to 12.87 ± 0.42 mV in newborn animals (Sedláček & Macek, 1965). The mean membrane potential of cortical cell elements increases from 19.3 ± 2.03 mV in full-term fetuses up to 28.1 ± 2.64 mV in the cerebral cortex of newborn animals. These average values are derived from the apparent shift of maximal values of membrane potentials up to 90 mV, while the upper limit in term fetuses reaches only up to the 60 mV category of the histograms.

Very interesting changes were noted in cortical impedance, which, between term fetal and neonatal stages, decreased by more than 1 kΩ (Sedláček, 1967). This is a very important sign of the abolition of final critical hypoxia of brain tissue developed just before birth and eliminated during the establishment of pulmonary respiration.

The spontaneous cortical bioelectric activity in newborn guinea pigs manifests an increase of frequency and a decrease of amplitude, which may be characterized as a pattern of neonatal arousal reaction (Esquivel de Gallardo, Fleischman, & Ramirez de Arrelano, 1964; Sedláček, 1971a). The difference in parameters of the ISPO's is described by increased amplitude and decreased frequency of these infraslow waves (Fig. 2), which may in turn be considered as a manifestation of a higher degree of processes taking part in the generation of ISPO's on the surface of the cerebral cortex.

Into the group of quantitative changes must also be placed the parameters of somatosensory evoked cortical responses and the consistency of unconditioned motor reactions to strong acoustic stimulation.

In the qualitative group belong the differences in functional patterns between full-term fetuses and neonatal animals. The functions under consideration here are the morphology of cortical visually evoked responses (Sedláček, 1971a) and the change in the elaboration of conditioned acoustic reactions (Sedláček, 1968).

The neonatal cortical optic response is characterized by a biphasic spike complex with initial positivity. This complex is followed by slow positive-negative components. The mean latency of evoked response is relatively short (36.8 ± 2.70 msec), the peak latency of the initial positive spike is 45.5 ± 3.42 msec and of the initial negative spike, 61.3 ± 6.18 msec. The voltage of both spikes depends on the voltage of the first positive component. In about one-half of newborn animals the positive voltage was greater than the negative: + 196.5 ± 18.2 μV, − 133.5 ± 11.8 μV. In the other half the relation was reverse: + 157.2 ± 12.8 μV, − 219.2 ± 16.7 μV. The cortical evoked response in newborn animals was fully consistent whether stimulated with single flashes or with frequencies of 1 Hz.

The elaboration of conditioned reaction gave about 50% of positive conditioned responses of all trials. Either the same procedure was used as in full-term fetuses, or the acoustic conditioned signal was reinforced by electric stimulation of the auricle, evoking a shaking reaction of the head. The same score with the same conditioned reaction develops in infant rats only after 10–20 days of postnatal life (Sedláček, 1963).

D. Perinatal Changes

If we compared the gradual progress of fetal development of cortical parameters manifested during the last 2 weeks of pregnancy with the differences between full-term fetal and neonatal states (within the first 12 hours of extrauterine life), the slope of perinatal development would be very apparent.

The differences in the cortical functional characteristics of the brain within this time interval raise two important questions:

(1) When and within what time limits are these strong quantitative and qualitative changes realized? If we attain a satisfactory answer to this first question, then the second problem follows: (2) What are the causes of these changes?

The first question was studied in full-term fetuses aged around 67–68 days of gestation and divided into two groups. In the first group all of the conditions for the onset of lung respiration after the clamping of the umbilical cord were insured. In the second group the reverse condition was arranged: the fetus inspired the saline from the bath in the experimental chamber with resulting progressive hypoxia.

The changes in cortical functions were studied and compared in both groups, primarily during the first 10 minutes after the arrest of fetoplacental circulation.

With respect to the first question mentioned above, the results show that the main part of the fetal–neonatal difference in cortical characteristics disappears during a few minutes after the clamping of the umbilical cord in full-term fetuses delivered by cesarean section, provided the umbilical arrest evokes regular lung ventilation. That is documented by the slope increase of cortical steady potential (Fig. 5). The neonatal value of cortical steady potential reaches about 13 mV, which represents about 180% of term fetal value. About 160% of the full-term fetal value is reached during only 10 minutes of lung ventilation in the perinatal period.

A similar change of cortical steady potential was recorded in the mean value of membrane potentials of cortical cell elements.

Another change in the perinatal period concerns the ease of establishing the conditioned reaction (Sedláček *et al.*, 1964). The connection between the

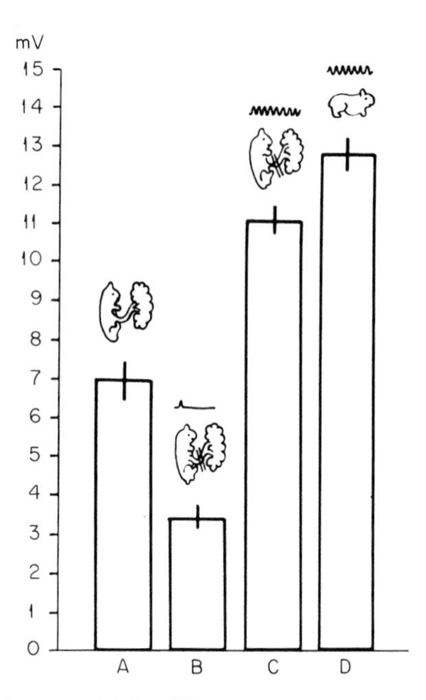

FIG. 5. Cortical steady potential in different conditions during the perinatal period. Ordinate: cortical steady potential in millivolts. (A) Normal full-term fetus before the clamping of cord; (B) full-term fetus 10 minutes after cord clamping without the onset of lung ventilation; (C) full-term fetus 10 minutes after the umbilical arrest followed by regular lung respiration; (D) normal newborn animal. Columns, mean ±SE.

acoustic conditioned (CS) and electrical unconditioned stimuli (UCS) was ineffective in full-term fetuses with an *intact* fetoplacental circulation. After clamping the umbilical cord, followed by about 1 hour of lung ventilation, positive conditioned reactions were registered in 50% of all trials. This degree of conditioning is practically the same as in normal newborn animals during the first postnatal day (Fig. 6) (Sedláček, 1963).

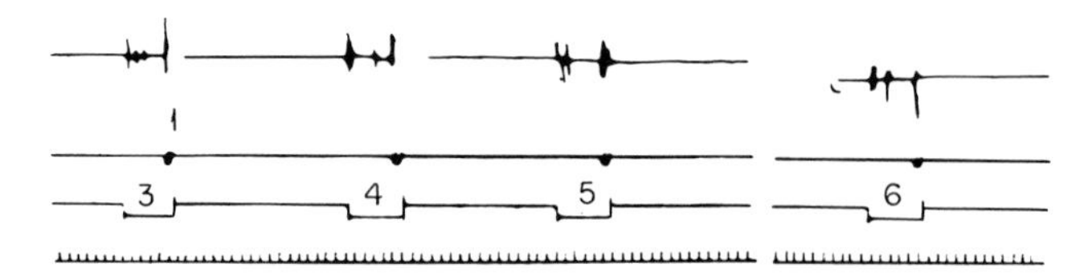

FIG. 6. A part of elaboration of a conditioned reaction in full-term guinea pig fetus 60 minutes after the clamping of umbilical cord and the onset of regular lung ventilation. Lines up to down: fetal motor reaction, mark of unconditioned electric stimulation of neck skin, mark of conditioned acoustic stimulus; time in seconds.

Very apparent changes are observed in the morphology of the cortical optic evoked response (Sedláček, 1971a). In full-term fetuses, within several minutes after clamping of the umbilical cord and the onset of respiration, a new morphological component appears in the cortical optic response—an initial positive spike followed by a negative spike (Fig. 7). The increase of the positive voltage is related to a partial decrease of the negative voltage. A comparison of cortical responses in full-term fetuses before and after clamping of the umbilical cord and the onset of respiration showed that the latency of the initial positive spike is the same as the initial negative spike before the perinatal turning point.

E. Analysis of Perinatal Changes in Cerebral Cortex

The physiology of the perinatal period, which terminates with parturition of the fetus from its protective intrauterine environment, comprises the most important developmental period (Stave, 1970b). All mammalian fetuses, whether precocial or altricial, have one thing in common: by the time they are born they must all have developed circulatory and pulmonary systems which are fully capable of maintaining extrauterine existence. Even the cortical properties change in important ways during the culmination of fetal development.

The arrest of fetoplacental circulation is a crucial event which evokes a whole complex of biochemical and morphological changes, which evidently have very far-reaching functional consequences (Greenfield & Shepherd, 1953).

One of the first events is the onset of lung ventilation which changes

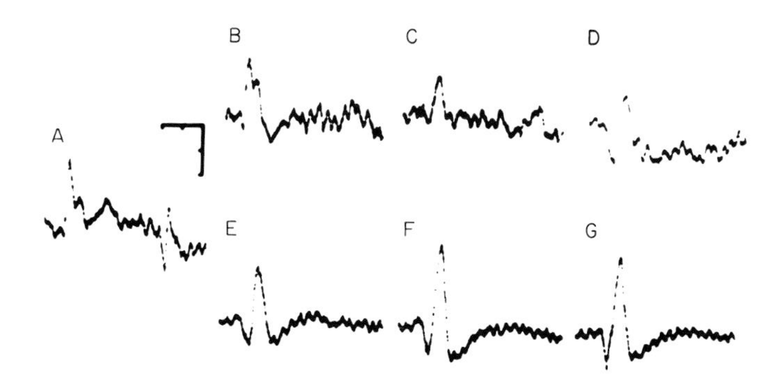

FIG. 7. The changes of cortical optic evoked response in full-term fetus after the umbilical arrest and the onset of lung respiration. (A) Normal fetal response before the clamping of umbilical cord; (B–G) responses after cord clamping. (B) .5 minute, (C) 1 minute, (D) 1.5 minutes; (E) 2.5 minutes; (F) 3.5 minutes; (G) 4.5 minutes. Calibrations: vertical, 50 uV per division, horizontal, 50 msec per division. Negativity upward.

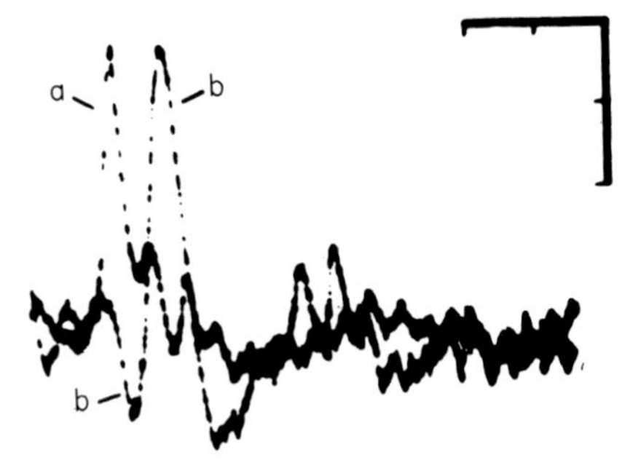

FIG. 8. Cortical optic evoked responses in full-term fetus before (a) and 3.5 minutes after the clamping of umbilical cord followed by the onset of lung respiration (b). Calibrations: vertical, 50 uV per division, horizontal, 50 msec per division. Negativity upward.

the oxygen saturation of systemic and cerebral blood and the pathways of blood distribution within the circulatory system (Born *et al.*, 1954). Disturbances in the onset and further development of lung respiration evoke regressive changes of functional parameters of the cerebral cortex. This is illustrated by the regression of cortical steady potential (Fig. 9), by similar changes in the mean value of cortical membrane potentials, and by a shift

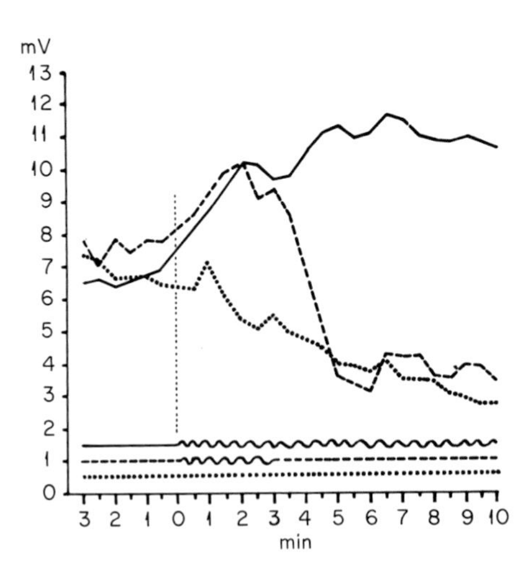

FIG. 9. Development of the cortical steady potential during perinatal changes in full-term fetuses of guinea pig. Abscissa: time in minutes before and after the clamping of the umbilical cord; ordinate: cortical steady potential in millivolts. Full line: full-term fetuses with normal onset of lung respiration; interrupted line: full-term fetuses with transient gasping effort; dotted line: full-term fetuses with aspiration of saline. Low lines: the schematic respiratory activity indicated in the same kind of lines as the upper curves.

to the right in the histograms (Fig. 10). These changes are accompanied by the disappearance of the cortical evoked responses in the visual as well as in the somatosensory fields.

Our preliminary (unpublished) investigations have shown that, in full-term guinea pig fetuses delivered by cesarean section (i.e., without previous disturbance of placental circulation during natural uterine labor), the first gasp is usually evoked within 5–30 seconds after artificial clamping of the umbilical cord without any modification of further development of regular lung respiration. It is possible to discern two important events in the interval between clamping of the cord and the onset of effective regular lung respiration: (*1*) The first is a short-term and transient increase of hypoxia in brain tissue (Humphrey, 1953, 1964) before the first effective gasps occur from endogenous (pO_2, pCO_2, and pH in cerebral blood) and reflex stimulation of the CNS (Villee, 1960). The guinea pig is comparable to the sheep fetus,

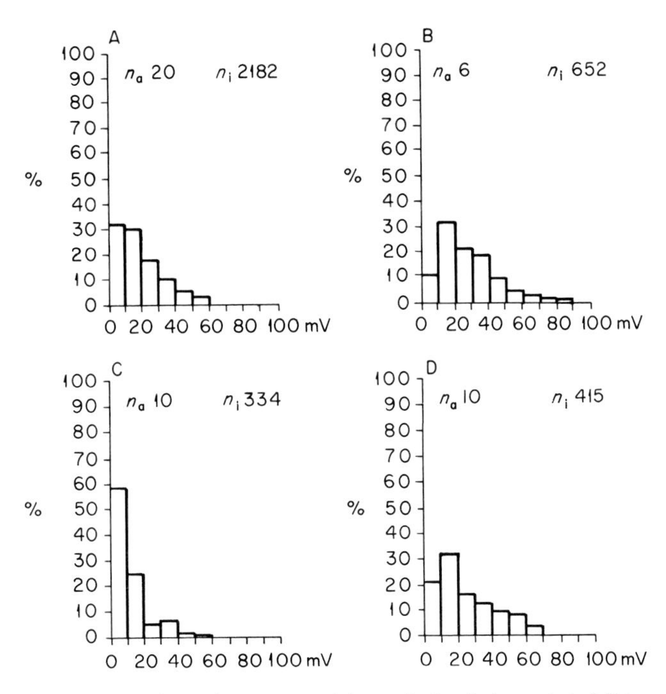

FIG. 10. Histograms of membrane potentials cortical cell elements in full-term fetuses in different perinatal conditions and in newborn guinea pigs. Abscissa: voltage categories in millivolts; ordinate: percentage of distribution of single values. (A) Full-term fetuses before the clamping of umbilical cord; (B) newborn guinea pigs; (C) full-term fetuses after 11 minutes of brain hypoxia; (D) full-term fetuses after 11 minutes of regular lung respiration. n_a = Number of animals; n_i = number of all single values of membrane potentials considered in the histogram.

in which the onset of respiration after the cord is clamped also develops in two steps: first, a strong gasping effort usually preceded by some degree of asphyxia and, second, the establishment of normal rhythmic breathing movements accompanied by a rise in arterial pO_2 from 25 mmHg up to 60 mmHg and by a fall in pCO_2 down to the fetal level (Dawes, 1968). This transient brain hypoxia must also be connected with the redistribution of the blood volume within systemic circulation after the umbilical arrest (Boda, Bélay, Eck, & Csernay, 1971). (2) The second event is an enormous influx of afferent stimulation, especially from the respiratory system (lungs and muscles), in connection with the initial pressing gasps. This effort first abolishes the fetal lung atelectasy (imperfect expansion of the fetal lung tissue at birth before the onset of respiratory movements), and then it passes into regular respiratory movements (Burns, 1963; Harned, 1970).

One of the main pathways of this afferent impulse bombardment is vagal input (Camproresi & Sant'Ambrogio, 1971; Woldring & Dirken, 1951). The vagal nerves mature at the moment of birth, and they act as input channels from aortic pressoreceptors (which reacts to hypoxia, hypercapnia, increase of H^+), and from inflation and deflation receptors activated during the initial inspiratory effort (Brady & Tooley, 1966; Young & Cottom, 1966).

It has been shown in full-term fetuses and in newborn guinea pigs that, at a certain stage, hypoxia has an activating effect upon cortical neurons (Figs. 11 and 12), and that the elimination of vagal input abolishes the important perinatal changes of cortical function. We observed that bilateral vagotomy is followed by the abolition of the initial positive spike in the cortical optic response (Sedláček, 1971a) (Fig. 13), as well as by the abolition of the conditioned reaction, whether or not respiration continues (Sedláček, 1968) (Fig. 14).

The relationship of hypoxia, especially of bilateral vagotomy, to changes in the acoustic conditioned reaction and the visual and somatosensory cortical responses suggests that the afferent input connected with the onset of lung respiration affects the functional state of the neonatal CNS in a predominantly nonspecific fashion which insures the establishment of activation (arousal) mechanisms.

This role of vagal afferentation from the respiratory apparatus for the functional state of the CNS has also been demonstrated in chick embryos during the last days of incubation after the onset of respiratory movements (Sedláček, 1964). In that case the state of vagal input also plays a positive or negative role in the elaboration of a simple conditioned reaction.

IV. Discussion

At the beginning of the discussion of our experimental results, we must emphasize a very important qualification related to ontogenetic research.

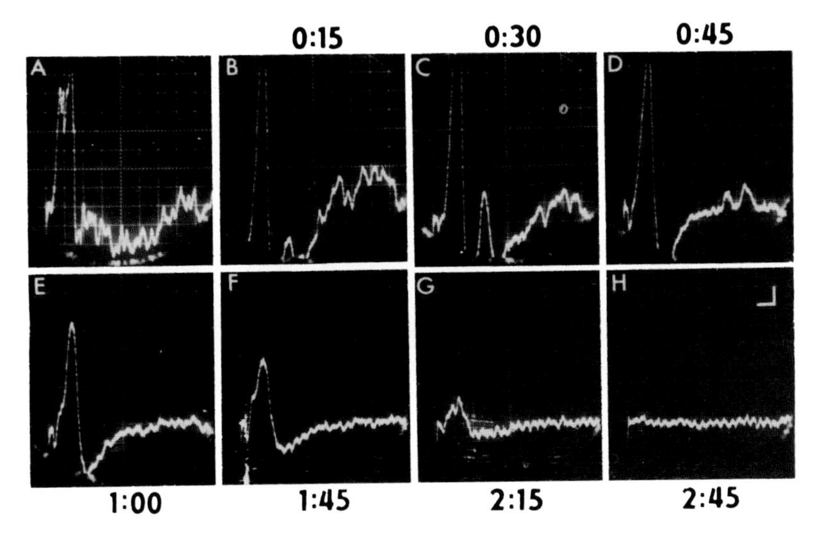

FIG. 11. Cortical somatosensory responses evoked by electrical stimulation of contralateral sciatic nerve in newborn guinea pig during the brain anoxia. (A) Normal response before the stop of artificial intratracheal respiration; (B–H) responses after the stop of respiration at intervals indicated in minutes: seconds. Calibrations: vertical, 50 uV; horizontal, 50 msec. Negativity upward.

While generalizations and hypotheses are necessary for the progress of our understanding of developmental processes, they should not be accepted as generalizable from one to another animal species without direct supporting evidence (Stave, 1970b).

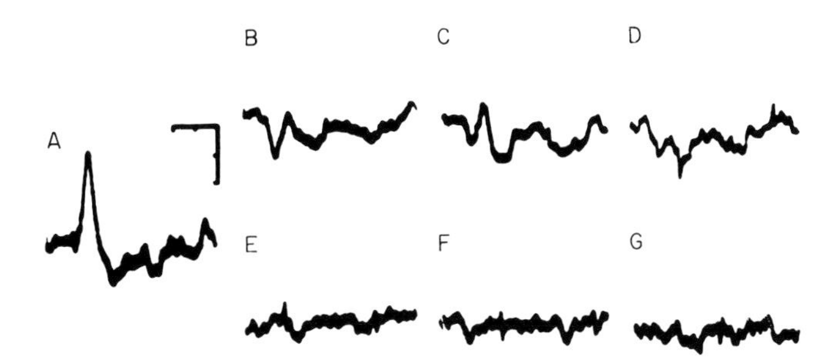

FIG. 12. The asphyctic changes of the morphology of cortical optic evoked response in full-term fetus after the clamping of umbilical cord and aspiration of saline during gasping effort. (A) Normal fetal response; (B–G) responses after the clamping of umbilical cord. (B) .5 minutes; (C) 1 minute; (D) 1.5 minutes; (E) 2.5 minutes; (F) 3.5 minutes; (G) 4.5 minutes. Calibrations: vertical, 50 uV per division; horizontal, 50 msec per division. Negativity upward.

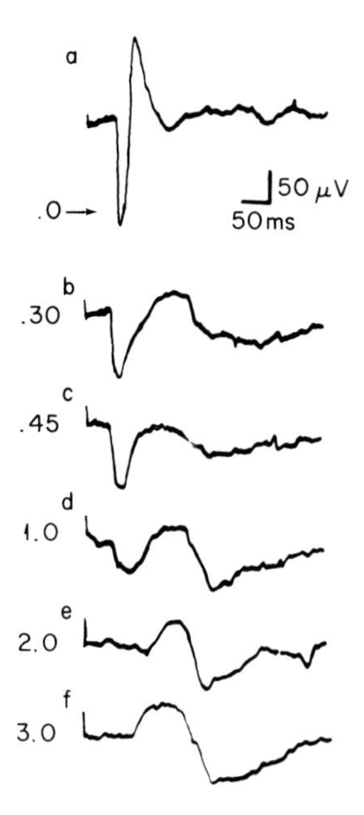

FIG. 13. Changes of cortical optic evoked response in newborn guinea pig after bilateral cervical vagotomy. (a) Normal neonatal response; (b–f) responses after vagotomy (horizontal arrow) at intervals indicated in minutes and seconds.

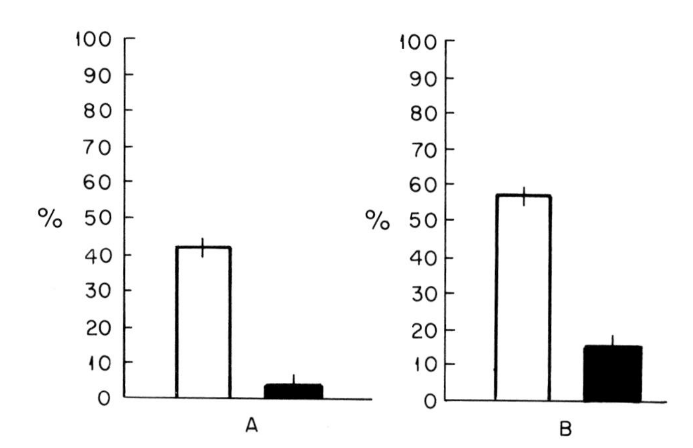

FIG. 14. Effect of bilateral cervical vagotomy upon the results of elaboration of acoustic conditioned reaction in full-term fetuses after the onset of lung respiration (A) and in newborn guinea pigs (B). Ordinate: percentage of conditioned reactions of all trials (mean ± se). White columns: animals after control ischiadectomy; black columns: animals after bilateral cervical vagotomy.

Three working hypotheses follow from the present results. The confirmation or contradiction of them shall be the aim of our further experimental study, with special attention to the analysis at other levels of organization (e.g., biochemical, physicochemical, etc.).

1. The first problem: The parameters of cortical function become transformed from the full-term fetal stage to the neonatal stage within several minutes after the arrest of fetoplacental circulation and the onset of lung ventilation. The capabilities of the CNS in newborn guinea pigs are so highly developed that they enable the neonate to be independent of the mother's care to a remarkable extent. This fact may only be the result of the finished process of maturation at the moment of birth, yet the functional manifestations of this high stage of maturation are quite different *before* and *after* clamping of the umbilical cord and onset of lung respiration.

We deduce from these functional differences between full-term fetuses and newborn animals that the *potential* capabilities resulting from fetal maturation of the CNS, especially the cerebral cortex, are partially suppressed by fetal conditions, especially within the last critical days before birth. This suppression is suddenly unmasked after some minutes during the perinatal period. These complex changes which occur during the perinatal crisis in mature full-term fetuses may be termed "neonatal arousal." During this time, when the respiratory effort begins, the fetus also manifests other signs of arousal: head turning and head shaking, movements of the eyelids, etc. (Dawes, 1968; Gesell, 1945). Similar arousal may be, after all, observed in other "dormant organs" *in utero*.

In support of this view of the perinatal complex, there are also interesting findings from another field. From the developmental point of view we can distinguish two types of enzymes, one of which becomes induced by the process of birth no matter whether parturition occurs physiologically or artificially (Stave, 1970a). This fact is connected with a repressive factor in the uterine environment from which release is obtained at birth, and which in turn triggers the initiation of enzyme activity at birth (Nemeth, 1963). This triggering is effective during normal, premature, or delayed parturition. It may also be supposed that the enzyme system must be mature to be triggered by birth conditions, but that the fetal conditions are unfavorable for the manifestation of its activity.

We know that the perinatal changes in the cortical parameters occur during a few minutes. It is important to elucidate whether the dynamics of perinatal changes in brain tissue, which may play the role of a triggering stimulus (pO_2, pCO_2, pH, activity of some essential functional enzyme systems, compartmentalization of brain tissue, etc.), correspond in their time scale to the course of changes in the functional and electrical properties of brain tissue.

2. The prolongation of the fetal period evidently causes a deterioration of fetal conditions, but the fetal damage evokes many premature reactions, e.g., respiratory movements, increase of fetal motility, defecation, etc. The second problem is: How early can an artificial change of suppressive fetal preterm conditions (artificial lung ventilation, artificial increase of vagal input, etc.) evoke the changes in the functional properties of the cerebral cortex usually observed in the perinatal period in the full-term fetus? In other words, at what stage of prenatal maturation does the conflict begin between the stage of maturation of brain tissue and the conditions of fetal existence?

3. The third problem: The rapidity with which the perinatal changes in the cerebral cortex take place precludes the participation of slow, gradual processes of morphological maturation (Armstrong-James & Johnson, 1970; Johnson & Armstrong-James, 1970). Another kind of change might be the restriction of the extracellular space, which may be realized within a short time limit. Such a change of the compartmentalization in brain tissue may increase the chance of contacts among a given neuronal population (as among nerve cells and glial elements) and may be of significance for the functional and electrophysiological state of the nervous systems (Vernadakis & Woodbury, 1965). It is difficult to assume that within minutes after clamping of the umbilical cord there could occur maturational changes such as an increase in synaptic contacts or an increase in the number of cell processes and/or synapses per unit volume of cortical tissue (Armstrong-James & Johnson, 1970), which characterize the long process of morphological maturation of the cerebral cortex (Åström, 1967; Scheibel & Scheibel, 1964). Therefore, we are inclined to divide the functional development of the cerebral cortex in the guinea pig into two essential phases: the first phase consists of the long-lasting gradual process of maturation of *morphological* and *chemical* architecture of the cerebral cortex, followed by corresponding *functional* manifestations. The concomitance is disconnected in the last days of the fetal period. The unfavorable preterm fetal physiological conditions begin to delay the functional manifestations of prior morphological and chemical maturation.

The second phase displays itself during the perinatal crisis, when the emergence into the extrauterine environment abolishes this delay from the first phase and triggers functional manifestations which are the natural bases of independent life.

Thus, the hazardous and critical perinatal period involves the release of functional relations in the central nervous system which must have been developed during the earlier prenatal period.

V. Conclusion

When comparing the CNS of precocial (guinea pig) and altricial (e.g., rat) newborn animals from the aspect mentioned above, it is possible to characterize the fundamental difference as follows: The CNS of the guinea pig becomes *aroused* into assuming a postnatally independent existence during parturition, while the CNS of the altricial newborn *develops* its independent existence only within a shorter or longer period of *postnatal* life.

A further study of the three problems mentioned immediately above should allow a more detailed analysis of the triggering of functional relationships in the neonatal nervous system.

We venture to conclude our essay by repeating some fundamental words from the Introduction to "The Physiology of the Newborn Infant" by C. A. Smith (1959): "The subject of neonatal physiology not only arouses interest because of the rapidly changing activities under study. . . . To understand the fundamentals of the newborn's life is the first step in helping it to survive [p. 4]."

VI. Summary

Some electrophysiological parameters of the cerebral cortex and some behavioral reactions were investigated in developing fetal and neonatal guinea pigs. Special attention was given to perinatal changes after umbilical arrest and the onset of lung respiration, which are the special features of the perinatal crisis.

1. The cortical steady potential, mean value of membrane potentials of cortical cells and cortical impedance all increase progressively until term, but they do not reach the values determined in normal newborn animals.

2. The primary evoked responses in the fetal cortex indicate the integrative function of visual and somatosensory afferent systems. Also, the motor reactions to strong acoustic stimuli prove the functional activity of the auditory system.

3. Within a few minutes of umbilical arrest and the onset of lung ventilation, the quantitative and qualitative differences between the full-term fetal and the neonatal cortex are erased. The qualitative perinatal changes are illustrated by progressive changes in the morphology of cortical evoked responses and by the capability for the formation of acoustic conditioned reactions.

4. Experimental analysis showed the important contribution which the oxygen supply and the vagal input (connected with the establishment of lung respiration) make to brain function. Both these factors seem to play an important role in the triggering of normal neonatal neural function.

5. The experimental results are discussed from the point of view of neonatal arousal in mature newborn animals.

Acknowledgment

I want to thank Dr. Gilbert Gottlieb for his help, suggestions, and for criticisms of the manuscript.

References

Amoroso, E. C. Placentation. In A. S. Parker (Ed.), *Marshall's physiology of reproduction.* London: Longmans, Green, 1952.

Armstrong-James, M., & Johnson, R. Quantitative studies of postnatal changes in synapses in rat superficial motor cerebral cortex. *Zeitschrift für Zellforschung und Mikroskopische Anatomie*, 1970, **110**, 559–568.

Asdell, S. A. *Patterns of mammalian reproduction.* Ithaca, N.Y.: Cornell University Press, 1946.

Åström, K. E. On the early development of the isocortex in fetal sheep. *Progress in Brain Research*, 1967, **26**, 1–59.

Avery, G. Responses of foetal guinea pigs prematurely delivered. *Genetic Psychology Monographs*, 1928, **3**, 248–331.

Barcroft, J., & Young, I. M. Oxygen in the blood emerging from the brain of post-mature rabbit. *Journal of Physiology (London)*, 1943, **102**, 25P–26P.

Basmajian, J. V., & Ranney, D. A. Chemomyelotomy: substitute for general anesthesia in experimental surgery. *Journal of Applied Physiology*, 1961, **16**, 386.

Becher, R. F., King, J. E., Marsh, R. H., & Wyrick, A. D. Intrauterine respiration in the rat fetus. *American Journal of Obstetrics and Gynecology*, 1964, **90**, 236–246.

Berfenstam, R. Gruppenmedizinische Fragen in der Kinderheilkunde. In G. Fanconi & A. Wallgren (Eds.), *Lehrbuch der pädiatrie.* Basel: Schwabe, 1967.

Bergström, R. M. Brain and muscle potentials from the intrauterine foetus in unnarcotized conscious animals. *Nature (London)*, 1962, **195**, 1004–1005. (a)

Bergström, R. M. Prenatal development of motor functions. *Annales Chirurgiae et Gynaecologiae Fenniae, Supplementum*, 1962, **112**. (b)

Bergström, R. M. A surgical technique for the study of brain muscle and EEG potentials in the foetus. *Annales Chirurgiae et Gynaecologiae Fenniae*, 1962, **51**, 504–510. (c)

Bergström, R. M. Development of EEG and unit electrical activity of the brain during ontogeny. In L. Jílek & S. Trojan (Eds.), *Ontogenesis of the brain.* Prague: Charles University Press, 1968.

Bergström, R. M., Hellström, P. E., & Stenberg, D. Über die Entwicklung der elektrischen Aktivität im Grosshirn des intrauterinen Meerschweinchenfetus. *Annales Chirurgiae et Gynaecologiae Fenniae*, 1962, **51**, 466–474.

Boda, D., Bélay, M., Eck, E., & Csernay, L. Blood distribution of the organs examined by ^{86}Rb uptake under intrauterine conditions and in the newborn in normal and hypoxic rabbits. *Biologia Neonatorum*, 1971, **18**, 71–77.

Born, G. V. R., Dawes, G. S., Mott, J. C., & Widdicombe, J. G. Changes in the heart and lungs at birth. *Cold Spring Harbor Symposia on Quantitative Biology*, 1954, **19**, 102–108

Brady, J. P., & Tooley, W. H. Cardiovascular and respiratory reflexes in the newborn. *Pediatric Clinics of North America*, 1966, **13**, 801–821.

Brück, K., & Wünnenberg, B. Über die Modi der Thermogenese beim neugeborenen Warmblüter, Untersuchungen an Meerschweinchen. *Pflügers Archiv für die Gesamte Physiologie des Menschen und der Tiere*, 1965, **282**, 362–375.

Bureš, J. The ontogenetic development of steady potential differences in the cerebral cortex in animals. *Electroencephalography and Clinical Neurophysiology*, 1957, **9**, 121–130.

Bureš, J., Eifková, E., & Mareš, P. Spreading depression and maturation of some forebrain structures in rats. In P. Kellaway & I. Petersen (Eds.), *Correlative studies in infancy*. New York: Grune & Stratton, 1964.

Burns, D. B. The central control of respiratory movements. *British Medical Bulletin*, 1963, **19**, 7–9.

Camproresi, E., & Sant'Ambrogio, G. Influences on the respiratory rhythm originating from the lung and the chest wall. *Pflügers Archiv*, 1971, **324**, 311–318.

Čapek, K., & Jelínek, J. The development of the control of water metabolism. I. The excretion of urine in young rats. *Physiologia Bohemoslovaca*, 1956, **5**, 91–96. (a)

Čapek, K., & Jelínek, J. The development of the control of water metabolism. II. The development of miction in puppies. *Physiologia Bohemoslovaca*, 1956, **5**, 97–102. (b)

Carmichael, L. An experimental study in the prenatal guinea-pig of the origin and development of reflexes and patterns behavior in relation to the stimulation of specific receptor areas during the period of active fetal life. *Genetic Psychology Monographs*, 1934, **16**, 337–491.

Crain, S. M., Peterson, E. R., & Bornstein, M. B. Formation of functional interneuronal connections between explants of various mammalian central nervous tissues during development *in vitro*. In G. E. W. Wolstenholme & M. O'Connor (Eds.), *Ciba foundation symposium on growth of the nervous system*. London: Churchill, 1968. Pp. 13–31.

Dawes, G. S. *Foetal and neonatal physiology*. Chicago: Yearbook Publ., 1968.

Deza, L., & Eidelberg, E. Development of cortical electrical activity in the rat. *Experimental Neurology*, 1967, **17**, 425–436.

Draper, R. L. The prenatal growth of the guinea pig. *Anatomical Record*, 1920, **18**, 369–392.

Esquivel de Gallardo, F. O., Fleischman, R. W., & Ramirez de Arrelano, M. I. R. Electroencephalogram of the monkey fetus in utero and changes in it at birth. *Experimental Neurology*, 1964, **9**, 73–84.

Flexner, L. B. Enzymatic and functional patterns of the developing mammalian brain. In H. Waelsch (Ed.), *Biochemistry of the developing nervous system*. New York: Academic Press. 1954.

Flexner, L. B., Tyler, D. B., & Gallant, L. J. Biochemical and physiological differentiation during morphogenesis. X. Onset of electrical activity in developing cerebral cortex of fetal guinea pig. *Journal of Neurophysiology*, 1950, **13**, 427–430.

Gesell, A. *The embryology of behavior*. New York: Harper, 1945.

Gottlieb, G. Ontogenesis of sensory function in birds and mammals. In E. Tobach, L. R. Aronson, & E. Shaw (Eds.), *Biopsychology of development*. New York: Academic Press, 1971. Pp. 67–128.

Greenfield, A. D. M., & Shepherd, J. T. Cardiovascular responses to asphyxia in the foetal guinea-pig. *Journal of Physiology* (*London*), 1953, **120**: 538–551.

Hahn, P. The changes of the oxygen consumption in rats during postnatal development and the relation of these changes on the temperature of external environment. *Physiologia Bohemoslovaca*, 1953, **2**, 373–380.

Hahn, P., Křeček, J., & Křečková, J. The development of thermoregulation. I. The development of thermoregulatory mechanisms in young rats. *Physiologia Bohemoslovaca*, 1956, **5**, 283–289.

Harned, H. S., Jr. Respiration and the respiratory system. In U. Stave (Ed.), *Physiology of the perinatal period.* New York: Meredith, 1970.

Holub, V. Developmental defects and inborn disturbances of the nervous system and muscles. In V. Pitha (Ed.), *Neurology of childhood.* Prague: Avicenum, 1963.

Humphrey, T. The relation of oxygen deprivation to fetal reflex arcs and the development of fetal behavior. *Journal of Psychology*, 1953, **35**, 3–43.

Humphrey, T. Some correlations between the appearance of human fetal reflexes and the development of the nervous system. *Progress in Brain Research*, 1964, **4**, 93–133.

Ibsen, H. L. Prenatal growth in guinea pig with special reference to environmental factors affecting weight at birth. *Journal of Experimental Zoology*, 1929, **51**, 51–91.

Jasper, H. H., Bridgman, C. S., & Carmichael, L. An ontogenetic study of cerebral electrical potentials in the guinea pig. *Journal of Experimental Psychology*, 1937, **21**, 63–71.

Johnson, R., & Armstrong-James, M. Morphology of superficial postnatal cerebral cortex with special reference to synapses. *Zeitschrift für Zellforschung und Mikroskopische Anatomie*, 1970, **110**, 540–558.

Křeček, J. 1971. The theory of critical developmental periods and postnatal development of endocrine functions. In E. Tobach, L. R. Aronson, & E. Shaw (Eds.), *Biopsychology of development.* New York: Academic Press, 1971. Pp. 233–248.

Lesný, I. *The clinical features of some congenital and early acquired diseases of the nervous system.* Prague: Avicenum, 1957.

Mourek, J., Himwich, W. A., Myslivecek, J., & Callison, D. A. The role of nutrition in the development of evoked cortical responses in rat. *Brain Research*, 1967, **6**, 241–251.

Nelson, W. E. An introduction to the medical problems of infants and children. In W. E. Nelson (Ed.), *Textbook of pediatrics.* Philadelphia: Saunders, 1966.

Nemeth, A. M. Initiation of enzyme formation by birth. *Annals of New York Academy of Sciences*, 1963, **111**, 199–202.

Ranck, J. B., & Windle, W. F. Brain damage in the monkey, Maccaca mulatta, by asphyxia neonatorum. *Experimental Neurology*, 1959, **1**, 130–153.

Scheibel, M. E., & Scheibel, A. B. Some structural and functional substrates of development in young cats. *Progress in Brain Research*, 1964, **9**, 6–25.

Scherrer, J., & Fourment, A. Electrocortical effects of sensory deprivation during development. *Progress in Brain Research*, 1964, **9**, 103–112.

Schwan, H. P. Electrical properties of tissues and cell suspensions. *Advances in Biological and Medical Physics*, 1957, **5**, 148–210.

Schwartze, H., Schwartze, P., & Schönfelder, J. Living fetuses of guinea pigs in acute experiments. *Biologia Neonatorum*, 1971, **17**, 238–248.

Sedláček, J. The principles of the development of reflex activity. *Acta Universitatis Carolinae, Medica*, 1961, **9**, 731–770.

Sedláček, J. The problems of the ontogenetic origin of the mechanism of temporary connection. *Acta Universitatis Carolinae, Medica*, 1963, **11**, 265–317.

Sedláček, J. Temporary connection in chick embryos and vagal deafferentation. *Physiologia Bohemoslovaca*, 1964, **13**, 421–424.

Sedláček, J. *Prenatal development of electrical properties of the cerebral tissue.* Prague: Academia, 1967.

Sedláček, J. Some problems of elaboration of a temporary connection in the prenatal period. *Progress in Brain Research*, 1968, **22**, 575–584.

Sedláček, J. Development of membrane potentials of cortical cell elements in guinea pig fetus. *Developmental Psychobiology*, 1969, **2**, 2–6.

Sedláček, J. Cortical responses to visual stimulation in the developing guinea pig during the prenatal and perinatal period. *Physiologia Bohemoslovaca*, 1971, **20**, 213–220. (a)

Sedláček, J. Development of the optic afferent system in chick embryos. *Advances in Psychobiology*, 1971, **5**, 195–237. (b)

Sedláček, J., Hlaváčková, V., & Švehlová, M. New findings on the formation of the temporary connection in the prenatal and perinatal period in the guinea pig. *Physiologia Bohemoslovaca*, 1964, **13**, 268–273.

Sedláček, J., & Macek, O. D.C. potential and high frequency impedance of the cerebral hemispheres in guinea pig fetuses in the perinatal period. *Physiologia Bohemoslovaca*, 1965, **14**, 371–378.

Sedláček, J., & Macek, O. Development of some basic electrical parameters of brain tissue in chick embryos. In L. Jílek & S. Trojan (Eds.), *Ontogenesis of the brain*. Prague: Charles University Press, 1968.

Shaffer, T. E. Preventive pediatrics. In W. E. Nelson (Ed.), *Textbook of pediatrics*. Philadelphia: Saunders, 1966.

Shelley, H. J. Glycogen reserves and their changes at birth. *British Medical Bulletin*, 1961, **17**, 137–143.

Smith, C. A. *The physiology of the newborn infant*. Oxford: Blackwell, 1959.

Stave, U. Enzyme development in the liver. In U. Stave (Ed.), *Physiology of the perinatal period*. New York: Meredith, 1970. (a)

Stave, U. Maturation, adaptation and tolerance. In U. Stave (Ed.), *Physiology of the perinatal period*. New York: Meredith, 1970. (b)

Stenberg, D. Analysis of the EEG of the guinea pig fetus. *Acta Physiologica Scandinavica*, 1968, **74**, 509–510.

Swenson, M. J. *Duke's physiology of domestic animals*. Ithaca, N.Y.: Cornell University Press, 1970.

Van Harreveld, A., & Schadé, J. P. Chloride movements in cerebral cortex after circulatory arrest and during spreading depression. *Journal of Cellular and Comparative Physiology*, 1959, **54**, 65–84.

Vernadakis, A., & Woodbury, D. M. Cellular and extracellular spaces in developing rat brain. *Archives of Neurology (Chicago)*, 1965, **12**, 284–293.

Villee, C. A. The role of anaerobic metabolism in fetal and neonatal survival. *Acta Psediatrica (Stockholm), Supplement*, 1960, **112**, 1–16.

Woldring, S., & Dirken, M. N. J. Site and extension of bulbar respiratory centre. *Journal of Neurophysiology*, 1951, **14**, 227–236.

Young, M., & Cottom, D. Arterial and venous blood pressure responses during a reduction in blood volume and hypoxia and hypercapnia in infants during the first two days of life. *Pediatrics*, 1966, **37**, 733–742.

AUTHOR INDEX

Numbers in italics refer to the pages on which the complete references are listed.

J

K

L

M

T

U

V

SUBJECT INDEX

N

O

P

R